W9-AEV-034

ANNUAL REVIEW OF NURSING RESEARCH

Volume 11, 1993

ANNUAL REVIEW OF NURSING RESEARCH

Volume 11, 1993

Joyce J. Fitzpatrick, Ph.D.
Joanne S. Stevenson, Ph.D.
Editors

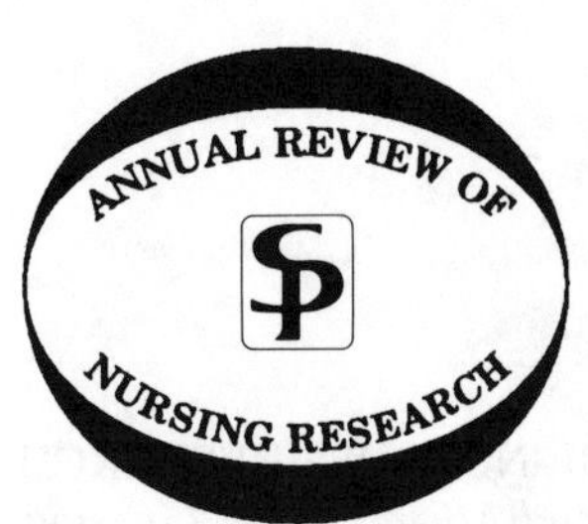

SPRINGER PUBLISHING COMPANY
New York

Order ANNUAL REVIEW OF NURSING RESEARCH, Volume 11, 1993, prior to publication and receive a 10% discount. An order coupon can be found at the back of this volume.

Springer Publishing Company, Inc.
536 Broadway
New York, NY 10012

93 94 95 96 97 / 5 4 3 2 1

ISBN-0-8261 8230-5
ISSN-0739-6686

ANNUAL REVIEW OF NURSING RESEARCH is indexed in *Cumulative Index to Nursing and Allied Health Literature and Index Medicus.*

Printed in the United States of America

Contents

Preface

This eleventh volume of the *Annual Review of Nursing Research* (ARNR) series marks the beginning of our second decade of publication. The 1980s was an era of expansion in nursing scholarship. It is our expectation that in the coming decade we will witness an increase in both the depth and breadth of nursing research. As this occurs, the content areas under review should be more clearly and narrowly defined. Chapters in Volume 11 represent an initial effort toward this goal.

In Part I, Research on Nursing Practice, we have included a focus on patient/client symptoms. Marquis Foreman reviews research on acute confusional states; Barbara Holtzclaw describes research on shivering; Kathleen Potempa's review is focused on research of chronic fatigue; Marylin Dodd reviews research on side effects of cancer chemotherapy; and Nancy Hester describes research on pain in children.

Part II, Research on Nursing Care Delivery, includes the following chapters: Patient Care Outcomes Related to Management of Symptoms by Sue Hegyvary, and the Role of Nurse Researchers Employed in Clinical Settings by Karin Kirchhoff. The Nursing Education section, Part III, includes a chapter by Claire Andrews and Carol Davis on nurse-midwifery education. Part IV, Research on the Profession, includes a chapter by Joan Turner on AIDS-Related Knowledge, Attitudes, and Risk for Infection Among Nurses.

Part V serves as a category for chapters that do not easily fit the content theme of Part I or the categories included in the other components. In this volume, Part V includes: Family Unit Focused Research by Ann L. Whall and Carol J. Loveland-Cherry; Opiate Abuse in Pregnancy by Cathy Strachan Lindenberg and Anne B. Keith; Alcohol and Drug Abuse by Eleanor J. Sullivan and Sandra M. Handley; and Patient Falls in Health Care Institutions by Janice M. Morse.

A new Advisory Board has participated in launching the new decade. We are pleased to welcome new Board members Violet Barkauskas, Marie Cowan, Claire Fagin, Suzanne Feetham, Phyllis Giovannetti, Kathleen McCormick, Jane Norbeck, and Christine Tanner. Continuing Advisory Board members Ada Sue Hinshaw and Harriet Werley will provide continuity from the previous Board. Roma Lee Taunton, coeditor of volumes 4 through 10, now joins us as an Advisory Board member. Our Advisory Board members play a major role in setting directions for the future, as well as recommending authors, chapters, and reviewers for each volume. Joanne S. Stevenson has joined me as a coeditor for Volumes 11 through 13.

Although there are many new ARNR team members working with us to start the new decade, we would be remiss in not acknowledging the ongoing support of key staff members at Case Western Reserve University. Nikki Polis continues as a member of the editorial staff, and we have the assistance of a number of support staff members.

As a celebration of the first decade of the ARNR series, a special International State of the Science Congress was held in Washington, DC, in August 1992. Nurse leaders from around the world joined together; examplars of the significant strides in nursing research were presented in several plenary sessions. A special volume in the ARNR series, Proceedings of the State of the Science Congress, will be published in 1994. Because the Congress was cosponsored by several national and regional professional nursing organizations, the Proceedings' publication will include a broader scope of content, with particular emphasis on nursing research and its clinical applications.

We look forward to your continuing involvement in this important series. Please let us know your ideas.

JOYCE J. FITZPATRICK
Senior Editor

Contributors

Claire M. Andrews, Ph.D.
Frances Payne Bolton School of Nursing
Case Western Reserve University
Cleveland, OH

Carol E. Davis, Ph.D.
College of Nursing
University of South Carolina
Columbia, SC

Marylin J. Dodd, Ph.D.
School of Nursing
University of California, San Francisco
San Francisco, CA

Marquis D. Foreman, Ph.D.
College of Nursing
University of Illinois at Chicago
Chicago, IL

Sandra M. Handley, Ph.D.
School of Nursing
University of Kansas Medical Center
Kansas City, KS

Sue T. Hegyvary, Ph.D.
School of Nursing
University of Washington
Seattle, WA

Nancy O. Hester, Ph.D.
School of Nursing
University of Colorado Health Sciences Center
Denver, CO

Barbara J. Holtzclaw, Ph.D.
School of Nursing
University of Texas
Health Sciences Center at San Antonio
San Antonio, TX

Anne B. Keith, Ph.D.
School of Nursing
University of Southern Maine
Portland, ME

Karin T. Kirchhoff, Ph.D.
College of Nursing and University Hospital
University of Utah
Salt Lake City, UT

Cathy Strachan Lindenberg, Dr.P-H.
College of Nursing
University of Massachusetts, Boston
Boston, MA

Carol J. Loveland-Cherry, Ph.D.
School of Nursing
University of Michigan
Ann Arbor, MI

Janice M. Morse, Ph.D.
School of Nursing
Pennsylvania State University
University Park, PA

Kathleen M. Potempa, D.N.Sc.
College of Nursing
University of Illinois at Chicago
Chicago, IL

Eleanor J. Sullivan, Ph.D.
School of Nursing
University of Kansas
Medical Center
Kansas City, KS

Joan G. Turner, D.S.N.
School of Nursing
University of Alabama
at Birmingham
Birmingham, AL

Ann L. Whall, Ph.D.
School of Nursing
University of Michigan
Ann Arbor, MI

Forthcoming

ANNUAL REVIEW OF
NURSING RESEARCH, Volume 12

Tentative Contents

PART I

Research on Nursing Practice

Chapter 1

Acute Confusion in the Elderly

MARQUIS D. FOREMAN
COLLEGE OF NURSING
UNIVERSITY OF ILLINOIS AT CHICAGO

CONTENTS

The history of acute confusion dates back 2,500 years to the writings of Hippocrates (Lipowski, 1990), but knowledge about the condition remains incomplete. Too often acute confusion in elderly individuals has been ignored. Elderly patients have at times been perceived as uninteresting, unimportant, unworthy, and beyond help (Foreman, 1986; Francis & Kapoor, 1990; Lipowski, 1990). Historically, aging has been considered synonymous with cognitive decline; thus, the occurrence of acute confusion was thought inevitable and beyond the influence of health care professionals. Additionally, the distinction was not made between acute reversible conditions and chronic states with permanent impairment. During the past 15 years, the notions and attitudes about the elderly and acute confusion have changed. As a result, there has been increasing attention to this condition within the clinical and research literature.

Clinical anecdotes about acutely confused patients and debates about nomenclature proliferate in the literature. The research about acute confusion is primarily descriptive in nature; experimental investigations about the causes and treatment of acute confusional states are few. The purposes of this review are to (a) critically review the research on acute confusion in the elderly; (b) summarize and integrate this literature, (c) highlight unresolved issues in the study of acute confusion, (d) identify gaps in the knowledge of this condition, (e) specify the implications of this knowledge for nursing practice, and (f) recommend future directions for research.

Literature for this review was identified using multiple techniques: (a) ancestry (tracking citations from publications), (b) computerized abstracting services, (c) hand bibliographic searches of *Dissertation Abstracts* and *Masters Abstracts,* and (d) written and telephone communication with investigators (internationally) known to have studied or be studying within this substantive area. The substantive area was defined as encompassing any of the following terms: *acute brain failure, acute brain syndrome, acute cerebral insufficiency, acute mental status change, acute organic psychosis, acute organic reaction, acute organic syndrome, agitated confusional state, altered mental status, cerebral insufficiency syndrome, delirium, dystergastic reaction, exogenous psychoses, intensive care unit delirium, intensive care unit psychosis, metabolic encephalopathy, organic brain syndrome, postcardiotomy delirium, postcardiotomy psychosis, pseudosenility, reversible cognitive dysfunction, reversible dementia, reversible toxic psychosis, subacute befuddlement, sundown syndrome, toxic confusional state, toxic delirious reaction, toxic encephalopathy, toxic-metabolic encephalopathy, toxic psychosis,* or *transient cognitive impairment.*

Criteria for inclusion in this review stipulated that the source had to be (a) research or data based, (b) written in English, and (c) conducted using adult samples. Most samples, however, were of older adults ($\geq$ 65 years of age). Because impaired cognition attributable to alcohol ingestion or intoxication is by definition different from the phenomenon of interest (delirium vs. delirium tremens) this literature was excluded from review. Both published and unpublished works were reviewed. The literature resulting from these searches and sampling strategies is reviewed subsequently. To facilitate this review, the literature about acute confusion was divided into two foci: conceptual and clinical. Topics related to each focus are discussed.

CONCEPTUAL ISSUES IN THE STUDY OF ACUTE CONFUSION

Conceptual issues in the study of acute confusion pose serious obstacles to integrating the body of information into a comprehensive body of knowledge. The main conceptual issues include (a) beliefs about acute confusion, (b) the lexicon, and (c) the nature of acute confusional states.

Beliefs About Acute Confusion

Beliefs are foundational to the study of any phenomenon. Beliefs influence the perception of a phenomenon, and, consequently, determine what are considered legitimate and significant areas of study relative to that phenomenon. Beliefs also can facilitate or obscure the understanding of a phenomenon. Historically, the beliefs about acute confusional states in the elderly have served to delay understanding.

Although it has been demonstrated that cognitive decline is not an inevitable concomitant of aging (Rowe & Khan, 1987), cognitive decline remains an expectation of aging (Brady, 1987), as acutely confused behavior fits the stereotype many individuals have of the elderly. Consequently, it is only recently that cognitive decline generally and acute confusion specifically have been considered legitimate areas of study (Foreman, 1986).

Beliefs, as reflected by perceptions of acute confusion, were examined by Wolanin (1973), who reviewed descriptions of the behavior of acutely confused patients found in hospital records of older patients. Wolanin found that descriptions of acutely confused behavior varied by discipline. Physicians used terms such as "poor historian," "forgetful," "poor memory," "cannot understand directions," and "incoherent" to describe acutely confused patients. Wolanin interpreted these behaviors as indicators of impaired intellectual functioning or indicators of cognitive inaccessibility—a characteristic of these patients interfering with the physician's instrumental function of diagnosis. Conversely, nurses noted behaviors such as "uncooperative," "combative," "hostile," "difficult to manage," "belligerent," and "agitated" to describe patients, many of whom may have been acutely confused. The problem with the chart review method is that it is not possible to know if these patients were or were not acutely confused.

Conversely, the attitudes of the professionals in using the language noted in the chart reviews seemed concerned primarily with their compromised ability to function as a professional rather than with the patients. Others have noted this professional ethnocentrism as well (Ludwick & Scott, 1991; Ludwick, Scott, & O'Toole, 1991; Morgan, 1985).

Another pervasive belief is that acute confusion equates with agitation, hyperactivity, and uncooperativeness (Lipowski, 1983b). One consequence of this association is that hypoactive and cooperative confused patients escape detection, treatment, and study. Yet, by definition, it is agreed that the behavioral manifestations of acute confusion vary between the extremes of hypoactivity and hyperactivity (American Psychiatric Association, 1987; Foreman, 1991; Liposwki, 1983a). Recent evidence suggests that these behavioral manifestations of acute confusion are a function of the etiologic agent(s) and not the acute confusional state per se (Neelon, Champagne, & Moore, 1989). It seems evident that for advancement to be made in the understanding of this phenomenon, the beliefs about acute confusion must be examined critically.

Lexicon of Acute Confusion

Nomenclature. The study of acute confusional states is confounded by its lexicon (Foreman, 1986; Francis & Kapoor, 1990; Lipowski, 1983a). A long-standing debate has existed as to which term—*acute confusion, delirium,* or *transient cognitive impairment*—is the diagnostic label that would lead to appropriate diagnosis and treatment of this condition. As noted earlier, numerous overlapping, and inconsistently used and defined terms are used interchangeably as synonyms. Whether the differences among these terms are ones of semantics or subtle variations in phenomena awaits data and interpretation (Foreman, 1991).

Throughout this chapter *acute confusion* will be used. This term requires no translation for bedside practitioners, and does not connote etiology. Additionally, the term acute confusion represents more closely what is observed clinically by nurses—a syndrome versus a single disease state (Vermeersch, 1991).

Definition of Terms. In this review the following terms are defined:

Acute confusion is a transient state of cognitive impairment: it is a syndrome manifested by simultaneous disturbances of consciousness, attention, perception, memory, thinking, orientation, and psychomotor behavior that develop abruptly and fluctuate diurnally (Foreman, 1991). The primary deficit is one of attention.

Cognition is comprised of three components: perception, memory, and thinking (Lipowski, 1983a).

Cognitive impairment is a class of states of dysfunctional cognition of which there are two main types: (a) global cognitive impairment in which all three components of cognition are simultaneously impaired (e.g., delirium); and (b) specific global impairment in which only one or predominately one component of cognition is impaired (e.g., amnestic disorder or organic hallucinosis) (Lipowski, 1990).

Delirium is a transient state of global cognitive impairment. The diagnostic criteria for delirium are (a) reduced ability to maintain attention to external stimuli and to shift appropriately attention to new external stimuli; (b) disorganized thinking; and (c) at least two of the following: (a) reduced level of consciousness; (b) perceptual disturbances; (c) disturbance of the sleep-wake cycle; (d) increased or decreased psychomotor behavior; (e) disorientation to person, place, or time; or (f) memory impairment. These clinical features of delirium develop over a short period (usually hours to days) and tend to fluctuate diurnally (American Psychiatric Association, 1987).

Mental status is the thinking sphere of behavior including sensorium and cognitive functions. Components of mental status include state of consciousness, attention, orientation, memory, calculation, abstraction, judgment, insight, use of language, general knowledge, personal appearance, and thought form, content, and process (Foreman, 1987; Fraser, 1988; Strub & Black, 1985).

The Nature of Acute Confusion

The major feature of acute confusion appears to be its transiency. Because this is a post hoc determination, differentiating acute confusion from other more chronic forms is problematic. Although consensus regarding nomenclature is lacking, there is agreement about the fundamental nature of acute confusion (American Psychiatric Association, 1987; Foreman, 1986, 1989, 1991; Nagley & Dever, 1988; Williams et al., 1979, 1985a, 1985b). The onset is acute or subacute depending on cause, whereas the course is short with diurnal fluctuations in symptoms. It gets worse at night and on awakening, and lasts from several hours to less than 1 month. Patients have reduced awareness, impaired attention span, and fluctuating levels of alertness. They exhibit impaired orientation and memory; thinking is disorganized, and perceptions are distorted. They are distracted easily, have disturbed or reversed sleep-wake cycles, and may be hyperkinetic or hypokinetic. (Foreman, 1986). The features of the condition are useful for differentiating acute confusion from chronic forms of cognitive impairment, such as the dementias (Foreman, 1986; Foreman & Grabowski, 1991). However, validation of these clinical features has received limited scientific study (Foreman, 1991).

Foreman (1991) identified five dimensions of acute confusion that approximated those identified in the literature. The five factors (cognition, orientation, motoric behavior, memory, and higher integrative functions) accounted for only one-third of the variance in confused behavior, indicating that there is much more to acute confusion than is represented by these five factors. However, these five factors were extremely sensitive and specific in identifying a state of acute confusion (Foreman, 1991), whereas those aspects most often used by practicing nurses—alertness and orientation (Brady, 1987; Rasmussen & Creason, 1991)—were not diagnostic of acute confusion (Foreman, 1991).

The variable manifestations of acute confusion across individuals and the fluctuating nature of the condition within one person across time increases the complexity of the phenomenon (Foreman, 1986). There is some speculation that this variability is a function of the underlying etiologic agent(s), or that there are subtypes or different patterns of acute confusion (Lipowski, 1983a; Neelon et al., 1989). Lipowski (1983a) described three variants of acute confusion based on the behavior, verbal and nonverbal, exhibited by the individual. The three variants are hyperkinetic, hypokinetic, and mixed. The hyperkinetic variant is the "classic" representation of the acutely confused patient and is characterized by hyperarousal of the autonomic system, psychomotor hyperactivity, marked excitability, and a tendency toward hallucinations. Conversely, the hypokinetic variant is often misdiagnosed as it conflicts with the stereotypic notion of acute confusion. The hypokinetic variant is characterized by reduced psychomotor activity, lethargy, somnolence, apathy, and reduced arousal and excitability. The mixed variant involved a fluctuating state between these two variants.

Neelon et al. (1989) identified three patterns of acute confusion, with manifestations reflecting underlying causal agents. The first pattern, "cognitive restricted," results from environmental challenges such as sensory deprivation or overload typical of acute care hospitals. The second pattern, "physiologic instability," has fluctuating symptomatology and arises from pathophysiologic states such as hypoxemia. The third pattern, "metabolic instability," is manifested by motor symptoms typically observed in encephalopathies and results from the toxic challenges of impaired hepatic or renal function, or from the adverse effects of multiple pharmacologic agents (prescribed and over the counter).

Obtaining knowledge about the nature of this condition is obstructed by designs that fail to reflect its central aspects. For example, many study designs were cross-sectional and rarely included multiple daily observations of patients, yet diurnal fluctuations of behavior are a hallmark of acute confusion.

The literature on acute confusion is largely atheoretic; one exception is the work of Neelon et al. (1985, 1989, 1991, 1992) who applied a human information-processing approach to the study of acute confusion.

Cumulatively, the beliefs, lexicon, and nature of acute confusion pose serious obstacles to the development of knowledge about this problem (Foreman, 1991; Lipowski, 1983a, 1990; Vermeersch, 1991). The professional focus of the beliefs, the semantic muddle, and the largely atheoretic study of acute confusion have led to what has been referred to as "conceptual chaos" (Foreman, 1991). This state of conceptual chaos undermines the search for knowledge about acute confusion. For knowledge development and innovation in patient care issues to progress, conceptual clarity must occur.

CLINICAL ISSUES IN THE STUDY OF ACUTE CONFUSION

The clinical issues in the study of acute confusion pose serious obstacles to the application to practice and further generation of knowledge of the condition. The clinical issues discussed in this section include (a) methods for detecting acute confusional states, (b) the etiologic basis of acute confusion, (c) the epidemiology of acute confusion, (d) outcomes of acute confusion, and (e) the care of patients who are acutely confused or have the potential to be.

Methods for Detecting Acute Confusion

Detection of acute confusion is often the only indication of physical illness in the elderly (Foreman, 1984, 1986; Francis & Kapoor, 1990; Lipowski, 1990). Therefore, it is important to diagnose. However, most cases of acute confusion escape detection (Cameron, Thomas, Mulvihill, & Bronheim, 1987; Gehi, Weltz, Strain, & Jacobs, 1980).

The haphazard and incomplete assessment of cognitive function by physicians and nurses leads to underdetection of acute confusion. In studying nurses, 43% (Lucas & Folstein, 1980) and 72% (Palmateer & McCartney, 1985) of the cases of acute confusion were not identified in hospitalized elders. Similar findings exist with samples of physicians. Thirty percent (DePaulo & Folstein, 1978) to 79% (Garcia, Tweedy, & Blass, 1984; McCartney & Palmateer, 1985) of cases were not recognized. These investigators concluded that the underdetection occurred because clinicians did not use standardized methods of cognitive assessment. No study was located that tested the hypothesis that routine use of standardized and systematic methods of evaluation improved the accuracy and timeliness of detecting acute confusion.

Methods have been developed to detect accurately and promptly patients who are acutely confused. However, there are competing requirements of maintaining psychometric rigor while maintaining clinical feasibility and patient acceptability. Some maintain that an acceptable instrument must be a screen and also usable to monitor cognitive function over time (Foreman, 1991; Vermeersch, 1991). However, it might be better to have two valid instruments rather than one.

Instruments currently used for detecting acute confusion fall into the following categories: (a) mental status questionnaires, (b) symptom checklists, (c) clinical interviews, and (d) psychomotor tests (Fraser, 1988; Levkoff, Liptzin, Cleary, & Evans, 1991; Nelson, Fogel, & Faust, 1986).

Mental status questionnaires, also known as bedside cognitive screening instruments are preferred by physicians. Several variants of the mental status questionnaire (Kahn, Goldfarb, Pollack, & Peck, 1960) were designed to have these qualities: sufficiently sensitive to detect a minor problem in cognitive function, sufficiently specific to exclude the fringes of normal functioning, able to characterize the specific nature of the impairment (e.g., acute confusion vs. dementia vs. depression), while remaining clinically feasible (i.e., acceptable to the patient, and quick and easy to administer and interpret by clinicians). The most frequently used mental status questionnaires are Pfeiffer's (1975) Short Portable Mental Status Questionnaire (SPMSQ), Folstein's (Folstein, Folstein, & McHugh, (1975) Mini-Mental State Examination (MMSE), and Jacobs' (Jacobs, Bernhard, Delgado, & Strain, 1977) Cognitive Capacity Screening Examination (CCSE). Although these questionnaires are considered the best available, only a dichotomous discrimination of patients is possible (i.e., discrimination between impaired and not impaired). Finer discriminations are not reliable (Foreman, 1987; Smyer, Hofland, & Jonas, 1979).

Numerous validation studies (see Table 1.1) of these instruments have been conducted with samples of individuals of varying racial (white, black, Hispanic); residential (community residing, hospitalized and institutionalized); health status (healthy, or with medical, neurologic, or psychiatric illnesses); and socioeconomic backgrounds. Findings of these studies made clear that the diagnostic precision of mental status questionnaires is limited (Anthony, LeResche, Niaz, Von Korff, & Folstein, 1982; Levkoff et al., 1991; Smyer et al., 1979; Wolber, Romaniuk, Eastman, & Robinson, 1984). It is difficult to establish whether this lack of diagnostic precision was a function of the properties of the instruments (i.e., of invalidity and unreliability) or of the acute confusion (i.e., of instability).

Also of concern with mental status questionnaires is the consolidation of findings into a composite or total score. This procedure reduces information and implies that attentional, memory, language, and other deficits are all equivalent. To surmount this concern, Kiernan, Mueller, Langston, and Van Dyke (1987) developed the Neurobehavioral Cognitive Status Examination

Table 1.1 Validation Studies of the Various Instruments for Detecting Acute Confusion

Short Portable Mental Status Questionnaire (Pfeiffer, 1975)
- Anthony, LeResche, Niaz, Von Korff, & Folstein, 1982
- Dalton, Pederson, Blom, & Holmes, 1987
- Erkinjuntti, Sulkava, Wikstrom, & Autio, 1987
- Fillenbaum & Smyer, 1981
- Foreman, 1987
- Haglund & Schukit, 1976
- Pfeiffer, 1975
- Smyer, Hofland, & Jonas, 1979
- Wolber, Romaniuk, Eastman, & Robinson, 1984

Mini-Mental State Examination (Folstein, Folstein, & McHugh, 1975)
- Bird, Canino, Stipec, & Shrout, 1987
- Bleecker, Bolla-Wilson, Kawas, & Agnew, 1988
- Dick, Guiloff, Stewart, Blackstock, Bielawska, & Marsden, 1984
- Escobar, Burnam, Karno, Forsythe, Landsverk, & Golding, 1986
- Fillenbaum, Hughes, Heyman, George, & Blazer, 1988
- Folstein, Folstein, & McHugh, 1975
- Foreman, 1987
- Jorm, Scott, Henderson, & Kay, 1988
- Magaziner, Bassett, & Hebel, 1987
- O'Connor, Pollitt, Hyde, Miller, Brook, & Reiss, 1989
- O'Connor, Pollitt, Treasure, Brook, & Reiss, 1989
- Paveza, Cohen, Blaser, & Hagopian, 1990
- Teng & Chui, 1987
- Teng, Chui, Schneider, & Metzger, 1987

Cognitive Capacity Screening Examination (Jacobs, Bernard, Delgado, & Strain, 1977)
- Foreman, 1987
- Gehi, Weltz, Strain, & Jacobs, 1980
- Jacobs, Bernard, Delgado, & Strain, 1977
- Kaufman, Weinberger, Strain, & Jacobs, 1979
- Omer, Foldes, Toby, & Menczel, 1983
- Strain, Fulop, Lebovits, Ginsberg, Robinson, Stern, Charap, & Gany, 1988
- Webster, Scott, Nunn, McNeer, & Varnell, 1984

Neurobehavioral Cognitive Status Examination (Kiernan, Mueller, Langston, & van Dyck, 1987)
- Kiernan, Mueller, Langston, & van Dyck, 1987
- Schwamm, van Dyck, Kiernan, Merrin, & Mueller, 1987

Confusion Assessment Method (Inouye, van Dyck, Alessi, Balkin, Siegal, & Horwitz, 1990)
- Foreman, Pompei, Lee, Ross, & Rudberg, 1991
- Inouye, van Dyck, Alessi, Balkin, Siegal, & Horwitz, 1990

Table 1.1 *(continued)*

Clinical Assessment of Confusion-A (Vermeersch 1990)
Foreman, 1989, 1991
Foreman, Pompei, Lee, Ross, & Rudberg, 1991
Kautz, Cheung, & Walker, 1991
Vermeersch, 1990

Neecham Confusion Scale (Neelon, Champagne, & McConnell, 1985)
Neelon, Champagne, & McConnell, 1985
Neelon, Champagne, McConnell, Carlson, & Funk, 1991, 1992
Miller, 1991
Siemsen, Miller, Newman, & Lucas, 1992

(NCSE) in which the multiple domains of cognitive function are evaluated independently, and a profile of function is generated. The NCSE provides greater and more specific information to the clinician; a cognitive profile is generated of the individual's cognitive abilities and disabilities that is said to be specific to the neuropsychiatric condition (e.g., senile dementia of the Alzheimer's type or hepatic encephalopathy) (Kiernan et al., 1987). Psychometric studies are acceptable (Kiernan et al., 1987; Schwamm et al., 1987), and results are promising. Additional limitations of the NCSE are that testing requires greater time to complete than other mental status questionnaires and poses considerable burden for the more impaired.

Other concerns about mental status questionnaires are that (a) performance is strongly influenced by age, educational level, ethnicity, and language (Bird, Canino, Stipec, & Shrout, 1987; Bleecker, Bolla-Wilson, Kawas, & Agnew, 1988; Escobar, Burnam, Karno, Forsythe, Landsverk, & Golding, 1986; Fillenbaum, Hughes, Heyman, George, & Blazer, 1988; Folstein et al., 1975; Jorm, Scott, Henderson, & Kay, 1988; Magaziner, Bassett, & Hebel, 1987). Older, more poorly educated minority persons whose primary language is not English perform less well; (b) distinction cannot be made between acute and chronic impairment; (c) all aspects of acute confusion are not measured by mental status questionnaires (e.g., psychomotor behavior, perceptual disturbances); and (d) responses are heavily verbal, and, thus cannot be used with nonverbal persons (e.g., those intubated and aphasic) (Foreman, 1987; Levkoff et al., 1991; Smyer et al., 1979; Wolber et al., 1984). More recently, Levkoff and colleagues (1991) and Vermeersch (1991) have questioned the validity of mental status questionnaires because they are based on antiquated (e.g., organic brain syndromes) rather than on contemporary (e.g., transient cognitive impairment) conceptualizations.

Behavioral, psychomotor, and symptom rating scales were developed to surmount many of the preceding identified limitations of mental status questionnaires. Instruments in these categories depend on the observations rather than the testing of acutely confused patients. Several instruments in this category exist: (a) the Confusion Rating Scale (Williams, Ward, & Campbell, 1988); (b) the Clinical Assessment of Confusion—A (Vermeersch, 1990); (c) the Delirium Rating Scale (Trzepacz, Baker, & Greenhouse, 1988); (d) the Confusion Assessment Method (Inouye, van Dyke, Alessi, Balkin, Siegal, & Horwitz, 1990); (e) the Neecham Confusion Scale (Neelon, Champagne, & McConnell, 1985); (f) the Delirium Symptom Interview (Albert et al., 1992); (g) the hand-held tachistoscope (Pauker, Folstein, & Moran, 1978); and (h) the Trailmaking Tests A and B (Reitan, 1958). These instruments were designed to detect acute confusion rather than some other phenomenon such as "mental status"; reflect objectively and consistently the essential aspects of acute confusion; accurately and promptly identify confusional behavior in all patients, especialy those not able to be evaluated using a questionnaire or interview format (e.g., individuals who are noncommunicative, persons who have sensory or physical impairments, and those in whom behavior changes rapidly or in whom manifestations of cognitive problems might be subtle); minimize the response burden on the patient; and facilitate use by nonpsychiatrically trained clinicians.

Despite good intentions and fairly rigorous validation testing, limitations of measurement persist. Many of the scales rely on clinical judgments for assessment, scoring, and interpretation, thus introducing subjectivity and unreliability (Kautz, Cheung, & Walker, 1991; Levkoff et al., 1991). Many of the behaviors to be observed are not specific to acute confusion (e.g., slurred speech, demanding behavior, and restlessness); therefore specificity is low (Foreman, Pompei, Lee, Ross, & Rudberg, 1991). Some procedures in these scales cannot be performed by acutely confused patients because such individuals cannot attend to directions (Anthony et al., 1985; Levkoff et al., 1991; Trzepacz et al., 1988). Educational and age biases persist (Pauker et al., 1978). Not all aspects of acute confusion are measured by the instruments, and the distinction cannot be made between acute and chronic conditions (Levkoff et al., 1991). Hence the need for additional valid and reliable instruments persists. Future instrument development should be deductive rather than empirical to ensure inclusion of all essential features of the phenomenon of acute confusion (Cameron et al., 1987; Inouye et al., 1990; Johnson et al., 1990; Trzepacz et al., 1988). Intensive and rigorous clinical testing is needed to demonstrate minimization of respondent burden, utility with noncommunicative patients, clinical feasibility for monitoring of changes in patient status, and ease of administration and interpetation for clinicians. Vermeersch (1991) suggested that two types of instruments may be needed: one to detect the onset of acute confusion, and another to monitor and determine the severity of the acute confusion. To date, no such instrument(s) has been developed.

Etiologic Basis of Acute Confusion

Multiple and disparate methods have been used to study the etiologic basis of acute confusion. Yet, no study fully met the criteria necessary for reaching definitive conclusions regarding the causal mechanisms behind acute confusion. Correlational designs have been used almost exclusively in the study of this condition. Thus, much is known about the various conditions surrounding the genesis of acute confusion, but little definitive and incontrovertible knowledge exists about causal relationships. As it seems unlikely that all plausible rival hypotheses could be eliminated or controlled without trivialization, it is improbable that definitive, incontrovertible evidence of the causal relationships of acute confusion will be found.

Nonetheless, what has been discovered about the etiologic basis of acute confusion is relatively consistent. First, it is clear that patients who are older (Blachy & Starr, 1964; Fields, MacKinzie, Charlson, & Perry, 1986; Golinger, Peet, & Tune, 1987; Jordan, Wilkinson, & Giuffre, 1991; Raway, 1991; Rockwood, 1989; Williams et al., 1979, 1985b); sicker (Blachy & Starr, 1964; Evans, 1987; Fields et al., 1986; Foreman, 1989; Francis, Martin, & Kapoor, 1990; Pompei, Foreman, Ross, Lee, & Rudberg, 1991; Rockwood, 1989); and cognitively impaired (Evans, 1987; Gustafson et al., 1988; Koponen, Hurri, Stenback, & Reikkinen, 1987; Koponen, Hurri, Stenback, Matilla, Soininen, & Riekkinen, 1989; Pompei et al., 1991; Rockwood, 1989) are more vulnerable to acute confusion during hospitalization.

Second, acute confusion generally has multiple rather than single causes (Foreman, 1989; Francis et al., 1990; Jolley, 1981) that span the spectrum of human illnesses. Hence, shifts in physiologic parameters are not perceived as clinically significant. This lack of perceived clinical significance emanates from lack of knowledge about precise limits of normal physiologic functioning, pharmacotherapeutics specific to the elderly, and interactive effects of medications. Thus, what is perceived as a situation within normal limits may in fact be an abnormal clinical state with accompanying acute confusion.

Third, there is general agreement about the most prevalent conditions associated with the genesis and presence of acute confusion. Although the designs of the studies failed to meet criteria for making definitive causal inferences, authors generally interpreted the relationships between these conditions and acute confusion as causal. Various pharmacologic agents were the most frequently identified cause of acute confusion (Foreman, 1989; Francis et al., 1990), especially agents with anticholinergic properties (Berrgren et al., 1987; Blazer, Federspiel, Raya, & Schaffner, 1983; Brannstrom, Gustafson, Norberg, & Winblad, 1989; Dellasega, 1990; Dickson, 1991; Golinger et al., 1987; Miller, Richardson, Jyu, Lemay, Hiscock, & Keegan, 1988; Mondimore, Damlouji, Folstein, & Tune, 1983; Purdie, Honigman, & Rosen, 1981; Summers, 1978; Tune, Holland, Folstein, Damlouji, Gardner, & Coyle, 1981), or those that have central nervous system effects (Berrgren et al., 1987; Brannstrom et al., 1989; Dellasega, 1990; Dickson, 1991; Purdie et al., 1981; Savageau et al., 1982; Sirois, 1988). The second most prevalent identified etiology was infection (Blank & Perry, 1984; Dickson, 1991; Francis et al., 1990; Levkoff et al., 1988; Morse & Litin, 1971; Purdie et al., 1981; Rabins & Folstein, 1982; Rockwood, 1989; Sadler, 1981), especially urinary tract and respiratory infections. However, it is unknown if the causal mechanism is a function of the infective agent or the hyperthermic response to the infective process. Fluid (Egerton & Kay, 1964; Francis et al., 1990; Gardner, 1984; Seymour, Henschke, Cape, & Campbell, 1980) and electrolyte imbalances, especially sodium (Dickson, 1991; Foreman, 1989; Francis et al., 1990; Morse & Litin, 1969; Purdie et al., 1981; Rockwood, 1989), and potassium (Foreman, 1989; Morse & Litin, 1969; Sirios, 1988), were identified as the third most common cause of acute confusion. Metabolic disturbances such as azotemia, alterations in pH, and nutritional deficiencies are the fourth most common cause (Dickson, 1991; Foreman, 1989; Francis et al., 1990; Gardner, 1984; Levkoff et al., 1988; Morse & Litin, 1969; Neelon et al., 1991; Rockwood, 1989).

It also has been shown that the etiologic basis of acute confusion varies across the trajectory of illnesses (Quinless, Cassese, & Atherton, 1985; Williams et al., 1985b); the nature of the health problem (i.e., medical vs. surgical); and the setting (Dellasega, 1990; Roberts & Lincoln, 1988). However, it is unclear whether this variability was entirely a function of the phenomenon itself or an artifact of the assessment techniques used to describe the phenomenon. Variables that were significant in studies with univariate designs dropped out when examined with multivariate designs (e.g., PaO_2). Also, some variables were significant for some patient populations and not for others (e.g., hypothermia and hemorrhage for surgical patients). Hence, there is disagreement as to whether the study of acute confusion should occur within narrowly defined patient populations (e.g., elderly patients undergoing surgery for traumatic hip fracture) or within more general populations (e.g., general medical patients). Those favoring narrow populations wish to control competing hypotheses, whereas the others asserted that acute confusion has universal characteristics; studies of narrow medical diagnostic categories may generate artifacts specific to that medical diagnostic category.

Debate continues about the relationships between sensory impairment, the environment, and acute confusion. Some argued that the relationship between sensory impairment and acute confusion is causal, whereas others insisted it is coincidental. Extremes in environmental characteristics are common with acute confusion, but it is not known if environmental factors are causative.

Epidemiology of Acute Confusion

The reported incidence and prevalence rates of acute confusion varied widely from a low of 8% in postoperative patients just before discharge from the hospital (Williams et al., 1979) to a high of 85% in terminally ill cancer patients (Massie, Holland, & Glass, 1983). This disparity in incidence and prevalence rates resulted from variability in the conceptual definition, measurement, precision of diagnostic criteria, diagnostic aids, and diagnostician. Generally, the more conservative the conception and operation, and the more sensitive and specific the measures, the lower the estimates of prevalence and incidence (e.g., studies of delirium diagnosed by a psychiatrist using the *Diagnostic and Statistic Manual*, 3rd ed., rev., criteria for delirium (Cameron et al., 1987; Inouye et al., 1990; Johnson et al., 1989; Trzepacz et al., 1988) are low). More liberal methods were associated with higher estimates of prevalence and incidence. Additionally, the presentation and manifestation of acute confusion among individuals and within an individual across time, methods of case finding, setting, and patient population influenced the findings about the incidence and prevalence of acute confusion.

Prevalence on Admission to the Hospital. The prevalence of acute confusion on admission to acute care hospitals has not been studied widely, but the findings of the few studies are consistent. Williams et al. (1979) reported a prevalence of 16% at admission for surgical repair of traumatic hip fracture. More recently, a prevalence of 16% also was reported in a sample of general medical patients (Francis et al., 1990) and surgical patients (Wanich, Sullivan, Gottleib, & Johnson, 1991). There has been speculation that acute confusion at admission results from the underlying health condition for which the individual was hospitalized (Foreman, 1989, 1991).

Incidence During Hospitalization. During hospitalization, the incidence of acute confusion ranged from 6% (Francis et al., 1990) to 55% (Chisholm, Deniston, Igrisan, & Barbus, 1982). Typically, the incidence ranges between 20% and 40% (e.g., Cavanaugh, 1983; Foreman, 1989, 1991; Neelon et al., 1991; Roberts & Lincoln, 1988; Schor et al., 1990; Williams et al., 1979, 1985a, 1985b). As mentioned previously, some of the variability in the incidence may be explained by methodological inconsistencies. However, assuming that the true incidence of acute confusion during hospitalization is much greater than that upon admission, it would be logical to conclude that many cases of acute confusion are iatrogenic or nosocomial in nature, and, therefore, preventable (Foreman, 1989, 1991). Nevertheless, Foreman,

Thies, and Anderson (1991) found no differences in various physiologic parameters between patients who were admitted acutely confused and those who became acutely confused later in the course of hospitalization.

Postoperative Incidence. Estimates of the postoperative incidence of acute confusion ranged from 15% in the first 24 hours after surgery (Jordan et al., 1991; Summers, 1978) to a high of 72% in cardiac surgery patients (Sadler, 1981). The cause of the acute confusion has been attributed to intraoperative hypotension (Quinless et al., 1985), profound intraoperative and postoperative hypothermia (Gardner, 1984; Sadler, 1981; Wragg, Dimsdale, Moser, Daily, Dembitsky, & Archbold, 1988), hemorrhage (Morse & Litin, 1969, 1971; Savageau, Stantor, Jenkins, & Klein, 1982), and the anticholinergic effect of various medications (Berrgren et al., 1987; Blazer et al., 1983; Brannstrom et al., 1989; Dellasega, 1990; Dickson, 1991; Golinger et al., 1987; Mondimore et al., 1983; Purdie et al., 1981; Summers, 1978; Tune et al., 1981).

Historically, the incidence of acute confusion was reported as higher in surgical than medical patients (Levkoff, Besdine, & Wetle, 1986), which may reflect a more conservative surgical attitude. However, recent data (Pompei et al., 1991) indicated that the incidence of acute confusion is the lowest in patients undergoing elective general surgical procedures (approximately 10% to 20% incidence), moderate in patients with general medical conditions (approximately 22% to 50%), and highest in patients with critical (requiring immediate medical or surgical intervention) or terminal illness (approximately 58% to 85%).

Incidence at Discharge From the Hospital. It seems reasonable that discharge from the hospital would occur only after the resolution of the acute confusion. However, such is not the case. Furstenberg and Mezey (1987) reported 29% of elderly patients admitted for the surgical repair of a fractured hip were discharged while acutely confused. Although the exact figure is unknown, Rogers et al. (1989) reported many of the subjects they studied remained acutely confused at the time of discharge. Dellasega (1990) reported that 46% of elderly patients admitted to a visiting nurse service had some degree of acute confusion.

Onset and Duration of Acute Confusion. The onset of acute confusion during hospitalization occurs shortly after admission (Berrgren et al., 1987; Chisholm et al., 1982; Egerton & Kay, 1964; Foreman, 1989, 1991; Johns, Large, Masterton, & Dudley, 1974; Morse & Litin, 1971; Pompei et al., 1991; Raway, 1991; Wanich et al., 1991; Williams et al., 1979; Wragg et al., 1988). Onset has been reported to range from the first 24 hr to the 6th day of hospitalization. Modal day of onset across studies is day 2, or between 24 and 48 hr of hospitalization. Few instances of the onset of acute confusion have been reported beyond the 6th day of hospitalization.

Controversy continues relative to the time of onset of acute confusion. Lipowski (1989) maintains that acute confusion often begins at night. Engel (1989), however, contends that it is not so, but that acutely confused patients, "whose level of awareness is already impaired, are likely to become further disoriented, frightened, and disturbed in the dark and quiet of the night, and hence behave in ways more likely to attract the attention of the staff" (p. 264).

Scant information was available about the duration of a state of acute confusion. Gustafson et al. (1991) recently reported the duration of acute confusion in patients postsurgery for the repair of hip fracture as less than 7 days. Pompei et al. (1991) reported the modal duration of an acute confusional state as approximately 3 to 4 days; cases of acute confusion lasting 7 days were rare.

Although desirable, more precise conclusions about the incidence, prevalence, onset, and duration of acute confusion are not possible. This imprecision is a result of methods that vary among studies and that are incongruent with the characteristics of the phenomenon. First, because the methods and criteria for case finding vary, what has been identified as acute confusion in one study may not be in another. Also, varying methods of detection were associated with varying degrees of sensitivity and specificity; more sensitive and specific methods were able to detect acute confusion sooner than those that are less sensitive and specific. As a result, different methods generated different findings about the incidence and prevalence of acute confusion.

Because it is agreed that acute confusion is dynamic (i.e., the clinical features fluctuate over the course of a day), multiple measurements over a 24-hr period would be expected. However, most investigators assessed the patients once per day (e.g., Foreman, 1989, 1991) and others measured acute confusion every other day (e.g., Williams et al., 1985). With widely spaced data points it is difficult to draw valid and reliable conclusions about the dynamic nature of acute confusion. Although more frequent measurements would provide more complete information about acute confusion, more frequent measurements are intrusive, add to respondent burden, lead to higher rates of subject attrition and misclassification (false positives owing to fatigue and false negatives owing to learning effects). Unobtrusive techniques might be helpful to improve sensitivity and specificity of measurement.

Outcomes of Acute Confusion

Findings about outcomes of acute confusion consistently showed that acute confusion is a marker of poor prognosis (Dickson, 1991; Eagles, Beattie, Restall, Rawlinson, Hagen, & Ashcroft, 1990; Fields, MacKenzie, Charlson, & Sax, 1986; Flint & Richards, 1956; Furstenberg & Mezey, 1987; Levkoff et al., 1986, 1988; Pompei et al., 1991; Rabins & Folstein, 1982; Rogers et al., 1989; Schor et al., 1990; Thomas, Cameron, & Fahs, 1988; Trzepacz, Teague, & Lipowski, 1985; Weddington, 1982). Outcomes included length of hospital stay, morbidity, mortality (inhospital and posthospitalization), and discharge disposition.

The length of hospitalization is protracted for patients experiencing some degree of acute confusion while hospitalized. Overall, patients with acute confusion were hospitalized about twice as long as nonconfused patients. This is true in recent as well as older studies, and in studies of both surgical and medical patients. Pompei et al. (1991) found that nonconfused elderly patients were hospitalized the same number of days as the diagnostic-related groups (DRG) reimbursement coverage. Conversely, patients who met specific criteria for acute confusion were hospitalized 4 days more than allowable by DRG. Schor et al (1991) reported similar findings.

Mortality rates for acutely confused patients were consistent across studies. Acutely confusioned elders were 3 to 5 times more likely to die than those who were not. Pompei et al. (1991) reported an inhospital mortality rate of 14% for acutely confused patients and less than 5% for comparable patients; in the 3 months following discharge from hospital the rates were 24% versus 10%, respectively. Schor et al. (1991) reported similar mortality rates: 26% versus 9%, and Rogers et al. (1989) reported 54% versus 15%.

Morbidity was higher in patients who were acutely confused. Acutely confused patients were more likely to experience adverse reactions to treatment, complications from the original illness(es), have a more protracted recuperative phase, and were less likely to return to preillness level of function (both cognitive and physical). Thus, acute confusion was a major reason for the nursing home placement of these patients (Zarit & Zarit, 1983).

Some argue that it was not the acute confusional state per se that resulted in poorer outcomes, but that acutely confused patients were more severely ill. However, in the study of Pompei et al. (1991), severity of illness failed to explain the variance in outcomes experienced by acutely confused patients. Hence, it may be impossible to conclude how morbidity and acute confusion are related. Does the acute confusion precipitate greater comorbidity; is greater morbidity reflective of greater physiologic instability that in turn is the cause of the acute confusion; or is there some interactive relationship between these two events? Further research is warranted.

Care of Patients Who are Acutely Confused

Intervention studies to prevent or manage acute confusion are few (Bay, Kupferschmidt, Opperwall, & Speer, 1988; Budd & Brown, 1974; Chatham, 1978; Fields et al., 1986; Gustafson et al., 1991; Langland & Panicucci, 1982; Lazarus & Hagens, 1968; Miller, 1991; Moore, 1977; Moore et al.,

1991; Nagley, 1986; Owens & Hutelmyer, 1982; Wanich et al., 1991; Williams et al., 1985b). Most interventions, especially those conducted by nurse investigators, have manipulated psychosocial variables, testing the influence of such strategies as providing orientation, clarification, and meaning to the patient's immediate environment (Bay et al., 1988; Budd & Brown, 1974; Chatham, 1978; Langland & Panicucci, 1982; Wanich et al., 1991; Williams et al., 1985b), continuity between patient and caregiver (Williams et al., 1985b), and anticipatory information about acute confusion (Owens & Hutelmyer, 1982). These strategies alone led to a lower incidence of acute confusion, fewer complications, a shorter hospitalization, and lessened the physiologic response to the experience. However, the incidence and consequences of acute confusion persisted at significant levels. Hence, it seems reasonable that these psychosocially oriented interventions are a necessary but insufficient intervention for acute confusion. Similarly, Gustafson et al. (1991) tested an intervention that was primarily physiologically based (e.g., oxygen therapy to prevent/minimize hypoxia and prevent perioperative hypotension). This intervention also led to a reduction in the incidence and severity of acute confusion, shortened the duration of the event, minimized complications, and shortened the length of hospitalization. Mortality and disposition on discharge were unaffected, and the incidence of acute confusion remained high, although reduced. As with psychosocial strategies, purely physiologically based interventions appear insufficient treatments for acute confusion. Interventions that incorporate both physiologic and psychosocial strategies seem a reasonable approach for future research.

Lived Experience of Acute Confusion

Acute confusion has been studied from the professionals', that is, the outsiders' perspectives. No accounts exist of the lived experience of acute confusion. Although such study is vital, many previously acutely confused elders are unable to recall the event; still others find it too unsettling to discuss it with others (Foreman, 1990). Yet, without insight into the subjective meaning and experience of acute confusion, a comprehensive understanding of this phenomenon may not be attainable. Qualitative or phenomenologic research into acute confusional states could provide valuable insights.

DIRECTIONS FOR FUTURE RESEARCH

Much remains unknown about acute confusion. It is clear that this is a prevalent and life-threatening condition among the elderly ill. Little theoretic or conceptual development has occurred, yet conceptualization is basic to knowledge generation. Thus, for any appreciable progress to occur in knowledge development relative to acute confusion, theoretic and conceptual efforts must increase and conceptual clarity must be achieved.

Some semblance of consensus must be reached relative to nomenclature to facilitate the communication of ideas. At a minimum, investigators must make explicit the conceptual and operational definitions and assumptions foundational to the study of acute confusion.

Cumulatively, the beliefs, lexicon, and nature of acute confusion pose serious obstacles to the development of knowledge about this important health problem (Foreman, 1991; Lipowski, 1983a, 1990; Vermeersch, 1991).

The nature of acute confusion also remains unclear because study designs fail to incorporate fundamental characteristics of acute confusion. For example, investigators ignore diurnal fluctuations in symptomatology. Studies must be designed to examine all variables causally implicated in the pathogenesis of acute confusion. Hence, designs should be (a) multivariate to include variables that incorporate relevant physiologic, psychologic, sociologic, and environmental factors; (b) continuous to capture the diurnal fluctuation of symptomatology; and (c) time series to follow elderly individuals not only across the trajectory of illness but through recovery to "health," and across all health care delivery settings. Interactive effects must be examined. Clinical, as opposed to statistical, significance also must be considered. Designs should incorporate sensitive and specific methods of measurement to determine precisely the nature and severity of cognitive deficits that comprise the phenomenon called acute confusion.

Additionally, phenomenologic approaches to the study of acute confusion must be undertaken to complement the knowledge gained through more traditional research approaches. Such study is difficult, but without insight into the human experience of acute confusion, it is doubtful that a comprehensive understanding of this phenomenon can be attained, or that effective methods of caring for such individuals can be devised.

Although considerable energies have been spent in developing measures for detecting acute confusion, there is need for improvement. The search continues for instrumentation that is (a) practical—easy to administer and interpret, nonburdensome for respondents, thus permitting frequent administrations, and effective in mute patients; (b) sensitive and specific—producing few false-positive or -negative misclassifications, and resistant to cultural, racial, and educational effects; and (c) discriminating—able to detect minor cognitive deficits, distinguish acute confusion from dementia and depression, and detect acute confusion superimposed on dementia or depression.

The incidence and prevalence of acute confusion is well documented, but little is known about the natural history of acute confusion. Yet information about timing and duration is crucial for developing cost-effective and efficacious interventions. Definitive information about the causes rather than correlates of acute confusion is needed. Accurate and clinically useful models or profiles of patients at risk for developing acute confusion, and profiles or models of patients who are resistant to acute confusion are needed. These predictive models or profiles should be able to be individualized, and should provide direction for preventing and managing patients with acute confusion.

ACKNOWLEDGMENTS

The assistance of Li-fen Wu, MS, RN, doctoral student, College of Nursing, University of Illinois-Chicago, in the preparation of this manuscript is acknowledged. Additionally, comments by Patricia E. H. Vermeersch, PhD, are greatly appreciated.

REFERENCES

Albert, M. S., Levkoff, S. E. Reilly, C., Liptzin, B., Pilgrim, D., Cleary, P. D., Evans, D., & Rowe, J. W. (1992). The Delirium Symptom Interview: An interview for the detection of delirium symptoms in hospitalized patients. *Journal of Geriatric Psychiatry and Neurology, 5,* 14–21.

American Psychiatric Association (1987). *The diagnostic and statistical manual of mental disorders* (3rd ed., rev.). Washington, DC: Author.

Anthony, J. C., LeResche, L., Niaz, U., Von Korff, M. R., & Folstein, M. F. (1982). Limits of the "Mini-Mental State" as a screening test for dementia and delirium among hospitalized patients. *Psychological Medicine, 12,* 397–408.

Anthony, J. C., LeResche, L. A., Von Korff, M. R., Niaz, U., & Folstein, M. F. (1985). Screening for delirium on a general medical ward: The tachistoscope and a global accessibility rating. *General Hospital Psychiatry, 7,* 36–42.

Bay, E. J., Kupferschmidt, B., Opperwall, B. J., & Speer, J. (1988). Effect of the family visit on the patient's mental status. *Focus on Critical Care, 15*(1), 10–16.

Berrgren, D., Gustafson, Y., Eriksson, B., Bucht, G., Hansson, L. I., Reiz, S., & Winblad, B. (1987). Postoperative confusion after anesthesia in elderly patients with femoral neck fractures. *Anesthesia and Analgesia, 66,* 497–504.

Bird, H. R., Canino, G., Stipec, M. R., & Shrout, P. (1987). Use of the Mini-Mental State Examination in a probability sample of a Hispanic population. *Journal of Nervous and Mental Disease, 175,* 731–737.

Blachy, P. H., & Starr, A. (1964). Post-cardiotomy delirium. *American Journal of Psychiatry, 121,* 371–375.

Blank, K., & Perry, S. (1984). Relationship of psychological process during delirium to outcome. *American Journal of Psychiatry, 141,* 843–847.

Blazer, D. G., Federspiel, C. F., Ray, W. A., & Schaffner, W. (1983). The risk of anticholinergic toxicity in the elderly: A study of prescribing practices in two populations. *Journal of Gerontology, 38,* 31–35.

Bleecker, M. L., Bolla-Wilson, K., Kawas, C., & Agnew, J, (1988). Age-specific norms for the Mini-Mental: State exam.. *Neurology, 38,* 1565–1568.

Brady, P. B. (1987). Labeling of confusion in the elderly. *Journal of Gerontological Nursing, 13*(6), 29–32.

Brannstrom, B., Gustafson, Y., Norberg, A., & Winblad, B. (1989). Problems of basic nursing care in acutely confused and non-confused hip-fracture patients. *Scandinavian Journal of Caring Science, 3*(1), 27–34.

Budd, S., & Brown, W. (1974). Effect of a reorientation technique on postcardiotomy delirium. *Nursing Research, 23,* 341–348.

Cameron, D. J., Thomas, R. I., Mulvihill, M., & Bronheim, H. (1987). Delirium: A test of the Diagnostic and Statistical Manual III criteria on medical in patients. *Journal of the American Geriatrics Society, 35,* 1007–1010.

Cavanaugh, S. (1983). The prevalence of emotional and cognitive dysfunction in a general medical population: Using the MMSE, GHQ, and BDI. *General Hospital Psychiatry, 5,* 15–24.

Chatham, M. A. (1978). The effect of family involvement on patients' manifestations of postcardiotomy psychosis. *Heart & Lung, 7,* 995–999.

Chisholm, S. E., Deniston, O. L., Igrisan, R. M., & Barbus, A. J. (1982). Prevalence of confusion in elderly hospitalized patients. *Journal of Gerontological Nursing, 8*(2), 87–96.

Dalton, J. E., Pederson, S. L., Blom, B. E., & Holmes, N. R. (1987). Diagnostic errors using the Short Portable Mental Status Questionnaire with a mixed clinical population. *Journal of Gerontology, 42,* 512–514.

Dellasega, C. (1990). *The prevalence of cognitive impairment in a cohort of elderly admission to the Visiting Nurse Association of Cleveland.* Unpublished manuscript, Pennsylvania State University, School of Nursing, University Park, PA.

DePaulo, J. R., Jr., & Folstein, M. F. (1978). Psychiatric disturbances in neurological patients: Detection, recognition, and hospital course. *Annals of Neurology, 4,* 225–228.

Dick, J. P. R., Guiloff, R. J., Stewart, A., Blackstock, J., Bielawska, C., Paul, E., & Marsden, C. D. (1984). Mini-Mental State Examination in neurological patients. *Journal of Neurology, Neurosurgery, and Psychiatry, 47,* 496–499.

Dickson, L. R. (1991). Hypoalbuminemia in delirium. *Psychosomatics, 32,* 317–323.

Eagles, J. M., Beattie, J. A. G., Restall, D. B., Rawlinson, F., Hagen, S., & Ashcroft, G. W. (1990). Relation between cognitive impairment and early death in the elderly. *British Medical Journal, 300,* 239–240.

Egerton, N., & Kay, J. H. (1964). Psychological disturbances associated with open heart surgery. *British Journal of Psychiatry, 110,* 433–439.

Engel, G. L. (1989). Delirium in the elderly patient [Letter to the editor]. *New England Journal of Medicine, 321,* 264.

Erkinjuntti, T., Sulkava, R., Wikstrom, J., & Autio, L. (1987). Short Portable Mental Status Questionnaire as a screening test for dementia and delirium among the elderly. *Journal of the American Geriatrics Society, 35,* 412–416.

Escobar, J. I., Burnam, A., Karno, M., Forsythe, A., Landsverk, J., & Golding, J. M. (1986). Use of the Mini-Mental State Examination (MMSE) in a community population of mixed ethnicity: Cultural and linguistic artifacts. *Journal of Nervous and Mental Disease, 174,* 607–614.

Evans, L. K. (1987). Sundown syndrome in institutionalized elderly. *Journal of American Geriatrics Society, 35,* 101–108.

Fields, S. D., MacKenzie, R., Charlson, M. E., & Perry, S. W. (1986). Reversibility of cognitive impairment in medical inpatients. *Archives of Internal Medicine, 146,* 1593–1596.

Fields, S. D., MacKenzie, R., Charlson, M. E., & Sax, F. L. (1986). Cognitive impairment. Can it predict the course of hospitalized patients? *Journal of the American Geriatrics Society, 34,* 579–585.

Fillenbaum, G. G., Hughes, D. C., Heyman, A., George, L. K., & Blazer, D. G. (1988). Relationship of health and demographic characteristics to Mini-Mental State Examination score among community residents. *Psychological Medicine, 18,* 719–726.

Fillenbaum, G. G., & Smyer, M. A. (1981). The development, validity, and reliability of the OARS Multidimensional Functional Assessment Questionnaire. *Journal of Gerontology, 36,* 428–434.

Flint, F. J., & Richards, S. M. (1956). Organic basis of confusional states in the elderly. *British Medical Journal, 2,* 1537–1539.

Folstein, M. F., Folstein, S. E., & McHugh, P. R. (1975). "Mini-Mental State": A practical guide for grading the cognitive state of patients for the clinician. *Journal of Psychiatric Research, 12,* 189–198.

Foreman, M. D. (1984). Acute confusional states in the elderly: An algorithm. *Dimensions of Critical Care Nursing, 3,* 207–215.

Foreman, M. D. (1986). Acute confusional states in the hospitalized elderly: A research dilemma. *Nursing Research, 35,* 34–38.

Foreman, M. D. (1987). Reliability and validity of mental status questionnaires in elderly hospitalized patients. *Nursing Research, 36,* 216–220.

Foreman, M. D. (1989). Confusion in the hospitalized elderly: Incidence, onset, and associated factors. *Research in Nursing & Health, 12,* 21–29.

Foreman, M. D. (1990). *The meaning and experience of acute confusion.* Unpublished manuscript, University of Illinois at Chicago, College of Nursing, Chicago.

Foreman, M. D. (1991). The cognitive and behavioral nature of acute confusional states. *Scholarly Inquiry for Nursing Practice, 5*(1), 3–16.

Foreman, M. D., & Grabowski, R. (1991). *Cognitive impairment in the elderly: A diagnostic dilemma.* Unpublished manuscript, University of Illinois at Chicago, College of Nursing, Chicago.

Foreman, M. D., Pompei, P., Lee, B. J., Ross, R., & Rudberg, M. A. (1991). *Detecting delirium in the hospitalized elderly.* Unpublished manuscript, University of Illinois at Chicago, College of Nursing, Chicago.

Foreman, M. D., Thies, S., & Anderson, M. A. (1991). *Adverse consequences of hospitalization for acute illness in the elderly.* Unpublished manuscript, University of Illinois at Chicago, College of Nursing, Chicago.

Francis, J., & Kapoor, W. N. (1990). Delirium in hospitalized elderly. *Journal of General Internal Medicine, 5,* 65–79.

Francis, J., Martin, D., & Kapoor, W. N. (1990). A prospective study of delirium in hospitalized elderly. *Journal of the American Medical Association, 263,* 1097–1101.

Fraser, M. (1988). Selecting an instrument to measure mental status and consciousness. In M. Frank-Stromborg (Ed.), *Instruments for clinical nursing research* (pp. 47–78). Norwalk, CT: Appleton & Lange.

Furstenberg, A. L., & Mezey, M. D. (1987). Mental impairment of elderly hospitalized hip fracture patients. *Comprehensive Gerontology, 1,* 80–85.

Garcia, C. A., Tweedy, J. R., & Blass, J. P. (1984). Underdiagnosis of cognitive impairment in a rehabilitation setting. *Journal of the American Geriatrics Society, 32,* 339–342.

Gardner, J. (1984). Post-operative confusion in elderly hip surgical patients. *Australian Journal of Advanced Nursing, 1*(3), 6–10.

Gehi, M., Weltz, N., Strain, J. J., & Jacobs, J. (1980). Is there a need for admission and discharge cognitive screening for the medically ill? *General Hospital Psychiatry, 3,* 186–191.

Golinger, R. C., Peet, T., & Tune, L. E. (1987). Association of elevated plasma anticholinergic activity with delirium in surgical patients. *American Journal of Psychiatry, 144,* 1218–1220.

Gustafson, Y., Berrgren, D., Brannstrom, B., Bucht, G., Norberg, A., Hansson, L. A, & Winblad, B. (1988). Acute confusional states in elderly patients treated for femoral neck fracture. *Journal of the American Geriatrics Society, 36,* 525–530.

Gustafson, Y., Brannstrom, B., Berggren, D., Ragnarsson, J. I., Sigaard, J., Bucht, G., Reiz, S., Norberg, A., & Winblad, B. (1991). A geriatric-anesthesiologic program to reduce acute confusional states in elderly patients treated for femoral neck fractures. *Journal of the American Geriatrics Society, 39,* 655–662.

Haglund, R. M. J., & Schuckit, M. A. (1976). A clinical comparison of tests of organicity in elderly patients. *Journal of Gerontology, 31,* 654–659.

Inouye, S. K., van Dyck, C. H., Alessi, C. A., Balkin, S., Siegal, A. P., & Horwitz, R. I. (1990). Clarifying confusion: The Confusion Assessment Method. A new method for detection of delirium. *Annals of Internal Medicine, 113,* 941–948.

Jacobs, J. W., Bernard, M. R., Delgado, A., & Strain, J. J. (1977). Screening for organic mental syndromes in the medically ill. *Annals of Internal Medicine, 86,* 40–46.

Johns, M. W., Large, A. A., Masterton, J. P., & Dudley, H. A. F. (1974). Sleep deprivation and delirium after open heart surgery. *British Journal of Surgery, 61,* 377–381.

Johnson, J. C., Gottleib, G. L., Sullivan, E., Wanich, C., Kinosian, B., Forciea, M. A., Sims, R., & Hogue, C. (1990). Using DSM-III criteria to diagnose delirium in elderly general medical patients. *Journals of Gerontology: Medical Sciences, 45,* M113–M119.

Jolley, D. (1981). Acute confusional states in the elderly. In D. Coakley (Ed.), *Acute geriatric medicine* (pp. 175–189). London: Croom Helm.

Jordan, B. L., Wilkinson, C., & Giuffre, M. (1991). *Acute confusion in hospitalized elderly postoperative patients.* Unpublished manuscript. Dartmouth-Hitchcock Medical Center, Hanover, NH.

Jorm, A. F., Scott, R., Henderson, A. S., & Kay, D. W. K. (1988). Educational level differences on the Mini-Mental State: The role of test bias. *Psychological Medicine, 18,* 727–731.

Kahn, R. L., Goldfarb, A. I., Pollack, M., & Peck, A. (1960). Brief objective measures for the determination of mental status in the aged. *American Journal of Psychiatry, 117,* 326–328.

Kaufman, D. M., Weinberger, M., Strain, J. J., & Jacobs, J. W. (1979). Detection of cognitive deficits by a brief mental status examination: The Cognitive Capacity Screening Examination, a reappraisal and a review. *General Hospital Psychiatry, 3,* 247–255.

Kautz, D. D., Cheung, R. B., & Walker, M. K. (1991). *Practical assessment of subtle changes in cognition in hospitalized elders*. Unpublished manuscript, University of Kentucky, College of Nursing, Lexington, KY.

Kiernan, R. J., Mueller, J., Langston, J. W., & Van Dyke, C. (1987). The Neurobehavioral Cognitive Status Examination: A brief but differentiated approach to cognitive assessment. *Annals of Internal Medicine, 107,* 481–485.

Koponen, H., Hurri, L., Stenback, U., Matilla, E., Soininen, H., Riekkinen, & P. J. (1989). Computed tomography findings in delirium. *Journal of Nervous and Mental Disease, 177,* 226–231.

Koponen, H., Hurri, L., Stenback, U., & Riekkinen, P. J. (1987). Acute confusional states in the elderly: A radiological evaluation. *Acta Psychiatria Scandinavia, 76,* 726–731.

Langland, R. M., & Panicucci, C. L. (1982). Effects of touch on communication with elderly confused clients. *Journal of Gerontological Nursing, 8*(3), 152–155.

Lazarus, H. R., & Hagens, J. H. (1968). Prevention of psychosis following open-heart surgery. *American Journal of Psychiatry, 124,* 1190–1195.

Levkoff, S., Besdine, R., & Wetle, T. (1986). Acute confusional states (delirium) in the hospitalized elderly. *Annual Review of Gerontology and Geriatrics. 6,* 1–26.

Levkoff, S., Liptzin, B., Cleary, P., & Evans, D. (1991). Review of research instruments and techniques used to detect delirium. *International Psychogeriatrics, 3,* 251–268.

Levkoff, S. E., Safrana, C., Cleary, P. D., Gallop, J., & Phillips, R. S. (1988). Identification of factors associated with the diagnosis of delirium in elderly hospitalized patients. *Journal of the American Geriatrics Society, 36,* 1099–1104.

Lipowski, Z. J. (1983a). Transient cognitive disorders (delirium/acute confusional states in the elderly). *American Journal of Psychiatry, 140,* 1426–1436.

Lipowski, Z. J. (1983b). The need to integrate liaison psychiatry and geropsychiatry. *American Journal of Psychiatry, 140,* 1003–1005.

Lipowski, Z. J. (1989). Delirium in the elderly patient. *New England Journal of Medicine, 320,* 578–582.

Lipowski, Z. J. (1990). *Delirium: Acute confusional states*. New York: Oxford University Press.

Lucas, M. J., & Folstein, M. F. (1980). Nursing assessment of mental disorders on a general medical unit. *Journal of Psychiatric Nursing and Mental Health Services, 18,* 31–33.

Ludwick, R., & Scott, M. (1991). *Time, work and frustration: Perceptions of caring for confused patients*. Unpublished manuscript, Kent State University, Kent, OH.

Ludwick, R., Scott, M., & O'Toole, R. (1991). *Nurse recognition and reaction to patients' confusion*. Unpublished manuscript, Kent State University, Kent, OH.

Magaziner, J., Bassett, S. S., & Hebel, J. R. (1987). Predicting performance on the Mini-Mental State Examination: Use of age- and education-specific equations. *Journal of the American Geriatrics Society, 35,* 996–1000.

Massie, M. J., Holland, J., & Glass, E. (1983). Delirium in terminally ill cancer patients. *American Journal of Psychiatry, 140,* 1048–1050.

McCartney, J. R., & Palmateer, L. M. (1985). Assessment of cognitive deficit in geriatric patients: A study of physician behavior. *Journal of the American Geriatrics Society, 33,* 467–471.

Miller, J. (1991). *The environmental optimization intervention protocol*. Unpublished doctoral dissertation, Oregon Health Sciences University, School of Nursing, Portland, OR.

Miller, P. S., Richardson, J. S., Jyu, C. A., Lemay, J. S., Hiscock, M., & Keegan, D. L. (1988). Association of low serum anticholinergic levels and cognitive impairment in elderly presurgical patients. *American Journal of Psychiatry, 145,* 342–345.

Mondimore, F. M., Damlouji, N., Folstein, M. F., & Tune, L. (1983). Post-ECT confusional states associated with elevated serum anticholinergic levels. *American Journal of Psychiatry, 140,* 930–931.

Moore, D. P. (1977). Rapid treatment of delirium in critically ill patients. *American Journal of Psychiatry, 134,* 1431–1432.

Moore, K. A., Champagne, M. T., Neelon, V. J., & Bresler, L. E. (1991). *Primary nurse ratings of nursing care needs of elderly hospitalized medical patients.* Unpublished manuscript, University of North Carolina at Chapel Hill School of Nursing, Chapel Hill, NC.

Morgan, D. L. (1985). Nurses' perceptions of mental confusion in the elderly: Influence of resident and setting characteristics. *Journal of Health and Social Behavior, 26,* 102–112.

Morse, R. M., & Litin, E. M. (1969). Postoperative delirium: A study of etiologic factors. *American Operating Room Nurses Journal, 10*(11), 85–92.

Morse, R. M., & Litin, E. M. (1971). The anatomy of a delirium. *American Journal of Psychiatry, 128,* 143–148.

Nagley, S. J. (1986). Predicting and preventing confusion in your patients. *Journal of Gerontological Nursing, 12*(3), 27–31.

Nagley, S. J., & Dever, A. (1988). What we know about treating confusion. *Applied Nursing Research, 1,* 80–83.

Neelon, V. J., Champagne, M. T., & McConnell, E. S. (1985). *The Neecham Confusion Scale.* Unpublished manuscript, University of North Carolina at Chapel Hill School of Nursing, Chapel Hill, NC.

Neelon, V. J., Champagne, M. T., McConnell, E. S., Carlson, J. R., & Funk, S. G. (1992). Use of the Neecham Confusion Scale to assess acute confusional states of hospitalized older patients. In S. Funk, E. Tournquist, M. Champagne, & R. Wiese (Eds.), *Key aspects of eldercare: Managing falls, incontinence, and cognitive impairment* (pp. 278–289). New York: Springer Publishing Co.

Neelon, V. J., Champagne, M. T., McConnell, E. S., Carlson, J. R., & Funk, S. G. (1991). *Clinical correlations of the Neecham Confusion Scale in assessing cognitive status of the hospitalized older patient.* Unpublished manuscript, University of North Carolina at Chapel Hill School of Nursing, Chapel Hill, NC.

Neelon, V. J., Champagne, M. T., & Moore, K. A. (1989). *Acute confusion in hospitalized elders: Vertical and horizontal patterns of development—Implications for intervention.* Unpublished manuscript, University of North Carolina at Chapel Hill School of Nursing, Chapel Hill, NC.

Nelson, A., Fogel, B. S., & Faust, D. (1986). Bedside cognitive screening instruments: A critical assessment. *Journal of Nervous and Mental Disease, 174,* 73–83.

O'Connor, D. W., Pollitt, P. A., Hyde, J. B., Fellows, J. L., Miller, N. D., Brook, C. P. B., & Reiss, B. B. (1989). The reliability and validity of the Mini-Mental State in a British community survey. *Journal of Psychiatric Research, 23,* 87–96.

O'Connor, D. W., Pollitt, P. A., Treasure, F. P., Brook, C. P. B., & Reiss, B. B. (1989). The influence of education, social class, and sex on Mini-Mental State scores. *Psychological Medicine, 19,* 771–776.

Omer, H., Foldes, J., Toby, M., & Menczel, J. (1983). Screening for cognitive deficits in a sample of hospitalized geriatric patients: A re-evaluation of a brief mental status questionnaire. *Journal of the American Geriatrics Society, 31,* 266–268.

Owens, J. F., & Hutelmyer, C. M. (1982). The effect of pre-operative intervention on delirium in cardiac surgical patients. *Nursing Research, 31,* 60–62.

Palmateer, L. M., & McCartney, J. R. (1985). Do nurses know when patients have cognitive deficits? *Journal of Gerontological Nursing, 11*(2), 6–16.

Pauker, N. E., Folstein, M. F., & Moran, T. H. (1978). The clinical utility of the hand-held tachistoscope. *Journal of Nervous and Mental Disease, 166,* 126–129.

Paveza, G. L., Cohen, D., Blaser, C. J., & Hagopian, M. (1990). A brief form of the Mini-Mental State Examination for use in community care settings. *Behavior, Health, and Aging, 1,* 133–139.

Pfeiffer, E. (1975). A Short Portable Mental Status Questionnaire for the assessment of organic brain deficit in elderly patients. *Journal of the American Geriatrics Society, 23,* 433–441.

Pompei, P., Foreman, M. D., Ross, R., Lee, B. J., & Rudberg, M. A. (1991). *Early detection, evaluation, and treatment of delirium in the hospitalized elderly.* Unpublished manuscript, University of Chicago, Chicago.

Purdie, F. R., Honigman, B., & Rosen, P. (1981). Acute organic brain syndrome: A review of 100 cases. *Annals of Emergency Medicine, 10,* 455–461.

Quinless, F. W., Cassese, M., & Atherton, N. (1985). The effect of selected pre-operative, intraoperative, and postoperative variables on the development of postcardiotomy psychosis in patients undergoing open heart surgery. *Heart & Lung, 14,* 334–341.

Rabins, P. V., & Folstein, M. F. (1982). Delirium and dementia: Diagnostic criteria and fatality rates. *British Journal of Psychiatry, 140,* 149–153.

Rasmussen, B. H., & Creason, N. S. (1991). Nurses' perception of the phenomenon confusion in elderly hospitalized patients. *Vard Norden, 1,* 5–12.

Raway, B. (1991). *Acute confusion in two types of elderly hip surgery patients.* Unpublished manuscript, The Catholic University of America, Washington, DC.

Reitan, R. M. (1958). Validity of the trailmaking test as an indicator of organic brain damage. *Perceptual and Motor Skills, 8,* 271–276.

Roberts, B. L., & Lincoln, R. E. (1988). Cognitive disturbance in hospitalized elders. *Research in Nursing & Health, 11,* 309–319.

Rockwood, K. (1989). Acute confusion in elderly medical patients. *Journal of the American Geriatrics Society, 37,* 150–154.

Rogers, M. P., Liang, M. H., Daltroy, L. H., Eaton, H., Peteet, J., Wright, E., & Albert, M. (1989). Delirium after elective orthopedic surgery: Risk factors and natural history. *International Journal of Psychiatry in Medicine, 19,* 109–121.

Rowe, J. W., & Khan, R. L. (1987). Human aging: Usual and successful. *Science, 237,* 143–149.

Sadler, P. D. (1981). Incidence, degree, and duration of postcardiotomy delirium. *Heart & Lung, 10,* 1084–1092.

Savageau, J. A., Stanton, B. A., Jenkins, C. D., & Klein, M. D. (1982). Neuropsychological dysfunction following elective cardiac operation. *Journal of Thoracic and Cardiovascular Surgery, 84,* 585–594.

Schor, J., Levkoff, S. E., Liptzin, B., Cleary, P., Lipsitz, L., Pilgrim, D., Wetle, T., Reilly, K., Wei, J., Evans, D., & Rowe, J. W. (1990). Influence of delirium on hospital length of stay [Abstract]. *Journal of the American Geriatrics Society, 38,* A7.

Schwamm, L. H., Van Dyke, C., Kiernan, R. J., Merrin, E. L., & Mueller, J. (1987). The Neurobehavioral Cognitive Status Examination: Comparison with the Cognitive Capacity Screening examination and the Mini-Mental State Examination in a neurosurgical population. *Annals of Internal Medicine, 107,* 486–491.

Seymour, D. G., Henschke, P. J., Cape, R. D. T., & Campbell, A. J. (1980). Acute confusional states and dementia in the elderly: The role of dehydration/volume depletion, physical illness and age. *Age and Ageing, 9,* 137–146.

Siemsen, G. A., Miller, J., Newman, A., & Lucas, C. (1992). Predictive value of the Neecham Confusion Scale. In S. Funk, E. Tournquist, M. Champagne, & R. Wiese (Eds.), *Key aspects of eldercare: Managing falls, incontinence, and cognitive impairment* (pp. 289–299). New York: Springer Publishing Co.

Sirois, F. (1988). Delirium: 100 cases. *Canadian Journal of Psychiatry, 33,* 375–378.

Smyer, M. A., Hofland, B. F., & Jonas, E. A. (1979). Validity study of the Short Portable Mental Status Questionnaire for the elderly. *Journal of the American Geriatrics Society, 27,* 263–269.

Strain, J. J., Fulop, G., Lebovits, A., Ginsberg, B., Robinson, M., Stern, A., Charap, P., & Gany, F. (1988). Screening devices for diminished cognitive capacity. *General Hospital Psychiatry, 10,* 16–23.

Strub, R. L., & Black, F. W. (1985). *The mental status examination in neurology* (2nd ed.). Philadelphia: Davis.

Summers, W. K. (1978). A clinical method of estimating risk of drug induced delirium. *Life Sciences, 22,* 1511–1516.

Teng, E. L., & Chui, H. C. (1987). The modified Mini-Mental State (3MS) Examination. *Journal of Clinical Psychiatry, 48,* 314–318.

Teng, E. L., Chui, H. C., Schneider, L. S., & Metzger, L. E. (1987). Alzheimer's dementia: Performance on the Mini-Mental State Examination. *Journal of Consulting and Clinical Psychology, 55,* 96–100.

Thomas, R. I., Cameron, D. J., & Fahs, M. C. (1988). A prospective study of delirium and prolonged hospital stay. *Archives of General Psychiatry, 45,* 937–940.

Trzepacz, P. T., Baker, R. W., & Greenhouse, J. (1988). A symptom rating scale for delirium. *Psychiatry Research, 23,* 89–97.

Trzepacz, P. T., Teague, G. B., & Lipowski, Z. J. (1985). Delirium and other organic mental disorders in a general hospital. *General Hospital Psychiatry, 7,* 101–106.

Tune, L. E., Holland, A., Folstein, M. F., Damouji, N. F., Gardner, T. J., & Coyle, J. T. (1981). Association of postoperative delirium with raised serum levels of anticholinergic drugs. *Lancet,* 651–652.

Vermeersch, P. E. H. (1990). The Clinical Assessment of Confusion—A. *Applied Nursing Research, 3,* 128–133.

Vermeersch, P. E. H. (1991). Response to "The cognitive and behavioral nature of acute confusional states." *Scholarly Inquiry for Nursing Practice, 5,* 17–20.

Wanich, C., Sullivan-Marx, E., Gottlieb, G., & Johnson, J. (1992). *Functional status outcomes of a nursing intervention in hospitalized elderly. Image, 24,* 201–207.

Webster, J. S., Scott, R. R., Nunn, B., McNeer, M. F., & Varnell, N. (1984). A brief neuropsychological screening procedure that assesses left and right hemispheric function. *Journal of Clinical Psychology, 40,* 237–240.

Weddington, W. W., Jr. (1982). The mortality of delirium: An underappreciated problem. *Psychosomatics, 23,* 1232–1235.

Williams, M. A., Ward, S. E., & Campbell, E. B. (1988). Confusion: Testing versus observation. *Journal of Gerontological Nursing, 14*(1), 25–30.

Williams, M. A., Holloway, J. R., Winn, M. C., Wolanin, M. O., Lawler, M. L., Westwick, C. R., & Chin, M. H. (1979). Nursing activities and acute confusional states in elderly hip-fractured patients. *Nursing Research, 28,* 25–35.

Williams, M. A., Campbell, E. B., Raynor, W. J., Mlynarczyk, S. M., & Ward, S. E. (1985a). Reducing acute confusional states in elderly patients with hip fractures. *Research in Nursing & Health, 8,* 329–337.

Williams, M. A., Campbell, E. B., Raynor, W. W., Jr., Musholt, M. A., Mlynarczyk, S. M., & Crane, L. F. (1985b). Predictors of acute confusional states in hospitalized elderly patients. *Research in Nursing & Health, 8,* 31–40.

Wolanin, M. O. (1973). *Confusion in the elderly.* Paper presented at the Gerontological Research Conference, Blue Mountain Lake, NY.

Wolber, G., Romaniuk, M., Eastman, E., & Robinson, C. (1984). Validity of the Short Portable Mental Status Questionnaire with elderly psychiatric patients. *Journal of Consulting and Clinical Psychology, 52,* 712–713.

Wragg, R. E., Dimsdale, J. E., Moser, K. M., Daily, P. O., Dembitsky, W. P., & Archbold, C. (1988). Operative predictors of delirium after pulmonary thromboendarterectomy. *Journal of Thoracic and Cardiovascular Surgery, 96,* 524–529.

Zarit, S. H., & Zarit, J. M. (1983). Cognitive impairment. In P. M. Lewinsohn & L. Teri (Eds.), *Clinical geropsychiatry: New directions in assessment and treatment* (pp. 38–80). New York: Pergamon.

Chapter 2

The Shivering Response

Barbara J. Holtzclaw
School of Nursing
University of Texas Health Sciences Center-San Antonio

CONTENTS

Shivering is the primary defense against cold in humans beyond the first year of life. This seemingly innocuous response is so much a part of life that it is underestimated as a source of physical exertion and psychologic distress. Nurses and physicians usually are surprised to learn that vigorous shivering parallels moderate physical work in its energy expenditure. As evidence accumulates about the metabolic costs and sequelae of shivering in healthy persons, concern grows for those who are ill or physically frail. Physiologists have systematically studied shivering in animals and humans for nearly 40 years. By contrast, most medical and nursing research on the topic has occurred within the past decade. This integrative review is limited to human or primate studies. Much of what is known about the neural mechanisms of shivering was first elucidated from nonprimate animal models. These findings provide significant direction to human research. Discussion of shivering, for the purpose of this review, is limited to the thermoregulatory response and does not include transient tremors or "shivers" associated with fear, delight, or other sympathetic arousal. Shivering is defined as a protracted generalized course of involuntary contractions of skeletal muscles that are usually under voluntary control (Hemingway, 1963).

METHODS OF REVIEW

Research from nursing, medicine, and the biologic sciences was found through computerized and manual searches of *Index Medicus* and *Cumulative Index of Nursing and Allied Health Literature (CINAHL)*. Citations from 1970 to 1983 were manually searched, and those from 1983 to 1991 were searched by means of Silver Platter *Medline* and Silver Platter *CINAHL* interactive compact disk, read only memory (CD-ROM) program. *Biological Abstracts* were searched manually. Key words were often more successful than title searches in finding relevant literature. Shivering was often a variable in studies related to fever or rewarming. The terms *chills* or *rigors* were sometimes used instead of shivering. Early classic studies, some dating from the 1940s, were found by the "ancestry" approach. That is, previous generations of work were traced from references in more recent publications. Strom's chapter on thermoregulation (1960) and the chapter on shivering by Hemingway and Stuart (1963) included citations of studies that clarify the conceptual basis for subsequent work in shivering. Physiologic studies of animals and humans comprised the largest body of published research related to shivering. Before the 1980s, this work was located within the context of the more general topic of thermoregulation. An exception was Hemingway's (1963) comprehensive review of shivering, which continues to be cited as a time-honored reference. The physiologic studies cited provide scientific basis for clinical application by identifying neurologic pathways of shivering stimulus, dominance of skin receptors, patterns of shivering progression, and related metabolic expenditure.

The next largest group of published shivering-related studies is in the medical and nursing specialty of anesthesia. Most were related to incidental or induced hypothermia during surgery, but a smaller number were related to shivering associated with epidural anesthesia or birth. This review is limited to anesthesia citations involving problems for which both nurses and anesthetists share concern and control.

There is a paucity of research related to nursing actions to control shivering, although the problem is often addressed in the general nursing literature. The first published study was that of a nonpharmacologic measure, falling within the purview of independent nursing actions. In this pilot study researchers tested the effectiveness of extremity wraps to control shivering during surface cooling (Abbey et al., 1973). The same intervention was tested in a second study (Abbey & Close, 1979). In a comprehensive review (1982), Abbey clarified the scientific basis of the intervention used in these studies. The essential conceptual elements cited in this work provided a framework of nursing action for future studies and literature related to shivering (Holtzclaw, 1986; Rutledge & Holtzclaw, 1988; Holtzclaw, 1990a, 1990b, 1990c).

For purposes of the present review, research is grouped into five categories that have important clinical implications for nursing: (a) shivering as a primary thermoregulatory response includes citations that explain normal physiologic correlates and consequences; (b) shivering as a physiologic threat includes studies that provide evidence of adverse effects; (c) factors influencing shivering threshold includes studies central to prevention and control; (d) assessment of shivering includes reviews of measurements for clinical care and research; and (e) prevention and control of shivering includes studies with relevance to intervention.

SHIVERING AS A PRIMARY THERMOREGULATORY RESPONSE

Shivering plays an integral role in maintaining internal body temperatures within an optimum range (approximately 36.4°C–37.4°C) called the thermostatic "set point." When temperatures fall below this range, shivering provides heat-generating defense against the cold. Metabolic or nonshivering thermogenesis is of little significance to humans beyond infancy. Shivering is stimulated by functionally specific heat loss thermoreceptors in the skin, spinal cord, and brain. Thermosensory impulses are received at the preoptic area of the hypothalamus where they are functionally integrated. Deviations below the optimal set point activate the shivering center in the posterior hypothalamus (Hardy, 1980). Shivering is stimulated via the anterior spinal routes of the gamma efferent motor system to cause oscillation and friction of the fibrous muscle spindles of the fusimotor system (Sato, 1981). This rhythmic isotonic contraction of flexors and extensors against a constant load is *aerobic activity* requiring oxidative phosphorylation of glucose and fatty acids. These processes increase oxygen consumption three- to fivefold over resting values. Shivering generates significant amounts of heat but interferes with heat conservation. Muscle contractions actually promote heat loss by (a) creating convective currents from body movements, (b) increasing circulation to skin, and (c) perfusing cooler vascular beds.

Shivering as a Thermoregulatory Response to Fever

A comprehensive review of literature related to shivering should not overlook its relationship to fever. Shivering in fever is not caused by an actual heat deficit but by a "sensed" one. The pyrogen drives up the thermostatic set point to a higher level, causing a disparity between existing temperatures and those dictated by the set point (Stitt, Hardy, & Stolwijk, 1974). Shivering during the "chill phase" of fever is mediated by the same mechanisms as that from cooling, despite rising body temperatures. Shivering and vasoconstriction quickly raise body temperatures to the new set point level. During fever, heat loss from skin plays a predominant role in the febrile chill, with less cooling of skin necessary to stimulate shivering. This factor has great implications for nursing care to prevent shivering.

Nursing actions based on scientific knowledge can directly influence the onset, duration, and severity of the shivering response in febrile patients. Situations that promote heat loss abound in the clinical setting, yet many health care providers seem unaware of the incidence, severity, and threat of shivering to the patient. The extent to which shivering may compromise illness outcomes or increase morbidity is not known. There remain many untested interventions to diminish heat loss or promote conservation of heat in vulnerable patients.

SHIVERING AS A PHYSIOLOGIC THREAT

Metabolic Costs and Cardiorespiratory Sequelae

Vigorous shivering is fatiguing, even to healthy individuals who tolerate the energy expenditure as they do strenuous exercise. Metabolic costs of shivering activity were shown in young healthy males ($n = 9$), exposed while nude to changing temperatures ranging from 26°C to –3°C (Horvath, Spurr, Hutt, & Hamilton, 1956). Shivering was recorded by ballistocardiograph, ventilatory volumes were measured by a Tissot spirometer, and metabolic rate was determined by values from a Beckman analyzer for oxygen consumption (VO_2) and a Liston-Becker analyzer for carbon dioxide. During cooling, mean oxygen VO_2 increased gradually from a 228 ml/min baseline to a maximum of 674 ml/min, but VO_2 values rose significantly during shivering episodes. Carbon dioxide production followed a similar pattern with significant increases during shivering. Pairwise comparisons ($p < 0.05$) were used, but no statistical comparisons were made between the multiple repeated measures of VO_2.

Residual effects of profound oxygen demand during vigorous shivering include an oxygen debt that remains when muscular activity subsides. Large amounts of oxygen are consumed then with labored breathing and deep ventilation (Dowben, 1980). Horvath et al. (1956) found oxygen debt accounted for more than one-fifth the total oxygen expended during cold exposure. Moreover, the heat gained by shivering, when compared with heat content lost from cooling, showed an efficiency of about 11%. Shivering-related oxygen expenditure in healthy subjects is shown to equate to that of bicycle riding or shoveling snow (Newstead, 1987). Limits in the amount of heat that can be produced by shivering were demonstrated in healthy male subjects ($n = 16$) (Iampietro, Vaughan, Goldman, Kreider, Masucci, & Bass 1960) monitored during falling temperature and increasing wind velocity. Although values of 440 to 525 cal/hr were predicted from curves at higher temperatures, no subject achieved a greater heat production than 442 cal/hr, despite violent uncontrollable shivering. Highest levels of heat production occurred at low temperature and high wind speeds. This study was conducted with a small sample but in a carefully controlled laboratory situation. Measurements were made in a temperature and humidity controlled chamber, using a Tissot spirometer and Beckman oxygen analyzer. Descriptive rather than inferential statistical analyses were done.

Cardiorespiratory Consequences of Postoperative Shivering

The oxygen demand documented in healthy subjects who shiver raises reasonable concern for patients with hypoxemia or impaired cardiorespiratory systems. Yet the literature reveals little attention to the problem until postoperative shivering captured the interest of anesthesiology in the 1960s. Among the first published reports of postoperative shivering (Cohen, 1967), were observations that this activity markedly elevated VO_2 and lowered arterial oxygen saturation (SaO_2). Relationships between falling temperatures and metabolic expenditure were studied in adults (n = 24) undergoing elective surgery under general anesthesia (Roe, Goldberg, & Blair, 1966). When temperatures fell 0.2°C or more, subjects exhibited shivering, vasoconstriction, and VO_2 increases of 68%. When temperatures fell 0.3°C to 1.2°C, shivering activity raised VO_2 levels 92%. Relationships between shivering and SaO_2 were reported (Bay, Nunn, & Prys-Roberts, 1968) in general surgery patients (n = 24). Using t tests for comparison, the 10 who shivered had significantly lower SaO_2 values during shivering than at rest, and as compared with nonshivering patients. Interest in postoperative shivering grew as induced hypothermia for cardiovascular surgery became more common. Reliable instrumentation and continuous measurement during bypass and rewarming made it easier to study relationships between shivering and cardiorespiratory events. The metabolic analyzer, connected to the intake and outflow ports of the patient's mechanical ventilator, enabled sampling and analysis of inspired and exhaled gases. Geer and Holtzclaw (1986) used such a device to measure metabolic rate during postoperative shivering in 24 adult hypothermic cardiac bypass surgery patients. Shivering was monitored by electromyogram (EMG) and visually by ordinal scale of increasing cephalad-to-caudal progression (0 to 4). VO_2 increased significantly during stages 2 to 4, but was not matched by comparable increases in cardiac output (CO). Kaplan and Guffin (1985) cited similar findings in an abstract describing rewarming hypothermic cardiac surgery patients (n = 7). Despite being warmed to 37°C while on bypass, temperatures fell postbypass to a mean of 33.8°C accompanied by vigorous shivering. Cardiac output increased during shivering in two patients, but in the other five no change in CO occurred. Oxygen consumption doubled in all subjects, but oxygen delivery remained unchanged. This insufficient response to oxygen demand raises risk for hypoxemia in hemodynamically unstable patients.

Rapid rewarming after hypothermic bypass exacerbates problems related to rising metabolic rate. "Rewarming acidosis," originally blamed on the influx of fixed acids and metabolites from previously constricted vascular beds (Rosenfeld, 1963), is now believed to have respiratory origins as well. Sladen (1985) cited the problem of acute respiratory acidosis in nearly half the cardiac surgery patients studied (n = 75) during rapid rewarming. The investigator made no attempt to document shivering but emphasized the need to clarify its role. The same investigator, studying another group of 22 rewarming postoperative cardiac surgery patients, found 63% shivered (Sladen, Renaghan, Ashton, & Wyner, 1985). Among those who shivered, 60% developed acute respiratory acidosis, whereas none of the nonshivering group developed this problem. Other recent investigators showed that shivering suppression, ventilatory support, and measures to promote slow uniform warming of tissues prevented severe metabolic expenditure and acidosis during rewarming. Rodriguez, Weissman, Damask, Askanazi, Hyman, and Kinney (1983) demonstrated this effect in a study of 16 mechanically ventilated postoperative surgical patients. All were passively rewarmed with a sheet and thermal blanket: 8 were kept paralyzed with metocurine iodide, and 8 were given the standard treatment. The measurement of shivering in this study was imprecise, and did not estimate stages, levels, or severity. Investigators used visual observation to detect "gooseflesh" skin and descending episodic neck-to-pectoral muscular fibrillations, sometimes involving extremities. Subjects who were kept pharmacologically paralyzed did not shiver and were delayed in rewarming. Conversely, *t*-test comparisons show paralyzed subjects had lower oxygen consumption and myocardial oxygen consumption than controls. The sampling frame is not discussed, and it is not clear whether subjects were randomly assigned to treatment or control groups. Subjects in each group did not differ by age, weight, body surface area, or operative time. The article is widely cited because the investigators objectively measured and compared differences in metabolic expenditure between shivering and nonshivering patients.

Cardiorespiratory Consequences of Fever

Fever is recognized as a hypermetabolic state, but little attention is given to the role of febrile shivering in this process. The pyrogenic reaction is known to raise body temperature by increasing heat production, but specific contributions of cellular versus shivering thermogenesis are not clear. Consequences of febrile shivering are few. Calorimetric studies show that an increase of 1°C in body temperatures raises metabolic rate 10% to 13% (Beisel, Wannemacher & Neufeld, 1980). Palmes and Park (1965) studied temperature changes, shivering, and metabolic activity in healthy males ($n = 10$) with fever induced by typhoid vaccine. Study analyses consisted primarily of graphic comparisons and descriptive findings. Metabolic rate intensified during shivering, with VO_2 and degree of fever directly proportional to severity of shivering. Hyperventilation was driven by oxygen demand and had negligible effect on heat loss.

In a pilot and more extensive study, Holtzclaw (1990a, 1990b) examined consequences of drug-induced febrile shivering related to amphotericin B in anemic patients with cancer. Shivering was monitored in the pilot study by visual stages and in the second study by EMG. Heart rate and blood pressure were used to calculate rate pressure product (RPP), an index of myocardial oxygen consumption. In the second study, tympanic membrane (TM) temperatures were measured by hand-held light reflectance thermometer (Holtzclaw, 1990a). In both investigations, physiologic values were compared between intervals before, during, and after shivering by repeated measures analysis of variance. RPP was significantly higher during shivering episodes than either before or after in both studies. This demonstrated that although RPP and respiratory rate increased proportionally with TM temperature (Holtzclaw, 1990a), shivering raised it significantly higher.

Although the two studies had nearly identical aims, the pilot study was limited by several instrumentation problems. Temperature measurement could not be used as a variable in the pilot because clinical oral or rectal thermometers were considered hazardous to use with vigorously shivering patients who also had fragile mucous membranes. In the second study, investigators used TM thermometers with digital readout to obtain measurements. A similar problem in instrumentation in the pilot study was found in measurement of heart rate by auscultation and blood pressures from a wall-mounted mercury sphygmomanometer. Both modes of measurement are subject to observer error and problems with reliability, despite precautions in training and testing data collectors. Body movements during shivering interfere with clear ascultatory perception. The investigator improved measurement during the second study by using heart rate derived from the electrocardiograph and blood pressure obtained by automatic self-inflating cuff with digital readout.

The significance of shivering, febrile or otherwise, is probably not well appreciated among investigators who do not regularly deal with the topic. The absence of reference to shivering in a study of cardiovascular consequences and oxygen demands of fever is an example (Haupt & Rackow, 1983). The febrile state decreased left ventricular performance and myocardial oxygen consumption among patients in a critical care setting (n = 36). Hemodynamic measurements were continuously monitored, but no mention is made of the presence or absence of shivering. The investigators discussed possible sources of increased myocardial oxygen demand and tachycardia of fever with no consideration of the chill phase as a factor.

FACTORS INFLUENCING SHIVERING THRESHOLD

Shivering is stimulated by heat-loss sensors in the central nervous system and skin; however, those in skin are dominant. Skin thermoreceptors "lead" thermoregulatory responses to heat loss even though internal temperatures may remain constant. Three major factors appear to influence the threshold for shivering stimulus: the hypothalamic set-point range or threshold, tension of the muscle spindle, and gradients between skin and central temperatures. In situations in which heat loss and sympathetic stimulation occur concurrently, clear distinctions between cold-induced shivering and tremor may be more difficult to make (Goold, 1984; Sessler, Israel, Pozos, Pozos, & Rubinstein, 1988). Gradients between skin and core temperatures widen when patients are inadvertently or deliberately exposed to conditions of rapid heat loss, or during fever when the hypothalamic set point is reset to a higher level by effects of pyrogen.

Surface Cooling of Skin

Shivering from surface cooling ranges from transient chilling when a warm person is suddenly exposed to a cool environment to profound vigorous rigors that accompany induced hypothermia by surface cooling. The latter is generally induced by a cooling blanket, containing hollow coils of circulating coolant, which conducts heat away from the skin. Shivering is a compensatory mechanism to correct the discrepancy between falling skin temperatures with the hypothalamic set point.

Nielsen (1976) demonstrated the dominance of skin over core temperatures in eliciting changes in metabolic rate and shivering in six healthy males during warm and cool temperatures, while exercising, resting, or swimming in a flume of cold water. Large deviations in core temperature occurred with little effect on metabolic rate or shivering. These responses occurred only when the skin was cold and below tympanic membrane temperature. When skin was warmed above 34°C, low core temperature had no effect. The specific thermoreceptors in skin are not uniformly distributed (Hansel, 1970). Specific regions such as hands, feet, and face are more dominant in afferent influence. Research on specific nursing measures based on these principles is addressed in the section on prevention and control of shivering.

Central Cooling by Circulatory Heat Exchange

A major stimulus to shivering occurs after cardiac surgery to patients cooled to hypothermic levels by the cardiopulmonary bypass pump. Body temperatures are lowered below 30°C to reduce metabolic rate and oxygen demand during aortic cross-clamping. Unlike the hypothermic patient who is surface cooled, the centrally cooled bypass patient must rewarm from the "inside out." Deep interior regions are rewarmed by the bypass pump at the end of the procedure, but zones of poorly perfused superficial tissue remain cool and vasoconstricted. Steep temperature gradients between skin and core stimulate shivering as the patient emerges from effects of anesthesia and neuromuscular blocking. Although relationships of skin-to-core gradients and shivering have been studied in other groups, no published research that examined these effects in the centrally cooled patient was found. Gradients between central thermal zones were observed by Earp and Finlayson (1991) in a study of 14 postoperative cardiac surgery patients. Although pulmonary artery temperatures were higher than bladder temperatures immediately after bypass rewarming, reversal of the normal gradients occurred after shivering. The authors speculate that the hypermetabolic activities associated with shivering may contribute to this phenomenon.

Febrile Alteration of Set Point

Much of what is known about the origin of fever and its influence on humans has been discovered through animal studies. Animal studies have helped to clarify the pathways and effects of febrile study. Stitt, Hardy, and Stolwijk (1974) demonstrated in animal models the relationship of set-point reference and thermosensitivity during the chill phase of fever. Fever, once considered a pathologic condition, has been shown to have a role in host-defense response. Among the recently identified *endogenous pyrogens* are the cytokines known as the interleukins. Interleukin 1 is known to induce antibody formation by B lymphocytes, enhance mitogenesis of T lymphocytes, and activate lymphocytic response to antigen or mitogen. Biochemists and physiologists continue to clarify these roles (Kluger, 1991). Despite these potentially beneficial effects of fever, no known benefits relate to shivering. By contrast, the distress and energy expenditure from this response is well known (Beisel et al., 1980; Holtzclaw, 1990a, 1990b).

Emergence From Anesthesia

Postanesthetic recovery is a period of thermal instability for many patients. It is estimated that over half the patients undergoing general surgery experience core temperatures less than 36°C (Slotman, Jed, & Burchard, 1985). Emergence from anesthesia is known to produce other neurologic signs that resemble tremor similar to that of patients with spinal transection (Goold, 1984; Sessler et al., 1988). Cohen (1967) noted this phenomenon in patients receiving the halogenated hydrocarbon agent, halothane. Observations of muscle spasticity have been seen with other halogenated hydrocarbons and their isomers. Sessler et al. (1988) monitored rectal and mean skin temperatures and EMG in patients ($n = 9$) anesthetized with isoflurane (Forane). Visual shivering was rated, and EMG tracings from subjects were compared with those measured in other patients with cold-induced shivering and those with pathologic clonus from spinal cord transection. The investigators concluded from EMG comparisons, and lack of correlation between EMG activity and rectal temperature, that most spontaneous postanesthesia tremor seen after isoflurane is not thermoregulatory in nature. Findings of this study warrant further investigation to clarify the tremor/shiver controversy over whether the anesthetic or hypothermia is the cause. Clonic EMG tremors have been attributed to spinal reflex hyperactivity, caused by the action of the anesthetic to inhibit descending cortical control. This interpretation does not consider variations in cold-induced shivering manifested in humans that change from phase to phase. The initial tonic continuous contractions later change to more phasic clonic patterns (Kleinebeckel & Klussmann, 1990). Although acknowledging the persistent hypothermia in these subjects, the possibility of hypothermic suppression of thermoregulation is not addressed. Core temperatures below 34°C suppress thermoregulation (Strom, 1960). In such cases, skin sensation would fail to elicit shivering until more euthermic conditions were reached. The relationship of shivering to rectal temperature is not always a dependable correlate of shivering in the hypothermic patient, because the response is stimulated by integrated inputs from throughout the body. One problem with rectal temperatures reflecting dynamic changes in the hypothermic patient is that it lags behind pulmonary artery and tympanic membrane temperatures by 30 min or more (Azar, 1980). The question of statistical power for use of parametric tests with this small sample ($n = 9$) is not adequately justified. In the analysis, each muscle (eight per subject) is observed for 90 epochs, and considered as 720 observations. The assumption of independence for each observation is not met. McCulloch and Milne (1990) prospectively studied 30 patients undergoing minor elective procedures for incidence and duration of postanesthetic neurologic abnormalities in arousal state, muscle tone, deep tendon reflexes, and plantar reflex. Sustained clonus, shivering, intense muscular spasticity, and axillary temperatures were assessed. Patients receiving enflurane (Ethrane) had more transient neurologic signs than those receiving isoflurane (Forane). Temperature was unrelated to shivering.

Effects of Parturition

The precise mechanisms that cause shivering after childbirth are not known. Shivering is estimated to affect about 22% of normal vaginal deliveries (Jaameri, Jahkola, & Perttu, 1966) and may involve some elements of heat loss, pyrogenic response, or effects of anesthesia. Jaameri et al. (1966), compared 500 shivering patients with 500 controls and found few differences. Mean age of the shivering group was statistically higher, and there were more in that group with scanty amniotic fluid. An estimated 9.6% incidence of shivering occurs during the first stage of labor. Webb, James, and Wheeler (1981) found incidence tripled when epidural anesthesia was given, but warming the injectate made no difference in shivering incidence.

ASSESSMENT OF SHIVERING

Shivering activity is a difficult parameter to measure. The two methods most commonly found in the literature are EMG measurements and observed stages of shivering. Mechanical and palpation/sensation methods are less frequently reported. Oxygen consumption is cited by Hemingway (1963) as the most quantitative method of measuring shivering under controlled conditions, yet one particularly susceptible to nonshivering influences. For this reason, VO_2 is used more often in clinical studies as one of several indicators of shivering sequelae.

Electromyographic Measurement

Many investigators consider EMG to be the "gold standard" of shivering measurement. They are used with surface or needle electrodes in laboratory studies to measure action potentials from shivering muscles. Each type of electrode presents problems of its own. The intrusiveness and potential discomfort of needle electrodes make them undesirable for clinical application, and surface electrodes are plagued with problems of contact impedance of the skin. The bioelectric amplifier also must contend with difficult problems in obtaining small-amplitude biopotential signals from muscle contraction while ignoring 60-Hz interference from the environment. The local alternating current power source serving appliances, lighting, and electrical beds pervades the clinical area with electrical signals as much as a million times stronger than those being monitored (Applegate, 1988). Slight degrees of shivering are often difficult to differentiate from the bioelectrical activity from voluntary movement, respiratory activity, and cardiac conduction. Although the ease and objectivity of continuous EMG tracings are attractive for research use, this advantage is tempered by its inexactness as a measure of shivering intensity. Amplitude of EMG activity depends on the number of active motor units in the involved muscle and the frequency of their discharge. Therefore, variations in the size and placement of EMG electrodes can cause differences in measurements within and between subjects (Zuniga,

Truong, & Simons, 1970). Still other variations are caused by amplifier gains and settings within the monitoring equipment. Hemingway (1963) cites the lack of reproducibility as a major problem in using EMG to *quantify* shivering. Rectified or integrated EMG signals might reliably be used as arbitrary representations of shivering changes in a given subject within the same observation period. The use of EMG amplitude-frequency data in between observation or between subject comparisons has little meaning. The phasic pattern or rhythm of shivering has been used more successfully to document the incidence and stages of shivering (Hemingway, 1963). The continuous *tonic muscle activity* of the initial phases of shivering is different from the two other rhythms: *grouped* and *burstlike* patterns, seen during cold tremor in other species (Kleinebeckel & Klussmann, 1990). In humans, the initial phase is characterized by repetitive EMG activity preceding visible tremor. Later stages become more clonic in nature, occurring in groups or bursts. In 15 hypothermic cardiac surgery patients observed during rewarming, rapid phasic bursts of EMG activity in the 100- to 500-μV range were measured from the masseters. These signals occurred 3 to 50 min before the onset of visible shivering (Holtzclaw & Geer, 1986).

Mechanical Measurement

Shivering causes a tremor and physical vibration that is detectable by mechanical means. Although use of this method in clinical studies is negligible, the ballistocardiograph, accelerometer, pressure detectors, and piezoelectric crystals have been used in the laboratory. Alone, these measurements are not sufficient to differentiate between shivering and other physical movements. In combination with EMG to verify the typical phasic bursts of muscle contraction and visual observation to rule out nonshivering movements, mechanical methods are most useful to signal onset and intensity of shivering.

Palpatory Methods

Holtzclaw (1986) observed that palpable masseter vibrations referred to the mandibular ridge coincided with the EMG signals of nonvisible preshivering activity in a study of 15 hypothermic cardiac surgery patients. These vibrations were palpated as a mild mandibular "hum" to the examiner's fingers. As a consistent prodromal predictor of shivering this provided a clinical indicator as well as a method of identifying this stage of shivering for research. The method for palpating these vibrations is described in a review article (Holtzclaw, 1986) on postoperative shivering in which the researcher also reported the association between palpable and visible shivering and metabolic values. The study methods are minimally reported in the article, which focuses primarily on the physiologic and pharmacologic dynamics of shivering after cardiac surgery. Statistical comparisons of metabolic changes over time are decribed, showing little change during the mandibular hum, but significant change at the onset of visible shivering. The palpable mandibular hum was found to precede febrile shivering in the investigator's two subsequent studies (Holtzclaw, 1990a, 1990b). The need for a systematic protocol for palpation and training of data collectors to assure interrater reliability is emphasized by the author.

Visual Measurements

There is little standardization among published studies for visual observation of shivering severity. Shivering is often visually detected but poorly quantified in the research literature. Even when shivering sequelae are reported as carefully monitored variables, the measurement of shivering remains arbitrary. Hemingway demonstrated that shivering follows a cephalad-to-caudal progression, with earliest difficult-to-detect tremors beginning in the masseters and the most violent shivering including the extremities (1963). He and others developed some of the first visual scales for shivering by grading the tremor amplitude into levels of magnitude. Abbey et al. (1973) extended the work of Girling and Topliff (1966) by developing a clinical assessment scale for shivering severity based on stages of muscle involvement. Staged on an ordinal scale of 0 to 4, shivering was ranked as 0 = no evidence; 1 = palpable muscle tone in the masseters; 2 = palpable evidence of muscle tone in the pectorals; 3 = general continuous shivering without teeth chattering; and 4 = general continuous shivering with teeth chattering. Interrater reliability between data collectors was established and further validated by EMG. The scale was used in subsequent studies of shivering during surface cooling (Abbey & Close, 1979). It was adapted by Holtzclaw (1986) for use with postoperative cardiac patients by including the palpable mandibular hum, and modifying the teeth chattering criterion. The last change was made because all patients had endotracheal tubes, making teeth chattering difficult to differentiate from nonshivering "clenching" of teeth on the tubing. The scale was revised as follows: 0 = no visible or palpable shivering; 1 = palpable manidular vibration or electrocardiograph (ECG) artifact; 2 = visible fasciculation of the head or neck; 3 = visible fasciculation of the pectorals and trunk; and 4 = generalized shaking of the entire body, with or without teeth chattering. This scale was found reliable for shivering detection in its previsible stage. Verification of the mandibular "hum" by EMG lends support to its validity as a clinical predictor that might be useful to clinicians. Differentiation between stages 3 and 4 requires close observation, particularly when the patient is covered, as the trunk passively shakes the extremities during violent shivering. This shivering scale has been used in subsequent research with febrile patients (Holtzclaw, 1990a, 1990b).

PREVENTION AND CONTROL OF SHIVERING

By far, the greatest interest in shivering has been in determining measures to prevent or control the response. Literature falls into four categories of concern: shivering related to hypothermia, shivering related to anesthesia, febrile shivering, and postpartum shivering. There is some overlap in these categories. For example, there is some controversy over whether postanesthesia shivering is related to hypothermia or the effects of the anesthetic agent (Goold, 1984; Sessler et al., 1988).

Pharmacologic Measures

Nurses must often judge when and whether to administer drugs to alleviate shivering. Of major concern is the need to determine if the drug has eliminated shivering activity, or if it has merely alleviated the patient's awareness of shivering. Researchers evaluating effectiveness of shivering suppressent drugs provided important information to guide assessment and research. The most commonly used drugs to control shivering in current practice are neuromuscular blocking agents and narcotics. Although morphine and other opiates have been tested as shivering suppressants, meperidine hydrochloride has found greater acceptance. Although neuromuscular blockade guarantees the suppression of shivering by paralysis, it prolongs rewarming. Meperidine was effective in suppressing shivering in general surgery patients (n = 14) who received halogenated hydrocarbon anethesia (Macintyre, Pavlin, & Dwersteg, 1987). Shivering significantly increased VO_2 and carbon dioxide production, whereas meperidine suppressed visible postoperative shivering within 5 min of injection. Claybon and Hirsh (1980) found similar effects. Even when meperidine does not relieve shivering activity, it tends to diminish the patient's awareness of shivering and imparts a perception of warmth. Meperidine failed to ameliorate shivering during rewarming in 24 open heart surgery patients (Geer & Holtzclaw, 1986). Fifteen subjects shivered and showed significant increases in energy expenditure, despite treatment with meperidine and nitroprusside. Harris, Lawson, Cooper, and Ellis (1989), found intravenous meperidine no more effective than saline placebo in preventing shivering after epidural lidocaine anesthesia. Shivering related to epidural was not related to temperature, and was not ameliorated by any of the warming measures or meperidine. The authors concluded that this type of shivering may not be thermoregulatory in nature.

Meperidine has been tested as a shivering suppressant for shaking chills induced by pyrogenic drugs (Burks, Aisner, Fortner, & Wiernik, 1980). Nine patients were randomly assigned to treatment and 10 to placebo groups. Treatment was either intravenous meperidine, 25 to 60 mg ($M = 45$), or isotonic saline. Comparisons between groups showed significantly shorter duration of shivering among those receiving meperidine. Seven subjects were randomized during repeated infusions of amphotericin B; 19 chill reactions occurred and were treated with meperidine. The mean time for cessation of shivering was shorter in the treatment group. Fisher's exact tests and Student's *t*-tests of means were used for comparisons in the simple two-group comparative analyses. The type of analysis used for the repeated measures is not described and only the *p* values are cited. It is not clear whether the most severe reaction is used as the unit of analyses or if the repeated measures are inappropriately accumulated to enlarge the sample.

In two studies of the effectiveness of extremity wraps to reduce amphotericin B-induced shivering (Holtzclaw, 1990a, 1990b), patients were not deprived of routine meperidine to treat shivering. Instead, the amount of drug required for shivering was a dependent variable in these studies. In both studies, patients were randomly assigned to treatment or control conditions, and the amount of meperidine given during the amphotericin B infusion was compared between groups by independent-measures *t*-test. Patients with the wraps required less meperidine in both studies, although this finding was not statistically significant in the first study. Confounding variables that influenced meperidine administration were more carefully controlled in the second study. The investigator used inservice education to standardize criteria for meperidine administration before the second study, which essentially changed the way shivering suppressant drugs were given. Information to nurses included the pharmacodynamic nature and half-life properties of intravenous meperidine and the time that shivering generally occurred during the shiver-inducing infusion. These measures improved the drug's efficacy and decreased the total amount of drug needed by either group, but less meperidine was needed by the group with the physical intervention. The use of prostaglandin antagonists as shivering suppressants has not been fully examined. In a study involving physical measures, Abbey and Close (1979) found acetaminophen given 4 to 6 hours before hypothermia suppressed shivering.

Neuromuscular blockade provides the most effective arrest of shivering but must be confined to use with artificially ventilated patients. In hypothermic cardiac surgery patients, heat deficit is so great and heat distribution within the body so uneven that shivering is difficult to halt with narcotics or superficial rewarming. Rapid rewarming also poses circulatory and metabolic hazards. Instead, patients are kept paralyzed for longer periods to promote even heat distribution and prevent shivering. Zwischenberger, Kirsh, Dechert, Arnold, and Bartlett (1987) studied the effects of shivering on oxygen consumption in cardiac surgery patients (n = 33) randomized to either neuromuscular blockade with pancuronium bromide and metubine sulfate (n = 15) or to control conditions (n = 18). No measurement of shivering other than "observation" was described. Three patients with neuromuscular blockade shivered and were removed from the study, whereas six controls failed to shiver and were likewise not included in the sample. This reconfigured the groups to shivering nonparalyzed and nonshivering paralyzed subjects. The shivering group rewarmed more quickly (M = 4 h) than the paralyzed group (M = >6 h). The paralyzed group had lower minute oxygen consumption, carbon dioxide production, higher mixed venous oxygen saturation, and improved hemodynamic stability when values were compared by t-test with those of controls.

Physical Measures

Although numerous studies have tested physical measures to prevent and correct hypothermia, only about one-half of the investigators addressed the intervention's effects on shivering. The importance of specific cutaneous receptors as a shivering stimulus is well documented in controlled laboratory studies of humans (Collins, Easton, & Exton-Smith, 1981; Keatinge, Mason, Millard & Newstead, 1986) and primates (Murphy, Lipton, Loughran, Giesecke, 1984). In each, warming or cooling skin through radiation, convection or conduction, initiates or ameliorates shivering independent of central temperature. Dominance of particular regions such as the face or the extremities has been noted (Hensel, 1970; Mekjavic & Eiken, 1985).

Insulative Extremity Wraps. Based on the neurologic work by Hensel (1970) and others, Abbey developed a method of insulating the most dominant skin thermoreceptors while cooling patients to hypothermic levels. The interventions was tested in a pilot study (Abbey et al., 1973) carried out in several settings with intensive care unit patients (n = 15) cooled to reduce fever or cerebral edema. Hands and feet were protected with wraps of three layers of terry cloth toweling, and heat was conducted to the cooling blanket from the trunk. Visible shivering was graded by ordinal scale of severity (0–4) and temperatures by rectal probe. Shivering was anticipated in nearly all neurologically intact patients during hypothermic cooling, so no control group was used. Although data are reported descriptively, with no statistical analyses delineated, the findings are clinically significant. Wrapping the extremities lowered frank shivering incidence from the expected 94% to 100% down to 24% without use of any shiver-suppressant drugs.

The wrapping procedure was tested in a further study (Abbey & Close, 1979) of similar patients ($n = 35$), with bioinstruments to monitor EMG, ECG, and temperatures from auditory canal, rectum, and lateral thigh. This publication is an abstract and includes little detail about the characteristics of the subjects, except that 25 were neurosurgical and 10 nonneurosurgical patients. No statistical analyses are described other than levels of significance. With random assignment to two groups, those with extremity wraps experienced significantly less shivering than those not wrapped. The effects of integrated afferent inputs to shivering stimulus were supported in this study as no one temperature site predicted shivering.

This same intervention was found effective in preventing febrile shivering during amphotericin B administration (Holtzclaw, 1990a, 1990b). Rationale for the intervention was similar to that for surface cooling, even though in fever there was no heat deficit. The rising gradient between set point and environmental temperature tends to lower the threshold for shivering so that less cooling of skin is required to stimulate shivering. Even neutral or mildly cool room temperatures are sensed as very cold during a febrile chill. When randomly assigned subjects in the pilot ($n = 40$) and subsequent ($n = 20$) study were wrapped before infusion of the pyrogenic drug, they had significantly less shivering incidence and severity than controls (Holtzclaw, 1990a, 1990b). Whereas the pilot study was limited in many respects by use of visual and tactile observations for shivering assessment, interrater reliability was strengthened by training and testing data collectors. In the second study, continuous electromyographic monitoring was used. The efficacy of extremity wraps in reducing the need for shivering-suppressant drugs was investigated in both studies. Limited control over the amphotericin B protocol and criteria for narcotic administration confounded these findings in the pilot study. A standardized drug protocol for drug administration was used in the second study, and wrapped patients required significantly less narcotic for shivering relief.

Radiant Heat. Cutaneous receptors sense thermal variations before internal temperature changes occur and are dominant in initiating shivering. Conversely, radiant heat to skin can diminish the sensation of heat loss and suppress shivering, while making little change in deep body temperatures. In some studies, the radiant heat source was not directed to exposed skin, yet this is the only way to assess the effects of radiant heat appropriately. Use of radiant heat with the patient covered actually warms skin by conduction.

Continuous radiant heat was compared with warm blankets on postanesthetic shivering in 30 postpartum tubal ligation and cesarean section patients (Sharkey, Lipton, Murphy, & Giesecke, 1987). Mann-Whitney comparisons showed significantly less shivering duration and greater comfort in the radiant heat group. Joachimsson, Nystrom, and Tyden (1989) extensively tested use of a thermal ceiling to reduce shivering after hypothermic cardiac heart surgery. In a complicated design, patients were randomized to one of two groups. Group 1 (n = 12) were patients receiving various combinations of intravenous opiate and enflurane, who were mechanically ventilated. Group 2 (n = 16) were those who received epidural analgesia, general anesthesia with enflurane, and early extubation. All subjects were rewarmed with thermal ceilings. Shivering was determined by observed contractions and palpated muscular rigidity on a scale from 0 to 4. Radiant heat nearly eliminated postoperative shivering and reduced oxygen demand, regardless of anesthetic agent, allowing earlier extubation. Repeated measures analysis of variance was used over the first 4 postoperative hr to evaluate significant changes over time. Student's t-tests, with Bonferroni's adjustment for multiple use of the t-test, were used to compare physiologic measurements between groups. The effects of the thermal ceiling are almost incidental in this study, as most of the significant findings relate to the association between shivering and cardiorespiratory outcomes. When shivering was controlled, patients in either group were recovered with less pharmacologic treatment. In the group receiving inhalational anesthesia and opiates, intraoperative drugs caused persistent respiratory depression that necessitated mechanical ventilation for more than 10 hr postoperatively. The group receiving thoracic epidural analgesia and inhalational anesthesia were able to be extubated within 2 hr postoperatively. The investigators attribute the reduction in shivering to extended rewarming during the cardiopulmonary bypass and the use of the thermal ceiling during recovery.

No difference in postoperative shivering activity was found when radiant heat was used with or without pharmacologic intervention. Patients were covered with a warm blanket during recovery and a heat lamp (Emerson, Cambridge, MA) was applied when shivering was detected by EMG. Analysis of variance comparisons of shivering duration showed no significant difference between patients who received meperidine, fentanyl, or placebos of normal saline (Heffline, 1991).

Warmed Humidified Gases. Warmed anesthetic and inhalational gases have been studied with respect to hypothermia prevention, but their effects on shivering are not well documented. Pflug, Aasheim, Foster, and Martin (1978) compared adult abdominal surgery patients (n = 40) exposed to warmed, humidified gases during prolonged inhalation anesthesia with controls. Shivering was defined as muscular hyperactivity occurring only after the patient was conscious and excluded preconscious tremors of any kind.

Patients receiving warmed gases did not shiver, whereas one half of the control group shivered. TM and toe temperatures were significantly higher in the group receiving warmed gases throughout recovery. Only the great-toe temperature differed between shivering and nonshivering subjects. Although investigators concluded this difference (1.3°C) was inadequate to stimulate shivering, other studies show that heat-loss sensors on the feet are acutely sensitive to small changes in temperature (Abbey et al, 1973; Holtzclaw, 1990a, 1990b). The narrow classification of shivering activity limits generalization of this study.

Protective Garments and Drapes. Heat conservation during operative procedures has been studied with respect to preventing hypothermia, primarily by using wraps and coverings. Although few address postoperative shivering, a comparative study of 60 patients undergoing endarterectomy showed the complication to be less frequent when aluminized reflective blankets were added to routine surgical draping (Bourke, Wurm, Rosenberg, & Russell, 1984).

Warmed Epidural Injectate. Whether shivering after epidural anesthesia is thermally induced is not fully understood (Sessler & Ponte, 1990). Attempts to test this question by cooling or warming injectates have yielded variable results. If it is of thermal origin, it is unclear whether generalized heat loss or local cooling of the spinal cord is to blame. Ponte, Collett, and Walmsley (1986) warmed bupivacaine given as epidural anesthetic to 20 women for cesarean section, whereas 20 received room-temperature injectate. Warmed injectate reduced the shivering incidence significantly over controls. Harris et al. (1986), by contrast, found no difference in shivering when epidural anesthetic agent lidocaine was warmed to body temperature as compared with controls. Sessler and Ponte (1990) also found no relationship between temperature of the epidural injectate and the incidence of shivering in 10 nonpregnant volunteers subjected to cold and warm injectates. Cooling of skin temperature and vasoconstriction were found more influential in initiating shivering. Ogura, Fukuyama, and Nakagawa (1988) tested effects of warm irrigating fluid during and after transurethral prostatectomy in patients assigned either to warmed ($n = 62$) or room-temperature irrigating fluid ($n = 46$). Those with warmed irrigant had lower shivering incidence and less blood loss.

STRENGTHS AND LIMITATIONS OF EXISTING RESEARCH

Studies cited in this review varied widely in the type of instrumentation used and the control over threats to validity. Physiologic studies of both humans and animals usually involved elaborate shivering measurement with EMG recordings from several sites, and exercised the most rigorous control over extraneous variables. These studies often had small samples of fewer than 10 subjects. Reports included both graphic and numeric findings, although information about statistical analyses frequently was omitted. Investigators in anesthesia seldom used instrumentation for shivering measurement, and visual observation scales were not standardized. Although samples were among the largest in the studies reviewed, few justified the sample size or adequately described data analysis procedures. Chi-square was appropriately used by most comparative studies for nominal data. However, many investigators inappropriately used Student's *t*-test for multiple comparisons or two-group comparisons in which subjects contributed more than one score to the data. These methodologic flaws limit the conclusions one can draw from published reports and may explain divergent findings between studies. Studies by nurse researchers also suffered from small sample size, but gave considerable attention to design and control of intervening variables. Shivering measurements by EMG and visual scale had common levels of reference, and statistical analyses were appropriate to the design and level of measurement.

SUMMARY AND DIRECTIONS FOR FUTURE RESEARCH

Research related to shivering represents a chain of discovery, beginning with early animal studies in the biologic sciences. Neural mechanisms of shivering, afferent and efferent pathways, and the nature of thermoreceptors were discovered first in these laboratories. Physiologists have studied shivering in humans for the past 50 years, amassing a wealth of knowledge yet untapped by clinicians. The relatively recent research interest in postoperative shivering within anesthesiology grew with the advent of hypothermic cardiopulmonary bypass procedures. Although nurses have participated in interdisciplinary studies of shivering, the topic is a relatively new research interest for nursing, and few studies by nurses were found. Those found were studies of physical correlates and nonpharmacologic measures to prevent shivering. Many questions about shivering are yet unexplored. No studies were found in any discipline addressing the extent or tolerance of shivering in children. The phenomenon of postpartum shivering is virtually unexplored by nurses. Few studies have been done to describe shivering in weak or vulnerable groups such as the elderly or those with chronic disease. Groups at risk for sequelae from febrile shivering, such as those with acquired immune deficiency syndrome (AIDS) requiring pyrogenic drugs to treat opportunistic infection, have not been studied. Even though vasomotor responses can warm skin and are strongly modified by psychic factors, no studies have been done to explore relationships between pain, anxiety, and shivering. Nor have the subjective responses of shivering patients been detailed. Effects of hypnosis on shivering have only been studied in healthy subjects (Kissen, Reifler, and Thaler, 1964). In each of these situations questions of importance to nursing science are found. If shivering is accompanied by severe oxygen expenditure in healthy subjects, what effects are found in patients that are anemic, weak, or have respiratory problems? How does postoperative shivering affect recovery or the ability to return to activities of daily living? Could relaxation therapy and psychic imaging reduce shivering during surface cooling, pyrogenic drug infusions, or after childbirth? How effective would extremity wraps or radiant heat be in ameliorating febrile shivering during such procedures as plasmapheresis or prostaglandin E_2-induced termination of pregnancy?

Research is essential to identify patients at risk for shivering. Shivering often goes undetected in clinical situations; therefore, studies are needed to document the incidence and severity of shivering in a wide variety of conditions and age groups. One could predict that this group would include patients who are subjected to undue heat loss because of diminished subcutaneous fat, severe burns, or exposure during traumatic injuries. Considering the magnitude of energy expended by shivering, research to seek and test scientifically based interventions to prevent or control the response is long overdue.

REFERENCES

Abbey, J. C. (1982). Shivering and surface cooling. In C. M. Norris (Ed.), *Concept clarification in nursing* (pp. 223–242). Rockville, MD: Aspen.

Abbey, J. C., Andrews, C., Avigliano, K., Blossom, R., Bunke, B., Clark, E., Engberg, N., Healy, P., Peterson, J. Shirley, C., & Waers, C. (1973). A pilot study: The control of shivering during hypothermia by a clinical nursing measure. *Journal of Neurosurgical Nursing, 5*, 78–88.

Abbey, J. C., & Close, L. (1979). A study of control of shivering during hypothermia. *Communicating Nursing Research, 12*, 2–3.

Applegate, S. (1988). Electronics fundamentals: Common-mode rejection. *Biomedical Technology Today, 3*, 103–106.

Azar, I. (1980). Rectal temperature is best indicator of adequate rewarming during cardiopulmonary bypass. *Anesthesiology, 53*, 277–280.

Bay, J., Nunn, J. F., & Prys-Roberts, C. (1968). Factors influencing arterial pO_2 during recovery from anaesthesia. *British Journal of Anaesthesia, 40*, 398–407.

Beisel, W. R., Wannemacher, R. W., & Neufeld, H. A. (1980). Relation of fever to energy expenditure. In *Assessment of energy metabolism in health and disease:*

Report of the First Ross Conference on Medical Research (pp. 144–150). Columbus, OH: Ross Laboratories.

Bourke, D. L., Wurm, H., Rosenberg, M., & Russell, J. (1984). Intraoperative heat conservation using a reflective blanket. *Anesthesiology, 60,* 151–154.

Burks, C., Aisner I., Fortner, C. L., & Wiernik, P. H. (1980). Meperidine for the treatment of shaking chills and fever. *Archives of Internal Medicine, 140,* 483–484.

Claybon, L. E., & Hirsh, R. A. (1980). Meperidine arrests post-anesthesia shivering. *Anesthesiology, 53,* S180.

Cohen, M. (1967). An investigation into shivering following anaesthesia. *Proceedings of the Royal Society of Medicine, 60,* 752–753.

Collins, K. J., Easton, J. C., & Exton-Smith, A. N. (1981). Shivering thermogenesis and vasomotor responses with convective cooling in the elderly. *Journal of Physiology, 320,* 76P.

Darnall, R. A. (1987). The thermophysiology of the newborn infant. *Medical Instrumentation, 21,* 16–22.

Dowben, R. M. (1980). Contractility with special reference to skeletal muscle. In V. B. Mountcastle (Ed.), *Medical Physiology* (Vol. 1, pp. 107–109). St. Louis: Mosby.

Earp, J. K., & Finlayson, D. C. (1991). Relationship between urinary bladder and pulmonary artery temperatures: A preliminary study. *Heart & Lung, 20,* 265–270.

Geer, R. T., & Holtzclaw, B. J. (1986). Effects of increased oxygen consumption during rewarming after open heart surgery. *Anesthesiology, 65,* A525.

Girling, F., & Topliff, E. D. L. (1966). The effect of breathing 15%, 21%, and 100% oxygen on the shivering responses of nude human subjects at 10°C. *Canadian Journal of Physiological Pharmacology, 44,* 495–499.

Goold, J. E. (1984). Postoperative spasticity and shivering. *Anaesthesia, 39,* 35–38.

Hardy, J. D. (1980). Body temperature regulation. In V. A. Mountcastle (Ed.), *Medical physiology* (14th ed., pp. 1417–1456). St. Louis: C. V. Mosby.

Harris, M. M., Lawson, D., Cooper, C. M., & Ellis, J. (1989). Treatment of shivering after epidural lidocaine. *Regional Anesthesia, 14,* 13–28.

Haupt, M. T., & Rackow, E. C. (1983). Adverse effects of febrile state on cardiac performance. *American Heart Journal, 105,* 763–768.

Heffline, M. S. (1991). A comparative study of pharmacological versus nursing interventions in the treatment of postanesthesia shivering. *Journal of Post Anesthesia Nursing, 6,* 311–320.

Hemingway, A. (1963). Shivering. *Physiological Review, 43,* 397–422.

Hemingway, A., & Stuart, D. G. (1963). Shivering in man and animals. In J. D. Hardy (Ed.), *Temperature: Its use in science and industry* (Vol. 3, Part 3, pp. 407–427). New York: Reinhold.

Hensel, H. (1970). Temperature receptors in the skin. *In* J. D. Hardy, A. P. Gagge, & J. A. Stolwijk (Eds.), *Physiological and Behavioral Temperature Regulation* (pp. 442–453). Springfield, IL: Charles C. Thomas.

Holtzclaw, B. J. (1986). Postoperative shivering after cardiac surgery: A review. *Heart & Lung, 15* 292–302.

Holtzclaw, B. J. (1990a). Control of febrile shivering during amphotericin B therapy. *Oncology Nursing Forum, 17,* 521–524.

Holtzclaw, B. J. (1990b). Effects of extremity wraps to control drug induced shivering: A pilot study. *Nursing Research, 39,* 280–283.

Holtzclaw, B. J. (1990c). Shivering: A clinical nursing problem. *Nursing Clinics of North America, 25,* 977–986.

Holtzclaw, B. J., & Geer, R. T. (1986). Shivering after heart surgery: Assessment of metabolic effects. *Anesthesiology, 65,* A18.

Horvath, S. M., Spurr, G. B., Hutt, B. K., & Hamilton, I. H. (1956). Metabolic cost of shivering. *Journal of Applied Physiology, 8,* 595–602.

Iampietro, P. F., Vaughan, J. A., Goldman, R. F., Kreider, M. B., Masucci, F., & Bass, D. E. (1960). Heat production from shivering. *Journal of Applied Physiology, 15,* 632–634.

Jaameri, K. E. U., Jahkola, A., & Perttu, J. (1966). On shivering in association with normal delivery. *Acta Obstetricia et Gynecologica Scandinavica, 45,* 383–388.

Joachimsson, P. O., Nystrom, S. O., Tyden, H. (1989). Early extubation after coronary artery surgery in efficiently rewarmed patients: A postoperative comparison of opiate anesthesia versus inhalational anesthesia and thoracic epidural analgesia. *Journal of Cardiothoracic Anesthesia, 3,* 444–454.

Kaplan, J. A., & Guffin, A. V. (1985). Shivering and changes in mixed venous oxygen saturation after cardiac surgery. *Anesthesia & Analgesia, 64,* 235.

Keatinge, W. R., Mason, A. C., Millard, C. E., & Newstead, C. G. (1986). Effects of fluctuating skin temperature on thermoregulatory responses in man. *Journal of Physiology, 378,* 241–252.

Kissen, A. T., Reifler, C. B., & Thaler, V. H. (1964). Modification thermoregulatory responses to cold by hypnosis. *Journal of Applied Physiology, 19,* 1043–1050.

Kleinebeckel, D., & Klussmann, F. W. (1990). In E. Shonbaum & P. Lomax (Eds.), *Thermoregulation: Physiology and biochemistry* (pp. 235–253). New York: Pergamon Press.

Kluger, M. J. (1991). Fever: Role of pyrogens and cryogens. *Physiological Reviews, 71,* 93–127.

Macintyre, P. E., Pavlin, E. G., & Dwersteg, J. F. (1987). Effect of meperidine on oxygen consumption, carbon dioxide production, and respiratory gas exchange in postanesthesia shivering. *Anesthesia & Analgesia, 66,* 751–755.

McCulloch, P. R., & Milne, B. (1990). Neurological phenomena during emergence from enflurane or isofulrane anaesthesia. *Canadian Journal of Anaesthesia, 37,* 739–742.

Mekjavic, B., & Eiken, O. (1985). Inhibition of shivering in man by thermal stimulation of the facial area. *Acta Physiologica Scandinavica, 125,* 633–637.

Murphy, M. T., Lipton, J. M., Loughran, P., & Giesecke, A. H. (1984). Post anesthetic shivering in primates: Effects of low body temperature, skin warming and neurotransmitters. *Anesthesiology, 61,* A283.

Newstead, C. G. (1987). The relationship between ventilation and oxygen consumption in man is the same during both moderate exercise and shivering. *Journal of Physiology, 383,* 455–459.

Nielsen, B. (1976). Metabolic reactions to changes in core and skin temperature in man. *Acta Physiologica Scandinavica, 97,* 129–138.

Ogura, K., Fukuyama, T., & Nakagawa, K. (1988). The effects of warm irrigating fluid during and after transurethral prostatectomy. *Clinical Therapeutics, 10,* 20–21.

Palmes, E. D., & Park, C. R. (1965). The reguiation of body temperature during fever. *Archives of Environmental Health, 11,* 749–759.

Pflug, A. E., Aasheim, G. M., Foster, C., & Martin, R. W. (1978). Prevention of post-anaesthesia shivering. *Canadian Anaesthetists Society Journal, 25,* 43–49.

Ponte, J., Collett, B. J., & Walmsley, A. (1986). Anaesthetic temperature and shivering in epidural anaesthesia. *Acta Anaesthesiologia Scandinavica, 30,* 584–587.

Rodriguez, J. L., Weissman, C., Damask, M. C., Askanazi, J., Hyman, A. E., & Kinney, J. M. (1983). Physiologic requirements during rewarming: Suppression of the shivering response. *Critical Care Medicine, 11,* 490–497.

Roe, C. F., Goldberg, M. J., Blair, C. S., & Kinney, J. M. (1966). The influences of body temperature on early postoperative oxygen consumption. *Surgery, 60,* 85–92.

Rosenfeld, J. B. (1963). Acid-base and electrolyte disturbances in hypothermia. *American Journal of Cardiology, 12,* 678–682.

Rutledge, D. N., & Holtzclaw, B. J. (1988). Amphotericin B-induced shivering in cancer patients: A nursing approach. *Heart & Lung, 17,* 432–440.

Sato, H. (1981). Fusimotor modulation by spinal and skin temperature changes and its significance in cold shivering. *Experimental Neurology, 72,* 21.

Sessler, D. I., & Ponte, J. (1990). Shivering during epidural anesthesia. *Anesthesiology, 72,* 816–821.

Sessler, D. I., Israel, B. S., Pozos, R. S., Pozos, M., & Rubinstein, E. H. (1988). Spontaneous post-anesthetic tremor does not resemble thermoregulatory shivering. *Anesthesiology, 68,* 843–850.

Sharkey, M. B., Lipton, J. M., Murphy, M. T., & Giesecke, A. H. (1987). Inhibition of postanesthestic shivering with radiant heat. *Anesthesiology, 66,* 249–252.

Sladen, R. N. (1985). Temperature and ventilation after hypothermic cardiopulmonary bypass. *Anesthesia and Analgesia, 64,* 816–820.

Sladen, R. N., Renaghan, D., Ashton, J. P., & Wyner, J. (1985). Effect of shivering on mechanical ventilation after cardiac surgery. *Anesthesiology, 63,* 140A.

Slotman, G. J., Jed, E. H., & Burchard, K. W. (1985). Adverse effects of hypothermia in postoperative patients. *American Journal of Surgery, 149,* 495–501.

Stitt, J. T., Hardy, J. D., & Stolwijk, J. A. J. (1974). PGE_1 fever: Its effect on thermoregulation at different low ambient temperatures. *American Journal of Physiology, 227,* 622–629.

Strom, G. (1960). Central nervous regulation of body temperature. In J. Field, H. W. Magoun, & V. E. Hall (Eds.), *Handbook of Physiology: Neurophysiology* (Vol. 2, Section 1, 1173–1193). Washington DC: American Physiological Society.

Webb, P. J., James, F. M., & Wheeler, A. S. (1981). Shivering during epidural analgesia in women in labor. *Anesthesiology, 55,* 706–707.

Zuniga, E. N., Truong, X. T., & Simons, D. G. (1970). Effects of skin electrode position on averaged EMG potentials. *Archives of Physical Medicine & Rehabilitation, 51,* 264–272.

Zwischenberger, J. B., Kirsh, M. M., Dechert, R. E., Arnold, D. K., & Bartlett, R. H. (1987). Suppression of shivering decreases oxygen consumption and improves hemodynamic stability during postoperative rewarming. *Annals of Thoracic Surgery, 43,* 428–431.

Chapter 3

Chronic Fatigue

KATHLEEEN M. POTEMPA
COLLEGE OF NURSING
UNIVERSITY OF ILLINOIS AT CHICAGO

CONTENTS

Chronic fatigue is of interest to health professionals and lay people. Nursing and medicine have formally recognized the significance of chronic fatigue. The North American Nursing Diagnosis Association (NANDA) voted in 1988 to test fatigue clinically as a bona fide nursing diagnosis. Also in 1988, a panel of the Center for Disease Control (CDC) published guidelines for the diagnosis of the so-called chronic fatigue syndrome (Holmes et al., 1988).

The symptom of general fatigue and related feelings have been associated with several chronic illnesses and their treatments (Funk, Tornquist, Champagne, Copp, & Wiese, 1989). But because of the ubiquitous nature of the fatigue state, the study of the phenomenon has been complex and difficult. Clinical evaluation of fatigue in health care was begun by nurses in the 1970s with the study of patients with multiple sclerosis (Hart, 1978) and cancer (Haylock & Hart, 1979; McCorkle & Young, 1978). Since that time investigators of various disciplines have studied fatigue in clinical populations to determine symptom frequency, associated symptoms, and treatment strategies.

Today, a rapidly growing research focus is the cluster of fatigue-related symptoms observed in otherwise healthy individuals often, but not always, following a viral infection. Research also is expanding in the area of fatigue as a side effect of treatment or an effect of debilitating disease, such as cancer and acquired immune deficiency syndrome (AIDS). Thus, a striking feature of chronic fatigue is that it is a syndrome that occurs in various clinical states and is a sequela to many clinical treatments.

The purpose of this review is to provide an analysis of the conceptualization, phenomenology, and intervention strategies regarding chronic fatigue. Directions for further research are presented. Because chronic fatigue occurs in many clinical contexts, breadth of the literature to gather data sources for this review was sought. Literature of human subjects that related to fatigue, chronic fatigue, neurasthenia, D'Costa Syndrome, or Chronic Fatigue Syndrome, served as major key words for the search. Neurasthenia and D'Costa Syndrome were key words used prior to 1975 in the definition of chronic fatigue. Biological, nursing, medical, and psychological databases were used. Subheadings included words referring to the definition, mechanisms of, and treatment of the disorder in any clinical disease state. Published manuscripts and abstracts were retrieved. Finally, reference lists of manuscripts retrieved were scrutinized for articles missed in the primary searches. This method provided for a comprehensive review of the literature in chronic fatigue.

CONCEPTUALIZATION OF CHRONIC FATIGUE

Definition of Chronic Fatigue

Chronic fatigue has been defined as a decreased capacity to perform physical and mental work; overwhelming sustained exhaustion, lack of energy, and tiredness; and a combination of these (Potempa, 1989; Potempa, Lopez, Reid, & Lawson, 1986). Chronic fatigue is differentiated from acute fatigue both in duration and temporal relationship to an identifiable incident of energy expenditure (Piper, Lindsey, & Dodd, 1987; Potempa et al., 1986). Frequent episodes of acute fatigue may be part of the syndrome of chronic fatigue, whereas chronic fatigue is not considered the normal sequela of an acute bout of fatigue (Potempa et al., 1986).

Definition of Criteria

Major and minor criteria for the nursing diagnosis "chronic fatigue" and related factors have been defined by NANDA (Carpenito, 1992). According to NANDA guidelines, the major feature of chronic fatigue is verbalization, or self-report, of a sustained and significant lack of energy. These guidelines suggest that fatigue is a perception and that self-report is a major way of discerning its presence. Interestingly, the minor characteristics suggest more objective measures such as decreased concentration, task performance, and sexual activity as well as accident proneness. The framework provided by these guidelines has important implications for the way chronic fatigue is measured and diagnosed.

In contrast, one manifestation of chronic fatigue—the so-called chronic fatigue syndrome—is currently recognized as a distinct syndrome by the CDC with published criteria for making a clinical diagnosis (Holmes et al., 1988). The first major criterion, "Persistent or relapsing fatigue or easy fatigability that . . . does not resolve with bedrest . . . (and) is severe enough to reduce average daily activity by > 50%" (Holmes et al., 1988, p. 388) is strikingly similar to the defining characteristics listed by NANDA. However, the second major criterion, which requires the exclusion of other chronic clinical conditions and psychiatric diagnoses, is in contrast to NANDA guidelines in which it is assumed that there are many illnesses and treatments that are associated with chronic fatigue. Furthermore, the minor criteria of the CDC guidelines list symptoms commonly associated with an infectious process: mild fever, sore throat, painful lymph nodes, myalgia, headache, neuropsychologic complaints, and generalized fatigue. The literature is equivocal regarding the applicability of the CDC criteria, with some authors finding that strict application of recommended guidelines eliminates most cases of chronic fatigue seen in clinical practice (Lane, Matthews, & Manu, 1990; Valdini, Steinhardt, & Feldman, 1989).

From the earliest case studies, fatigue has been reported in a variety of contexts not just in association with a postinfectious condition (Straus, 1991). Although chronic fatigue is recognized as a disease by the CDC only under specified conditions and is recognized as a clinical symptom complex found in many clinical contexts by NANDA, the similarity of symptoms across clinical contexts suggests common mechanisms of the disorder. The elucidation of the mechanisms governing chronic fatigue and its associated symptoms will further clarify the definition and classification of chronic fatigue.

PHENOMENOLOGY OF CHRONIC FATIGUE SYMPTOMS

The phenomenology of a symptom includes information about where and when it typically occurs as well as its frequency, duration, associated symptoms, and relief patterns. These aspects of fatigue will be addressed for the phenomenon as reported in general clinical practice and in various specialized clinical populations.

Fatigue in General Clinical Practice

According to the National Ambulatory Medical Care Survey (1978), fatigue ranks seventh on the list of symptoms most frequently reported to medical practitioners, representing 10.5 million office visits and explaining 1.8% of all office visits. Studies have reported the estimated prevalence of fatigue in general medical practice to be 21% to 47% (Jerret, 1981; Kroenke, Wood, Mangelsdorff, Meier, & Powell, 1988; Morrison, 1980; Sugarman & Berg, 1984). However, there is some evidence to suggest that the sympton of tiredness is more prevalent than indicated by these studies of general practice. Banks, Beresford, Morrell, Walter, and Watkins (1975) reported that only 1 out of every 400 episodes of fatigue or tiredness experienced by young women was brought to the attention of a physician.

Chen (1986) analyzed fatigue data from the Health and Nutrition Education Survey from 1974 to 1975. He found that 14.3% of the men and 20.4% of women reported having significant fatigue. The risk evaluation performed indicated that women have a risk ratio that is 1.5 times greater than men. For men, significant correlates of fatigue were arthritis, asthma, emphysema, and anemia. For women, only arthritis and anemia were significantly related to chronic fatigue. Moreover, regardless of sex, subjects who were inactive had twice the risk of expressing chronic fatigue than active subjects. Also regardless of sex, the psychologic factors of depression, emotional stress, and anxiety were highly correlated with chronic fatigue. Thus, the concurrent presence of psychologic factors was the greatest risk factor in men and women for chronic fatigue. Furthermore, when sex, age, nutritional status, physical activity, and psychologic factors were considered together in regression analysis, only physical activity and psychological factors were significant predictors of chronic fatigue.

The limitations of these studies are the untested reliability and validity of measures used to assess fatigue and the poorly designed research designs used for determining prevalence of a symptom. The statistical estimation of sample size has never been employed in large-scale studies of chronic fatigue but is needed to determine true prevalence of a symptom from the known variance of the measures used.

Fatigue as a Postinfection Syndrome

Chronic fatigue was noted as a sequela to brucellosis (Evans, 1934). A subsequent prospective study by Spink (1951) found that 30 out of 65 patients with acute brucellosis had continued fatigue 1 year postinfection. In 17 of these 30 subjects, bacteriologic evidence of continued infection was observed, whereas in the remaining 13 subjects no apparent ongoing infectious process was found. In the study by Imboden, Canter, Cluff, and Trever (1959), 24 subjects with a history of brucellosis were divided into three groups: those who recovered from the acute infection without fatigue symptoms, those who had chronic fatigue for 6 months to 1 year after infection but were free of symptoms at the time of interview, and those who still had symptoms 2 or more years after the infection. Results indicated that the group that recovered acutely showed less psychologic disturbances than either chronic group, findings similar to Spink's (1951). The two chronic groups had lower self-concept and greater psychasthenia, depression, overt anxiety, morale loss, and neurotic scores than the group that recovered acutely. Although the psychologic tests were administered by psychologists who were blind to subject groups, interviewer bias may have resulted because of the nature of the content discussed.

Imboden, Canter, and Cluff (1961) studied soldiers infected during the Asian influenza epidemic of 1957 and found that fatigue became a chronic symptom in several subjects. The authors concluded that soldiers who took longer than 3 weeks to recover from the influenza had more preexisting depressive symptomatology than soldiers who recovered in less than 3 weeks.

The Epstein-Barr virus (EBV) infection has received widespread attention as a cause of chronic fatigue. Several case-report studies in the early to mid-1980s linked EBV infection with a chronic fatigue sequela (Jones et al., 1985; Morrison, 1980; Straus, 1988; Straus et al., 1985). All of these studies reported elevated serum antibodies to EBV antigens and linked EBV to chronic fatigue as the etiologic agent. But as Straus (1991) has pointed out, EBV may not be the causative agent for several reasons. First, EBV is highly prevalent in children and more than 90% of the adult American population has circulating antibodies to this virus. Second, subsequent case-control studies have shown a considerable overlap in antibody levels between fatigue-positive and fatigue-negative groups (Horwitz, Henle, Henle, Rudnick, & Latts, 1985). Finally, Holmes et al. (1987) reported higher levels of antibodies to several viruses in patients with chronic fatigue versus controls, not just higher titers for EBV. Instead of a single etiologic virus, this finding suggested a nonspecific immune activation in the so-called chronic fatigue syndrome.

The outbreak of respiratory influenza and accompanying fatigue in northern Nevada in the mid-1980s has implicated the herpes simplex virus HHV-6 as the initiating infection. Several follow-up studies of patients during this outbreak have appeared in the literature, all of which report fatigue as an overwhelming symptom that continued in many of these patients for years postinfection (Barnes, 1986; Daugherty et al., 1991; Holmes et al., 1987). Others have observed fatigue subsequent to other types of infection. Cohen and Hardin (1989) found that fatigue more than doubled from a retrospectively measured control phase in subjects who survived an acute infection with *Clostridium botulinum*. Chronic yeast infection with candida also has been implicated in the etiology of chronic fatigue (Truss, 1981).

Several recent studies have identified the association of depression with postinfectious chronic fatigue. Kruesi, Dale, and Straus (1989) studied 28 subjects who met the CDC criteria for the chronic fatigue syndrome and had no other known disorders. Psychiatric interview revealed a psychiatric diagnoses for 75% of the sample. These diagnoses included anxiety disorders and dysthymia including major depression. In all but two of the patients with concurrent psychiatric diagnosis, the onset of fatigue was retrospectively determined as occurring after the onset of the psychiatric symptoms. In this study, symptoms of fatigue needed to precede psychiatric symptoms by at least 1 year before fatigue was considered the first or prior diagnosis. Additionally, they noted that the relative rate of lifetime incidence of a major psychiatric diagnosis, which was estimated in this study as 75%, was considerably higher than the rate reported in other samples, for example, studies of diabetics or the general population.

Wessely and Powell (1989) compared a convenience sample of subjects with diagnosed postviral chronic fatigue, peripheral neuromuscular fatiguing illnesses (PN) (e.g., myasthenia gravis, myopathy, Guillan-Barré), or major depression. There were no differences in subjective fatigue between groups. When fatigue was excluded as a symptom in psychiatric assessment, 72% of chronic fatigue syndrome patients met criteria for a psychiatric diagnosis. Major depression applied to 47% of these cases, somatization disorder to 15%

of cases, and minor depression, phobic disorder, and generalized anxiety to the remaining 10%. Thirty-six percent of the (PN) group had psychiatric disorders. Mental fatigue and fatigability were equally common in the chronic fatigue syndrome and depression (DEP) groups but only occurred in PN subjects with psychiatric disorders. The authors concluded that the chronic fatigue syndrome groups most closely resembled the DEP affective symptom characteristics than the PN group. Likewise, Wood, Bentall, Gopfert, and Edwards (1991) compared 34 patients with chronic postviral fatigue and 24 patients with primary muscle disease (e.g., dystrophies) and found that 67% of chronic fatigue patients had major or minor anxiety and mood disorders, whereas the primary muscle disease group had a 16.5% comorbid incidence of major or minor anxiety and mood disorders. Manu et al. (1989) reported that 44% of a convenience sample of chronic fatigue patients had major depression on psychiatric interview. Of these 44%, the major depression preceded the onset of fatigue symptoms. Discriminate analysis revealed that variables from physical examination including electrocardiogram, exercise stress test results, viral serologic tests, liver function tests, complete blood count, and electolyte and thyroid function tests were poor discriminators of depressed/chronic fatigue versus chronic fatigue–only subjects. In contrast, Hickie, Lloyd, Wakefield, and Parker (1990) reported that although 50% of the patients with postinfectious chronic fatigue had comorbid major depression, the premorbid prevalence of major depression (12.5%) and total psychiatric disorder (24.5%) were no greater than the estimated level in other populations of patients with general medical disorders. The authors concluded that the psychologic disturbances were a likely consequence of, rather than an antecedent risk factor for, chronic fatigue.

A recent study has shown reduced basal glucocorticoid levels, low 24-hr urinary-free cortisol excretion, and elevated evening adrenocorticotropic hormone (ACTH) in patients with chronic fatigue syndrome compared with normal control subjects (Demitrack et al., 1991). In this same study, an increased sensitivity to ACTH with reduced maximal response to ACTH was also observed in the patients. Conclusions from this study were that a mild glucocorticoid deficiency or a deficiency of an arousal-producing neuropeptide such as cortisol-releasing hormone (CRH) may be related to the chronic fatigue syndrome. These results are particularly important because other disorders associated with fatigue and depressed mood, such as Cushing's disease and seasonal affective disorders, have also been associated with reduced CRH release (Kling et al., ,1991; Joseph-Vanderpool et al., 1991). It should also be noted that it is known that viral infections alter neurotransmitter and neuroendocrine regulation (Oldstone et al., 1982).

These data do not suggest that the so-called chronic fatigue syndrome is the result of an infection from a specific organism. In fact, a current hypothesis is that the symptom cluster associated with the chronic fatigue syndrome is due to an immune disorder secondary to an infection that may occur from any number of infectious organisms (Landay, Jessop, Lennette, & Levy, 1991). The association of psychologic problems, most often including major or minor anxiety and mood disorders, in the postinfectious form of chronic fatigue, is clear from the data. There is also beginning evidence to suggest that neuroendocrine mechanisms may be a common pathway linking the physical and affective symptoms associated with the chronic fatigue syndrome.

Fatigue in Pregnancy

Fatigue has been recognized as a common symptom of pregnancy and postpartum. Morrison (1980) found that pregnancy was the second most common cause of fatigue in general medical practice. Reeves, Potempa, and Gallo (1991) found that 90% of women less than 30 weeks pregnant (n = 30) reported fatigue that was serious enough to affect their daily lives. In studies by Fawcett and York (1986) and Reeves et al. (1991), fatigue was significantly associated with other self-reported negative mood states such as anger, anxiety, and depression. Reeves et al. (1991) also reported moderate correlations during early pregnancy between level of fatigue and age, nausea, weight gain, and feeling tired on awakening from sleep where the women with higher fatigue scores were younger, had more nausea, had less weight gain, and had less relief from sleep than women with lower fatigue scores. Also, this study reported that stamina, a measure of self-efficacy in the physical functioning domain, was associated with less fatigue and other negative mood states. Affonso, Lovett, Paul, and Sheptak (1990) reported that women had a high incidence of dysphoric mood, worrying, somatic and psychic anxiety, insomnia, fatigue, anger, and irritability across all periods of pregnancy studied. The authors concluded that these symptoms could not be explained solely on the basis of somatic discomforts associated with the pregnancy state, as these psychologic symptoms persisted throughout various stages of pregnancy and postpartum.

Because of relatively small sample sizes and lack of nonpregnant control subjects, conclusions about the true estimate of the prevalence of fatigue that is unique to pregnancy and postpartum cannot be made from these studies. The role of mediating factors in chronic fatigue such as stamina, age, and presence of nausea or sleep disturbances and related mood states in early pregnancy also is suggested, and needs further investigation throughout pregnancy and postpartum.

Fatigue in Postsurgical Patients

Fatigue in the postsurgical patient has been know clinically for many years. The fatigue in these patients has been conceptually related to the effects of starvation, sleep deprivation, bed rest, infection, and the results of anesthesia. A few studies have documented the reduced aerobic capacity and muscular efficiency in patients after surgery that has been related to bed rest and state of physical conditioning before surgery (Bassey & Fentem, 1974; Carswell, 1975). However, the empiric documentation of fatigue and proposed mechanisms has been otherwise poorly studied in postsurgical patients.

Recent studies have confirmed a reduction in muscular efficiency during low-level exercise after surgery as compared with presurgical measures (Zeiderman, Welchew, & Clark, 1990, 1991). In the later study, this reduced efficiency was greater in a group of subjects receiving epidural analgesia and was associated with greater subjective feelings of fatigue in these patients than in those patients receiving other types of anesthesia during surgery. These studies served to document that there is a greater energy expenditure for a given amount of physical work in the early recovery phase after surgery. The authors conclude that the increased effort required to perform simple tasks may contribute to the development of fatigue often seen in postsurgical patients. The role of anesthesia in the etiology and intensity of fatigue also is implicated but requires further investigation.

Fatigue in Cancer Patients

In cancer patients, chronic fatigue has been studied primarily as it relates to treatment. Eighteen reports since 1978 have described the prevalence, intensity, and, in some studies, the correlates of fatigue in cancer patients receiving chemotherapy (Adams, Quesada, & Gutterman, 1984; Blesch et al., 1991; Bloom et al., 1990; Cassileth, Lusk, & Bodenheimer, 1985; Cimprich, 1990; Davis, 1984; Fernsler, 1986; Jamar, 1989; Knoff, 1986; McCorkle & Quint-Benoliel, 1983; McCorkle & Young, 1978; Meyerowitz, Sparks, & Spears, 1979; Meyerowitz, Watkins, & Sparks, 1983; Nerenz, Love, & Leventhal, 1986; Pickard-Holley, 1991; Rhodes, Watson, & Hanson, 1988; Strauman, 1986; Walder, Lyver, & Wiernik, 1989). These studies can be collectively characterized as having small sample sizes, with only one notable exception being a study by Nerenz et al. (1986), which had 217 subjects. The prevalence estimates derived from several of these studies of fatigue in cancer patients undergoing chemotherapy is quite high, ranging from 80% to 99%. Severity of the symptom has not always been estimated, but in one study 64%

of those experiencing fatigue rated the fatigue as moderate to severe (Blesch et al., 1991). In this same study, the relationship of variables classified as biochemical, physiologic, and behavioral variables with fatigue intensity was evaluated. None of these correlations were significant except for duration of illness, mood disturbance scores, and the intensity of pain measure. The biochemical variables measured, including serum albumin, hemoglobin, hematocrit, electrolytes, muscle enzymes, and use of chemotherapeutic agents, were unrelated to fatigue. Only one study reported any relationship between fatigue and biochemical measures. Pickard-Holley (1991) reported a moderate covariation of amount of chemotherapy received and fatigue intensity ratings. Interestingly, in the few studies employing comparison groups, mean fatigue levels of patients were only slightly higher than those observed in control or comparison subjects. Although most of these studies can be criticized for failing to use multidimensional measures of fatigue, those that have employed such an approach have consistently reported moderate relationships between fatigue and negative mood states such as depression and anxiety. Although most studies have not been longitudinal, available data suggest that fatigue peaks and then wanes as therapy progresses.

Nine studies have been published regarding the effects of radiation therapy on the intensity and course of fatigue (Blesch et al., 1991; Bloom et al., 1990; Eardley, 1986; Haylock & Hart, 1979; King, Nail, Kreamer, Strohl, & Johnson, 1985; Kobashi-Schoot, Gerrit, Hanewald, Van Dam, & Bruning, 1985; Piper et al., 1989; Proctor, Karnahan, & Taylor, 1981; Quested, Malec, Harney, Kienker, & Romsaas, 1982). Similar to the studies of fatigue with chemotherapy, these studies had small sample sizes and no control groups. The prevalence of fatigue ranged from 50% to 100%, although Piper et al. (1989) reported that the fatigue was mild and intermittent. The effect of fatigue on daily activity performance has been poorly assessed, and existing studies have shown divergent results (Kobashi-Schoot et al., 1985; Quested et al., 1982). Fatigue appeared to peak and wane over the course of treatment. Correlates of fatigue included pain and depression (Kubricht, 1984; Piper, 1989). Fatigue has been related to the amount of rest required ($r = .58$), and differences in weekend patterns of fatigue or malaise were attributed to differences in dose of treatment.

These studies indicate that fatigue is significant in cancer patients receiving chemotherapy and radiation. However, the small sample sizes and lack of control groups preclude the conclusion that fatigue is more prevalent or intense during cancer treatment than in untreated patients or in healthy individuals. Possible modulating factors of fatigue identified were age, dose, and course of treatment; length of illness; level of pain and psychologic disturbances—all of which warrant further investigation.

Fatigue in Kidney Failure Requiring Dialysis

A few studies have investigated fatigue in patients with chronic kidney failure receiving dialysis. Cardenas and Kutner (1982) studied 137 patients on maintenance hemodialysis or peritoneal dialysis. All but two of the subjects were ambulatory without physical disabilities or limitations. Forty-two percent of the sample reported none to mild fatigue, 34% moderate fatigue, and 24% reported severe fatigue. The investigators reported that no relationships were observed between the level of fatigue and age, type of diagnosis or underlying disease, or any laboratory measure of fluid and electrolyte balance or kidney function including blood urea nitrogen or creatinine. Subjects receiving dialysis long term (more than 4 years) had less fatigue than subjects who were on dialysis less than 4 years. However, the number of subjects complaining of severe fatigue was equivalent between long- and short-term dialysis patients. The long-term subjects had higher self-reported levels of physical fitness than short-term dialysis subjects. Higher fatigue scores also were associated with higher depression ratings on the Zung self-report measure of depression. Srivastava (1989) studied 27 men and women undergoing hemodialysis. An index of physical performance indicated that subjects continued to perform at normal levels of activity despite their moderate fatigue ratings.

It can be concluded that subjective fatigue has been reported in subjects with chronic kidney failure receiving dialysis and that it has been associated with feelings of depression. The role of mediating factors, such as physical activity level as suggested by Cardenas and Kutner (1982), warrants further investigation. Also, the adaptation of long-term dialysis patients to fatigue and the factors influencing this process need to be investigated.

Fatigue in Multiple Sclerosis

Hart (1978) studied a convenience sample of 335 patients with multiple sclerosis (MS) and 30 healthy control subjects. MS subjects were divided into four groups according to level of disability. Significant differences were observed between control subjects and MS patients across disability groups. The higher disability groups also had higher fatigue scores than lower disability groups. Analysis of variance did not indicate differences in fatigue-related symptoms between healthy subjects and patients. However, authors indicated that anecdotal information suggested that patients were more likely to report "emotional stress" as causes of fatigue than controls. The most frequently reported strategy to reduce fatigue was an increase in naps and total sleep time. Limitations of this study include the differences in age distribution between patient and control groups and the retrospective assessment of fatigue, as the instrument chosen was designed to be a direct measure of fatigue as it is experienced. Krupp, Alvarez, La Rocca, and Scheinberg (1988) compared fatigue symptoms in 32 patients with MS to that experienced by 33 healthy control subjects. Patient and control subjects were similar with respect to age, geographic area, education, and sex distribution. Eighty-seven percent of MS patients reported frequent fatigue as compared with 51% in the controls. A significantly greater number of MS patients (65%) reported moderate to severe fatigue than did the control subjects (15%). There was a moderate correlation between fatigue severity and depression scores. There was no relationship between fatigue severity and degree of disability. Although this study showed significantly greater frequency and severity of fatigue in MS patients than in controls, control subjects also reported moderate to severe fatigue relatively frequently. This finding further supports the need for adequate control groups in evaluating the fatigue experience of patient groups. Likewise depression scores, although considerably higher in MS patients, were indicative of clinical depression in 12% of the control subjects.

INTERVENTIONS TO ALLEVIATE FATIGUE

The Role of Rest and Sleep

Rest and sleep is an intuitively logical approach to managing fatigue. Anecdotal evidence suggests that rest is a strategy often used in alleviating fatigue in cancer patients (Fernsler, 1986; Piper et al., 1989) and in pregnant women (Reeves et al., 1991). There is no systematic evidence to date that indicates that rest or sleep is an adequate intervention in chronic fatigue.

Aerobic Exercise and Physical Fitness

Exercise has been used as an intervention to reduce fatigue. Two intervention studies in cancer patients receiving treatment indicate that some form of physical activity, either aerobic training or physical therapy, improves fatigue and activity levels (MacVicar, Winningham, & Nickel, 1989; Quested et al., 1982). Quested et al. (1982) also found that stress management improved fatigue. However, because a shorter-term attention control group was employed, time-related attention as an intervening variable may have confounded treatment results.

The theoretic premise of exercise intervention studies can be further supported by evidence from studies where associations were observed between the level of physical fitness (Chen, 1986) or stamina (Reeves et al., 1991) and the degree of fatigue reported. Also, the data from these studies lend support to the theoretic scheme proposed by Potempa et al. (1986) where physical fitness is viewed as a physiologic factor that modulates the fatigue manifestations. However, the protective or modulating role of perceived stamina and physical fitness, vis-à-vis exercise training, needs to be further elucidated before clinical applications can be made.

Pharmacologic Treatments

Pharmacologic therapy for chronic fatigue has been used in a few clinical conditions. In chronic fatigue syndrome, Lloyd, Hickie, Wakefield, Boughton, and Dwyer (1990) reported improvement in subjective fatigue, commencement of work, and leisure activities in 43% of intravenous immunoglobulin-G drug-treated patients versus 12% of placebo-treated patients. However, Peterson et al. (1990) reported absolutely no benefit with intravenous immunoglobulin-G in a similar placebo-control trial. Acyclovir, an antiviral agent, also has been used to treat chronic fatigue syndrome with no apparent benefit (Straus et al., 1988). Amantadine, an anticholinergic drug, has been shown to reduce fatigue in some patients with MS (Cohen & Fisher, 1989; Murray, 1985; Rosenberg & Appenzeller, 1988).

RECOMMENDATIONS FOR FUTURE RESEARCH

It is clear from the research literature to date that chronic fatigue is a serious symptom that has been observed in many clinical contexts. This literature has been descriptive in nature employing unidimensional self-report measures of fatigue. Correlates of fatigue have included depression, emotional stress, anxiety, anger, total mood disturbance, younger age, and low physical fitness.

Measurement Issues

Self-Report Measures. Construct validity and reliability of measurement are major issues in fatigue research. Because fatigue has been defined as a perception, self-report measures of this perception have dominated the literature. The most frequently used self-report measure of fatigue is a symptom complaint of being tired, exhausted, or fatigued. This is particularly true in the literature related to the chronic fatigue syndrome, and fatigue prevalence studies in general clinical practice. Thus, our prevalence data on fatigue symptoms by and large have been based on subjective reports with unknown validity and reliability.

Other measures that have been used are visual analogue scale, the Pearson Byars Fatigue Feeling Checklist (Pearson, 1957), the Symptom Distress Scale (McCorkle & Young, 1978), the Rhoten Fatigue Scale (Rhoten, 1982) and the Profile of Mood States (McNair, Lorr, & Droppleman, 1971). The reliability data of these measures are acceptable. These measures have been collectively criticized, however, because they do not address fatigue as a multidimensional construct (Piper, 1989). Piper (1989) has developed a multidimensional fatigue instrument that assesses the following dimensions: temporal, intensity, affective, sensory, evaluative, associated symptoms, and relief patterns. This instrument has been evaluated with a relatively small number of patients with cancer, and more data are required to evaluate its psychometric properties and applications with confidence.

Objective Measures of Fatigue. Objective measures of performance rarely have been used in fatigue research. When measures of physical function have been used, the magnitude of observed relationships has not been stable across studies. Most studies have shown no relationship between level of fatigue and physical activity, disability, or performance. This may be due in part to the lack of standardized measures of physical functioning.

Other objective measures used in the evaluation of fatigue have included serologic data related to immune function, fluid and electrolyte balance, and organ function. These have been used in the diagnosis of the chronic fatigue syndrome or the evaluation of fatigue in cancer, pregnancy, and kidney disease. The assumption of these measures is that fatigue is a consequence of and directly related to the degree of infectious activity or organic dysfunction. However, most investigators have reported a weak association or no association between level of antibody activity or organic dysfunction and fatigue manifestations or disability. Level of physical disability cannot be objectively predicted from any putative measure of fatigue.

Future Research Directions

Several questions remain unanswered. If fatigue is a salient aspect of everyday life, what level of fatigue is normative, and when does the symptom become a disorder? The NANDA and CDC criteria offer a beginning framework for identifying the level at which chronic fatigue is a disorder to be treated. The limitation of the CDC-defining criteria is the exclusive application to the postinfectious form of chronic fatigue. The data clearly suggest that chronic fatigue occurs in many more contexts.

Available data suggest that there are more similarities than differences in how the symptom complex manifests across conditions. The validity of the CDC and NANDA guidelines needs to be assessed empirically with large-scale prospective studies.

The similarity of phenomenology of the primary fatigue symptom and related symptoms across clinical contexts is rather striking. For example, the comorbid occurrence of depression, anxiety, anger, and other mood disturbances with fatigue has been reported in all the clinical populations studied. Are personality and psychologic traits predisposing risk factors for chronic fatigue? Does chronic fatigue that is disabling cause or exacerbate psychologic problems? In other words, certain individuals may be prone to prolonged convalescence that manifests itself as chronic fatigue because of predisposing psychologic characteristics.

Chronic fatigue may not be a separate entity, but a pronounced psychomotor manifestation of depression. Because the biologic basis of fatigue and depression has not been well established, the assessment of these disorders is largely by subject self-report or observed behavioral manifestations. The possibility of common or at least associated biologic pathways for these disorders needs to be investigated. The role of glucocorticoid function in the etiology of fatigue in patients with chronic fatigue syndrome is a promising line of inquiry. Whether neuroendocrine dysfunction is also associated with the etiology of chronic fatigue in other clinical populations has not been investigated.

Studies to determine the efficacy of nursing interventions for chronic fatigue in its various clinical contexts are needed. To date, there are no known cures for chronic fatigue in any form, nor are there sufficient data to support any treatments for symptom control.

REFERENCES

Adams, F., Quesada, J. R., & Gutterman, J. U. (1984). Neuropsychiatric manifestations of human leukocyte interferon therapy in patients with cancer. *Journal of the American Medical Association, 151,* 938–941.

Affonso, D. D., Lovett, S., Paul, S. M., & Sheptak, S. (1990). A standardized interview that differentiates pregnancy and postpartum symptoms from perinatal clinical depression. *Birth, 17,* 121–130.

Banks, M. H., Beresford, S. A., Morrell, D. C., Walker, J. J., & Watkins, C. J. (1975). Factors influencing demand for primary medical care in women aged 20–44 years: A preliminary report. *International Journal of Epidemiology, 4,* 189–195.

Barnes, D. M. (1986). Mystery disease at Lake Tahoe challenges virologists and clinicians. *Science, 234,* 541–542.

Bassey, J., & Fentem, P. (1974). Extent of deterioration in physical condition during postoperative bedrest and its reversal by rehabilitation. *British Medical Journal, 4,* 194–196.

Blesch, K. S., Paice, J. A., Wickham, R., Harte, N., Schnoor, D. K., Purl, S., Rehwalt, M., Kopp, P. L., Manson, S., Coveny, S. B., McHale, M., & Cahill, M. (1991). Correlates of fatigue in people with breast or lung cancer. *Oncology Nursing Forum, 18*(1), 81–87.

Bloom, J. R., Gorsky, R. D., Fobair, P., Hoppe, R., Cox, R. S., Varghese, A., & Spiegel, D. (1990). Physical performance at work and at leisure: Validation of a measure of biological energy in survivors of Hodgkin's disease. *Journal of Psychosocial Oncology, 8*(1), 49–63.

Cardenas, D. D., & Kutner, N. G. (1982). The problem of fatigue in dialysis patients. *Nephron, 30,* 336–340.

Carpenito, L. J. (1992). *Nursing diagnosis: Applications for clinical practice*. Philadelphia: Lippincott.

Carswell, S. (1975). Changes in aerobic power in patients undergoing elective surgery. *Journal of Physiology [London], 251,* 42–43P.

Cassileth, B. P., Lusk, E. J., & Bodenheimer, B. J. (1985). Chemotherapeutic toxicity—the relationship between patients' pretreatment expectations and post-treatment results. *American Journal of Clinical Oncology, 8,* 419–425.

Chen, M. K. (1986). The epidemiology of self-perceived fatigue among adults. *Preventive Medicine, 15,* 74–81.

Cimprich, B. (1990). Attentional fatigue in the cancer patient. *Oncology Nursing Forum, 17*(Suppl. 2), 218.

Cohen, F., & Hardin, S. (1989). Fatigue in patients with catastrophic illness. In S. Funk, E. Tornquist, M. Champagne, L. Copp, & R. Wiese (Eds.), *Key aspects of comfort: Management of pain, fatigue, and nausea* (pp. 208–216). New York: Springer Publishing Co.

Cohen, R. A., & Fisher, M. (1989). Amantadine treatment of fatigue associated with multiple sclerosis. *Archives of Neurology, 46,* 676–680.

Daugherty, S. A., Henry, B. E., Peterson, D. L., Swarts, R. L., Bastien, S., & Thomas, R. S. (1991). Chronic fatigue syndrome in Northern Nevada. *Reviews of Infectious Diseases, 13* (Suppl. 1), S39–S44.

Davis, C. A. (1984). Interferon-induced fatigue. *Oncology Nursing Forum, 11,* 67.

Demitrack, M., Dale, J., Straus, S., Laue, L., Listwak, S., Kruesi, M., Chrousos, G., & Gold, P. (1991). Evidence for impaired activation of the hypothalamic-pituitary-adrenal axis in patients with chronic fatigue syndrome. *Journal of Clinical Endocrinology and Metabolism, 73,* 1224–1234.

Eardley, A. (1986). Patients and radiotherapy: Patients' experiences after discharge. *Radiography, 52,* 17–19.

Evans, A. C. (1934). Chronic brucellosis. *Journal of American Medical Association, 103,* 665.

Fawcett, J., & York, R. (1986). Spouses' physical and psychological symptoms during pregnancy and postpartum. *Nursing Research, 35,* 144–148.

Fernsler, J. (1986). A comparison of patient and nurse perceptions of patients self-care deficits associated with cancer chemotherapy. *Cancer Nursing, 9*(2), 50–57.

Funk, S., Tornquist, E., Champagne, M., Copp, L., & Wiese, R. (Eds.). (1989). *Key aspects of comfort: Management of pain, fatigue, and nausea.* New York: Springer Publishing Co.

Hart, L. K. (1978). Fatigue in the patient with multiple sclerosis. *Research in Nursing and Health, 1,* 147–157.

Haylock, P. J., & Hart, L. K. (1979). Fatigue in patients receiving localized radiation. *Cancer Nursing, 2,* 461–467.

Hickie, I., Lloyd, A., Wakefield, D., & Parker, G. (1990). The psychiatric status of patients with the chronic fatigue syndrome. *British Journal of Psychiatry, 156,* 534–540.

Holmes, G. P., Kaplan, J. E., Gantz, N. M., Komaroff, A. L., Schonberger, L. B., Straus, S. E., Jones, J. F., Dubois, R.E., Cunningham-Rundles, C., Pahwa, S., Tosato, G., Zegans, L. S., Purtilo, D. T., Brown, N., Schooley, R. T., & Brus, I. (1988). Chronic fatigue syndrome: A working case definition. *Annals of Internal Medicine, 108,* 387–389.

Holmes, G. P., Kaplan, J. E., Stewart, J. A., Hunt, B., Pinsky, P. F., & Schonberger, L. B. (1987). A cluster of patients with a chronic mononucleosis-type syndrome: Is Epstein-Barr virus the cause? *Journal of the American Medical Association, 257,* 2297–2302.

Horwitz, C. A., Henle, W., Henle, G., Rudnick, H., & Latts, E. (1985). Long-term serological follow-up of patients for Epstein-Barr virus after recovery from infectious mononucleosis. *Journal of Infectious Disease, 151,* 1150–1153.

Imboden, J. B., Canter, A., & Cluff, L. E. (1961). Convalescence and influenza: A study of the psychological and clinical determinants. *Archives of Internal Medicine, 108,* 393–399.

Imboden, J. B., Canter, A., Cluff, L. E., & Trever, R. W. (1959). Brucellosis: III. Psychologic aspects of delayed convalescence. *Archives of Internal Medicine, 103,* 406–414.

Jamar, S. (1989). Fatigue in women receiving chemotherapy for ovarian cancer. In S. Funk, E. Tornquist, M. Champagne, L. Copp, & R. Wiese (Eds.), *Key aspects of comfort: Management of pain, fatigue, and nausea* (pp. 224–228). New York: Springer Publishing Co.

Jerret, W. A. (1981). Lethargy in general practice. *Practitioner, 225,* 731–737.

Jones, J. F., Ray, C. G., Minnich, L. L., Hicks, M. J., Kibler, R., & Lucas, D. O. (1985). Evidence for active Epstein-Barr virus infection infection in patients with persistent, unexplained illnesses: Elevated anti-early antigen antibodies. *Annals of Internal Medicine, 102,* 1–7.

Joseph-Vanderpool, J., Rosenthal, N., Chrousos, G., Wehr, T. A., Skwera, R., Kasper, S., & Gold, P. W. (1991). Abnormal pituitary-adrenal responses to corticotropin-releasing hormone in patients with seasonal affective disorder: Clinical and pathophysiological implications. *Journal of Clinical Endocrinology and Metabolism, 72,* 1382–1387.

King, K. B., Nail, L. M., Kreamer, K., Strohl, R. A., & Johnson, J. E. (1985). Patients' descriptions of the experience of receiving radiation therapy. *Oncology Nursing Forum, 12*(4), 55–61.

Kling, M., Roy, A., Doran, A. R., Calabrese, J. R., Rubinow, D. R., Whitfield, H. J., May, C., Post, R. M., Chrousos, G. P., & Gold, P. W. (1991). Cerebrospinal fluid immunoreactive corticotropin-releasing hormone and adrenocorticotropic hormone secretion in Cushing's disease and major depression: Potential clinical implications. *Journal of Clinical Endocrinology and Metabolism, 72,* 260–271.

Knoff, M. T. (1986). Physical and psychological distress associated with adjuvant chemotherapy in women with breast cancer. *Journal of Clinical Oncology, 4,* 678–684.

Kobashi-Schoot, J. A., Gerrit, M. A., Hanewald, J. F., Van Dam, S. A., & Bruning, P. F. (1985). Assessment of malaise in cancer patients treated with radiotherapy. *Cancer Nursing, 8,* 306–313.

Kroenke, K., Wood, D. O., Mangelsdorff, D., Meier, N. J., & Powell, J. B. (1988). Chronic fatigue in primary care: Prevalence, patient characteristics, and outcome. *Journal of the American Medical Association, 260,* 929–934.

Kruesi, M. J., Dale, J., & Straus, S. E. (1989). Psychiatric diagnoses in patients who have chronic fatigue syndrome. *Journal of Clinical Psychiatry, 50,* 53–56.

Krupp, L. B., Alvarez, L. A., LaRocca, N. G., & Scheinberg, L. C. (1988). Fatigue in multiple sclerosis. *Archives of Neurology, 45,* 435–437.

Kubricht, D. A. (1984). Therapeutic self-care demands expressed by outpatients receiving external radiation therapy. *Cancer Nursing, 7*(1), 43–52.

Landay, A. L., Jessop, C., Lennette, E. T., & Levy, S. A. (1991). Chronic fatigue syndrome: Clinical condition associated with immune activation. *Lancet, 338,* 707–712.

Lane, T. J., Matthews, D. A., & Manu, P. (1990). The low yield of physical examinations and laboratory investigations of patients with chronic fatigue. *The American Journal of Medical Sciences, 299,* 313–318.

Lloyd, A., Hickie, I., Wakefield, D., Boughton, C., & Dwyer, J. (1990). A double-blind, placebo-controlled trial of intravenous immunoglobulin therapy in patients with chronic fatigue syndrome. *The American Journal of Medicine, 89,* 561–568.

MacVicar, M., Winningham, M., & Nickel, J. (1989). Effects of aerobic interval training on cancer patients' functional capacity. *Nursing Research, 38,* 348–351.

Manu, P., Matthews, D. A., Lane, T. J., Tennen, H., Hesselbrock, V., Mendola, R., & Affleck, G. (1989). Depression among patients with a chief complaint of chronic fatigue. *Journal of Affective Disorders, 17,* 165–172.

McCorkle, R., & Quint-Benoliel, J. (1983). Symptom distress, current concerns and mood disturbance after diagnosis of life-threatening disease. *Social Science Medicine, 17,* 431–438.

McCorkle, R., & Young, K. (1978). Development of a symptom distress scale. *Cancer Nursing, 1,* 373–378.

McNair, D. M., Lorr, M., & Droppleman, L. F. (1971). *POMS: Manual for profile of mood states*. San Diego: Educational and Industrial Testing Service.

Meyerowitz, B. E., Sparks, F. C., & Spears, I. K. (1979). Adjuvant chemotherapy for breast carcinoma. *Cancer, 43,* 1613–1618.

Meyerowitz, B. E., Watkins, I. K., & Sparks, F. C. (1983). Quality of life for breast cancer patients receiving adjuvant chemotherapy. *American Journal of Nursing, 83,* 232–235.

Morrison, J. D. (1980). Fatigue as a presenting complaint in family practice. *Journal of Family Practice, 10,* 795–801.

Murray, T. J. (1985). Amantadine therapy for fatigue in multiple sclerosis. *Le Journal Canadien Des Sciences Neurologiques, 12*(3), 251–254.

National Ambulatory Medical Care Survey: 1975 Summary. (1978). (United States Department of Health and Human Services Publication No. 78-1784). Washington, DC: U.S. Government Printing Office.

Nerenz, D. R., Love, R. R., & Leventhal, H. (1986). Psychological consequences of cancer chemotherapy for elderly patients. *Health Research, 20,* 961–976.

Oldstone, M., Sinha, Y., Blount, P., Tishon, A., Rodriquez, M., von-Wedel, R., & Lambert, P. W. (1982). Virus-induced alterations in homeostasis: Alterations in differentiated functions of infected cells in vivo. *Science, 218,* 1125–1127.

Pearson, R. G. (1957). Scale analysis of a fatigue checklist. *Journal of Applied Psychology, 41,* 186–191.

Peterson, P. K., Shepard, J., Macres, M., Schenck, C., Crosson, J., Rechtman, D., & Lurie, N. (1990). A controlled trial of intravenous immunoglobulin G in chronic fatigue syndrome. *The American Journal of Medicine, 89,* 554–560.

Pickard-Holley, S. (1991). Fatigue in cancer patients: A descriptive study. *Cancer Nursing, 14*(1), 13–19.

Piper, B. F. (1989). Fatigue: Current bases for practice. In S. Funk, E. Tornquist, M. Champagne, L. Copp, & R. Wiese, (Eds)., *Key aspects of comfort: Management of pain, fatigue, and nausea* (pp. 187–198). New York: Springer Publishing Co.

Piper. B. F., Lindsey, A. M., & Dodd, M. J. (1987). Fatigue mechanisms in cancer patients: Developing nursing theory. *Oncology Nursing Forum, 14*(6), 17–23.

Piper, B. F., Rieger, P. T., Brophy, L., Haeuber, D., Hood, L. E., Lyvet, A., & Sharp, E. (1989). Recent advances in the management of biotherapy related side effects: Fatigue. *Oncology Nursing Forum, 16*(Suppl. 6), 27–34.

Potempa, K. (1989). Fatigue: Directions for research and practice. In S. Funk, E. Tornquist, M. Champagne, L. Copp, & R. Wiese (Eds.), *Key aspects of comfort: Management of pain, fatigue, and nausea* (pp. 229–233). New York: Springer Publishing Co.

Potempa, K., Lopez, M., Reid, C., & Lawson, L. (1986). Chronic fatigue. *Image: Journal of Nursing Scholarship, 18,* 165–169.

Proctor, S. J., Karnahan, S., & Taylor, P. (1981). Depression as a component of post-cranial irradiation somnolence syndrome. *Lancet, 1,* 1215–1216.

Quested, K., Malec, J., Harney, R., Kienker, K., & Romsaas, E. (1982). Rehabilitation program for cancer related fatigue: An empirical study. *Archives of Physical Medicine and Rehabilitation, 63,* 532.

Reeves, N., Potempa, K. M., & Gallo, A. (1991). Fatigue in early pregnancy: An exploratory study. *Journal of Nurse-Midwifery, 36,* 303–309.

Rhodes, V. A., Watson, P. M., & Hanson, B. M. (1988). Patients' descriptions of the influence of tiredness and weakness on self-care abilities. *Cancer Nursing, 11,* 186–194.

Rhoten, D. (1982). Fatigue and the post-surgical patient. In C. M. Norris (Ed.), *Concept clarification in nursing* (pp. 277–300). Rockville, MD: Aspen Systems Corporation.

Rosenberg, G. A., & Appenzeller, O. (1988). Amantadine, fatigue, and multiple sclerosis. *Archives of Neurology, 45,* 1104–1106.

Spink, W. W. (1951). What is chronic brucellosis? *Annals of Internal Medicine, 35,* 358–374.

Srivastava, R. H. (1989). Fatigue in end-stage renal disease patients. In S. Funk, E. Tornquist, M. Champagne, L. Copp, & R. Wiese (Eds.), *Key aspects of comfort: Management of pain, fatigue, and nausea* (pp. 217–228). New York: Springer Publishing Co.

Strauman, J. J. (1986). Symptom distress in patients receiving phase I chemotherapy with taxol. *Oncology Nursing Forum, 13*(5), 40–43.

Straus, S. E. (1988). The chronic mononucleosis syndrome. *The Journal of Infectious Diseases, 157,* 405–412.

Straus, S. E. (1991). History of chronic fatigue syndrome. *Reviews of Infectious Disease, 13*(Suppl. 1), S2–S7.

Straus, S. E., Dale, J. K., Tobi, M., Lawley, T., Preble, O., Blaese, R. M., Hallahan, C., & Henle, W. (1988). Acyclovir treatment of the chronic fatigue syndrome: Lack of efficacy in the placebo-controlled trial. *New England Journal of Medicine, 319,* 1692–1698.

Straus, S. E., Tosato, G., Armstrong, G., Lawley, T., Preble, O. T., Henle, W., Davey, R., Pearson, G., Epstein, J., Brus, I., & Blaese, M. (1985). Persisting illness and fatigue in adults with evidence of Epstein-Barr virus infection. *Annals of Internal Medicine, 102,* 7–16.

Sugarman, J. R., & Berg, A. O. (1984). Evaluation of fatigue in a family practice. *Journal of Family Practice, 19,* 643–647.

Truss, C. O. (1981). The role of candida albicans in human illness. *Journal of Orthomolecular Psychiatry, 10,* 228–238.

Valdini, A., Steinhardt, S., & Feldman, E. (1989). Usefulness of a standard battery of laboratory tests in investigating chronic fatigue in adults. *Family Practice, 6,* 286–291.

Wadler, S., Lyver, A., & Wiernik, P. H. (1989). Clinical toxicities of the combination of 5-fluorouracil and recombinant interferon alfa-2a: An unusual toxicity profile. *Oncology Nursing Forum, 16*(Suppl. 6), 12–15.

Wessely, S., & Powell, R. (1989). Fatigue syndromes: A comparison of chronic "postviral" fatigue with neuromuscular and affective disorders. *Journal of Neurology, Neurosurgery, and Psychiatry, 52,* 940–948.

Wood, G. C., Bentall, R. P., Gopfert, M., & Edwards, R. H. (1991). A comparative psychiatric assessment of patients with chronic fatigue syndrome and muscle disease. *Psychological Medicine, 21,* 619–628.

Zeiderman, M., Welchew, E., & Clark, R. (1990). Changes in cardiovascular and muscle function associated with the development of postoperative fatigue. *British Journal of Surgery, 77,* 576–580.

Zeiderman, M., Welchew, E., & Clark, R. (1991). Influence of epidural analgesia upon postoperative fatigue. *British Journal of Surgery, 78,* 1457–1460.

Chapter 4

Side Effects of Cancer Chemotherapy

MARYLIN J. DODD
SCHOOL OF NURSING
UNIVERSITY OF CALIFORNIA, SAN FRANCISCO

CONTENTS

MANAGEMENT OF SIDE EFFECTS OF CANCER CHEMOTHERAPY

Cancer chemotherapy (CTX) drugs are given with the intent to cure, control, or palliate neoplasms (cancer). The CTX drugs destroy or damage not only cancer cells but also normal cells, resulting in adverse side effects. Much empiric work has been done describing CTX-induced side effects, with fewer studies having been conducted to prevent or manage side effects. This chapter includes a review of studies focused on managing side effects of CTX.

The search for this review was begun on the MEDLINE database covering the last 4 years. The key words of neoplasms, antineoplastic agents, and adverse effects resulted in more than 15,000 citations. Subsequent key words for inclusion were English language and studies involving humans only. The search was narrowed again by using the 48 side effects listed for 34 commonly prescribed chemotherapy drugs (Dodd, 1991). Each side effect was used in a search with the key word of antineoplastic agents. Pharmacologic studies (clinical drug trials) where one drug is compared with other drugs to test for the effectiveness of preventing or alleviating a CTX-induced side effect were excluded in the search because the focus of interest was nonpharmacologic treatments. Articles reporting experimental studies to prevent or manage the side effects of CTX involved only a few side effects. The predominant side effects reported were nausea and vomiting, mucositis/stomatitis, and hair loss. Studies of hair loss (alopecia) are not reviewed in this chapter. In 1989, the Federal Drug Administration prohibited the use of the scalp tourniquet and cooling devices while data are sought as to the safety of these products to treat hair loss. Broader-based intervention studies conducted by Dodd (1984, 1988) focused on enhancing self-care behaviors to prevent and manage CTX side effects. Names of authors known to be working on managing CTX side effects were searched. A manual search was conducted of journals (e.g., *Oncology Nursing Forum, Cancer Nursing, Seminars in Oncology Nursing*) believed to be highly relevant to the topic area and published longer than 4 years ago and up to 10 years back. Another purpose of the manual search was to ensure that all pertinent references from the MEDLINE search had been identified. Reference lists from key articles were used to expand the search. The time frame for this review is 1978 to the present.

The samples included in the studies must have been receiving CTX and not biologic response modifiers, colony-stimulating factors, hormonal therapy only, or a concurrent full course of radiation therapy. Although CTX was used in a limited way with bone marrow transplant (BMT) therapy (i.e., chemoradiation conditioning during the first 8 days of the BMT), the decision was made not to include BMT samples in this review because CTX has a limited role in BMT therapy. The samples included both adults and children as subjects/patients.

This review includes physiologic and psychologic symptoms only if they are attributable to the CTX the patient was receiving. Some of the physiologic symptoms are more directly related to the disease process (e.g., cancer cachexia), and some psychologic symptoms are more directly related to the cancer chemotherapy experience in toto and not to specific CTX drugs (e.g., anxiety). If the dependent (outcome) variables investigated in a study included at least one side effect of CTX, the study was reviewed.

Finally, regarding the criteria used for this review, the focus of this chapter is preventing or managing the side effects of CTX. Some of the interventions tested for the prevention or management of side effects were nurse initiated; some were not initiated by a nurse, but the intervention was within the scope of practice for nursing. As long as an intervention was judged to be within the scope of nursing practice, it was included in this review.

Nausea, Vomiting, and Retching

Although the symptoms of nausea, vomiting, and retching (N, V, & R) all arise from the central nervous system and are described frequently in tandem, it is important to note that they are actually three separate entities. Nausea is a subjective experience that has been described as an autonomic response (i.e., the conscious recognition of the need or desire to vomit) (Hogan, 1990). It is a very distressing feeling experienced in the back of the throat, the epigastrium, and frequently culminating in vomiting. Thirty percent to more than 75% of cancer patients who are receiving CTX experience vomiting (Needleman, 1987; Sallan & Cronin, 1985). Vomiting is the oral expulsion of the gastric contents that occurs as a result of positive changes in the intrathoracic pressure. The emetic center is composed of both the vomiting center and the chemoreceptor (CTZ) trigger zone and receives input from a variety of peripheral and central afferent sources (Seigel & Longo, 1981). The irritation to the CTZ is most frequently identified as the primary cause of CTX-induced nausea and vomiting (Borison, 1986). Retching is the attempt to vomit without oral expulsion. It is also called "dry heaves" (Rhodes, 1990). It is controlled by the respiratory center in the brainstem (Guyton, 1980). The frequency of retching has not been determined. Anticipatory nausea and vomiting (AN & V) is a learned conditioned response stimulated by something that occurs in association with the true stimulant (e.g., CTX). Through repeated pairings with CTX and its after effects, previously neutral stimuli (e.g., the sights, sounds, and odors of the treatment setting) acquire nausea- and emesis-eliciting properties (Redd & Hendler, 1984). Consequently, interventions targeted at the stimulus have reduced the incidence of AN & V. AN & V develops in approximately 33% of patients and usually occurs after the third or fourth cycle of CTX (Cotanch & Strum, 1987).

Interventions for Nausea, Vomiting, Retching, and Anticipatory Nausea and Vomiting

Most intervention studies have been conducted using behavioral techniques as the independent variable. The major types of behavioral techniques tested in these studies included hypnosis, progressive muscle relaxation training (PMRT) with guided imagery (GI), systematic desensitization, biofeedback combined with PMRT and GI, and distraction.

Although the point was made earlier that N, V, & R are separate entities, previous investigators have not treated them consistently as such. As a result the first part of this review includes studies that included N, V, & R either in combination or singularly. The second part of this review includes intervention studies conducted to prevent and alleviate AN & V. The rationale for the division of sections rests with the different mechanisms responsible for the occurrence of side effects.

Studies of Nausea, Vomiting, and Retching

There were 16 studies found in which investigators used some type of behavioral intervention to prevent or alleviate N, V, & R. Five additional studies were found that used nonbehavioral interventions to prevent or alleviate these side effects.

The emphasis in the behavioral intervention studies was more on managing or alleviating a side effect once it occurred rather than on preventing the side effects. One prevention study was found, but the investigators failed to do premeasures of the N, V, & R side effects (Burish, Carey, Krozely, & Greco, 1987).

The behavioral technique used by researchers in 7 of the 16 studies was PMRT with GI (Burish, Carey, Krozely, & Greco, 1987; Burish & Lyles, 1979; Carey & Burish, 1987; Cotanch, 1983; Cotanch & Strum, 1987; Lyles, Burish, Krozely, & Oldham, 1982; Scott, Donahue, Mastrovito, & Hakes, 1986). Included in these seven studies was a single case report that used only PMRT (Burish & Lyles, 1979) and another study that used PMRT with GI as well as other techniques (Scott et al., 1986). Three studies used hypnosis with specific suggestions and some form of imagery (Cotanch, Hockenberry, & Herman, 1985; Zeltzer, Kellerman, Ellenberg, & Dash, 1983; Zeltzer, LeBaron, & Zeltzer, 1984). For one of the three studies using hypnosis, a guided imagery component was included (Cotanch et al., 1985). For the other two studies with samples of children/adolescents using hypnosis, imagery protocol included having the children intensely involved in fantasy; then the therapist made specific suggestions (e.g., to relax, to feel safe, to have a good appetite) (Zeltzer et al., 1983, 1984). One of the hypnosis technique studies had a contrast group of supportive counseling that included distracting the child's attention away from the CTX experience (Zeltzer et al., 1984). Three additional studies used a distraction technique (Frank, 1985; Kolko & Rickard-Figueroa, 1985; LeBaron & Zeltzer, 1984).

In the Frank (1985) study, the adult sample was introduced to music therapy and guided imagery. These patients selected their music from several tapes and selected their scenic poster from several posters provided by the investigator. The investigator described her music tapes as "soft, slow, and sad." The reason for the sad theme was not given in the report.

The pediatric samples were introduced to two types of distraction: video games (Kolko & Rickard-Figueroa, 1985) and interactions with a therapist who directed the child's attention away from any thoughts or sensations related to nausea or vomiting (LeBaron & Zeltzer, 1984). The therapist used several methods to divert attention (e.g., playing games, telling stories). These methods were individualized for the child, but the investigators state that "all the methods had similar elements of diversion." Two additional studies were found that used biofeedback (measured by electromyography activity) in conjunction with PMRT with GI (Burish, Shartner, & Lyles, 1981; Shartner, Burish, & Carey, 1985).

The behavioral interventions were usually provided by the same therapist (clinical psychologist or nurse) over several sessions at a minimum or over the entire course of CTX. Providing interventions over the entire course of CTX was seen most often with single case studies. Audiotapes and pamphlets were provided in a few of the studies to augment the therapist but not to substitute for the patient-therapist sessions (Cotanch & Strum, 1987; Scott et al., 1986).

Most behavioral intervention studies measured nausea and vomiting as the dependent variable, although two studies measured only nausea (Burish et al., 1981; Carey & Burish, 1985), and other studies measured only vomiting (Zeltzer et al., 1983) and N, V, & R (Scott et al., 1986). None of these dependent variables were ever the only outcome or dependent variables of their respective studies. Other dependent variables frequently included were: "physiological arousal variables," that is, blood pressure, pulse, and respirations (BP,P,R), and electromyography activity (Burish & Lyles, 1979; Burish et al., 1981, 1987; Carey & Burish, 1987; Cotanch, 1983; Cotanch & Strum, 1987; Lyles et al., 1982; Scott et al., 1986; Shartner et al., 1985); affective states, anxiety, depression, and hostility (Burish & Lyles, 1979; Burish et al., 1981, 1987; Carey & Burish, 1987; Cotanch, 1983; Cotanch & Strum, 1987; Frank, 1985; Kolko & Rickard-Figueroa, 1985; Lyles et al., 1982; Shartner et al., 1985; Zeltzer et al., 1983); patients' expectations of antiemetic drugs and CTX (Carey & Burish, 1987); nutritional status and oral intake (Carey & Burish, 1987; Cotanch et al., 1985); caloric intake (Cotanch, 1983; Cotanch & Strum, 1987); anthropometric-skinfold measurements, and body weight (Cotanch, 1983; Cotanch & Strum, 1987); type and quality of antiemetic drugs (Burish et al., 1987; Cotanch, 1983; Cotanch et al., 1985); disruption in activities of daily living (LeBaron & Zeltzer, 1984); other side effects (Scott et al., 1986); locus of control (Zeltzer et al., 1983); and impact of illness and self-esteem (Zeltzer et al., 1983).

For the dependent variables other than N, V, & R, they were measured by standard methods (e.g., BP,P,R, intake and output), established instruments such as the State Trait Anxiety Inventory (STAI) by Speilberger (1970) (Cotanch, 1983; Cotanch & Strum, 1987; Frank, 1985; Kolko & Rickard-Figueroa, 1985; Zeltzer et al., 1983), Multiple Affect Adjective Checklist by Zuckerman, Lubin, Vogel, and Valerius (1964) (Burish & Lyles, 1979; Burish et al., 1987; Carey & Burish, 1987; Lyles et al., 1982), or investigator-developed Likert scales for anxiety (Burish & Lyles, 1979; Burish et al., 1981, 1987, Carey & Burish, 1987; Lyles et al., 1982; Shartner et al., 1985).

The theoretical frameworks used in these studies included physiology, emetic processes, and stress and adaptation. The earlier work in this area was done with single case reports and multiple sessions with one patient (Burish & Lyles, 1979; Burish et al., 1981). Of the 16 behavioral intervention studies that used behavioral techniques, 12 were conducted with adult samples and 4 with pediatric samples. From both the adult and pediatric samples, patients were often recruited to the study because they had experienced difficulties with N, V, & R during prior CTX (Carey & Burish, 1987; Cotanch, 1983; Cotanch et al., 1985; Frank, 1985; Kolko & Rickard-Figueroa, 1985; Zeltzer et al., 1983). Therefore, the interventions tested in these studies had an increased challenge to demonstrate significant improvement of N, V, & R.

The samples in this series of behavioral intervention studies have been heterogeneous in regard to having multiple types of cancer and consequently multiple types of CTX regimens. There were two exceptions to this heterogeneous pattern, a sample of adolescent leukemia patients (Kolko & Rickard-Figueroa, 1985) and a sample of women with ovarian cancer (Scott et al., 1986). The samples differed on where the patients were in their course of CTX (e.g., beginning CTX or several cycles into the CTX). Special sampling techniques were used to control extraneous variables known to influence the occurrence of N, V, & R. Investigators matched on age and CTX drugs (Zeltzer et al., 1984) and site of cancer and CTX drugs (Carey & Burish, 1987); stratified on the CTX emetogenicity (Burish et al., 1987) and antiemetic drug equivalents (Burish et al., 1987; Lyles et al., 1982); and a priori or controlled for the CTX regimen by adjusting the dependent variables in the data analysis (Carey & Burish, 1985; Lyles et al., 1982).

The predominant design used in this series of studies was quasi-experimental with repeated measures with the number of baseline (preintervention), intervention, and follow-up (without therapist providing the intervention) sessions varying with each study. Some studies lacked randomization (Cotanch, 1983; Frank, 1985; LeBaron & Zeltzer, 1984). In others, random assignment occurred after matching of the patients had occurred (Carey &

Burish, 1987), and one study described a "random selection process" that was unclear as to its meaning (Scott et al., 1986). Many of the studies lacked a control group (Cotanch, 1983; Frank, 1985; LeBaron & Zeltzer, 1984; Scott et al., 1986; Zeltzer et al., 1983). However, through multiple baseline measures, the investigators proposed that the "patients served as their own controls" (Cotanch, 1983; LeBaron & Zeltzer, 1984; Zeltzer et al., 1983). The single case reports tended to follow the patients over many sessions (e.g., 10 or 11 sessions) of CTX and perhaps to the completion of CTX. One small sample of adolescents (n = 3) did a variation on the repeated measures design by using a "combined multiple baseline across subjects design and an ABAB withdrawal design" (Kolko & Rickard-Figueroa, 1985). After the baseline measures were obtained the distraction technique of video games was introduced for several sessions, then withdrawn for several sessions, and then this pattern was repeated. Dependent variable measures occurred throughout all of these CTX sessions. The purpose of the follow-up sessions was to determine if the patient could maintain the effects of the intervention without the therapist. In another study, the withdrawal of the therapist was planned but did not occur because of the preference of the patients aged 10 to 18 years for the therapist to continue to provide the intervention (Le Baron & Zeltzer, 1984).

The instrument/techniques used to measure N, V, & R varied from self-report that was very congruent with the subjective nature of nausea to investigator-developed instruments (Frank, 1985; Kolko & Rickard-Figueroa, 1985; Scott et al., 1986) to established instruments (Cotanch, 1987). The self-report instruments used most often were in the Likert scale format (Burish et al., 1987, 1981; Carey & Burish, 1987; Cotanch et al., 1985; Cotanch & Strum, 1987; Frank, 1985; LeBaron & Zeltzer, 1984; Lyles et al., 1982; Shartner et al., 1985; Zeltzer et al., 1983). One investigator-developed instrument had many parameters of N, V, & R included as well as associated side effects (Scott et al., 1986). In contrast there was an absence of the description of instruments used to measure the patient's nausea and vomiting from the patient's, nurse's, and family member's perspectives (Cotanch, 1983). The source for the N, V, & R data included the patient, the nurse for both the pediatric and adult samples (Burish et al., 1987, 1981; Cotanch, 1983; Lyles et al., 1982; Scott et al., 1986), parents (LeBaron & Zeltzer, 1984; Zeltzer et al., 1983), family members (Cotanch, 1983), and an observer (Kolko & Rickard-Figueroa, 1985). The pediatric sample studies that used a parent for a source of their data did not specify who that parent was and if the parent remained constant throughout the study. The patients' self-report data were consistently gathered across all studies, and the other sources of data were used to corroborate the patients' self-report. Agreement among the patients', parents', and nurses' data was surprisingly high given the subjective nature of nausea. One group of investigators tried to have their adolescents complete diaries of vomiting episodes, but the compliance rate was less than 50% (Zeltzer et al., 1983).

Gard, Edwards, Harris, and McCormack (1988) raised an interesting measurement issue regarding the sensitizing effects of preintervention assessment on postintervention measures of nausea and vomiting. They conducted a study where *half* of their sample (n = 35) was asked to complete an inventory about the severity of side effects they experienced (including nausea and vomiting) following their most recent CTX session. The other half of the sample (n = 35) completed an inventory on parking conditions. Both of these inventories were completed in the clinic before CTX. Post-CTX measures (including nausea and vomiting) were completed by all patients at their homes and mailed back to the investigators. Patients in the experimental condition (severity of side effects at the premeasure) rated their nausea as more severe than controls (parking inventory at premeasure); no significant difference was reported for vomiting between the two groups. This finding for nausea would support the investigators' contention that the patients become sensitized to premeasures. Using this same issue of the sensitizing effects of preintervention assessment of nausea and vomiting, Burish and his colleagues (1987) conducted a study with 24 adult cancer patients where nausea was not mentioned to the experimental group at the preintervention assessment, but these patients were told that "the intervention (PMRT with GI) would help them recognize muscle tension in the body" (Burish et al., 1987, p. 44). This study demonstrated significant improvement in nausea and vomiting for the experimental group patients at the postintervention session. What remains unanswered in this study is if the sensitizing words of nausea and vomiting at the preintervention assessment would have the experimental group report more nausea and vomiting at the postintervention assessment and thereby nullify the effect of the intervention. Other studies in the area provided the answer in that nausea and vomiting were usually mentioned at the preintervention session and the PMRT with GI intervention resulted in significant improvement of nausea and vomiting at the postintervention session (Cotanch, 1983; Cotanch & Strum, 1987; Lyles et al., 1982).

There were several design issues raised in this series of studies. In some studies the repeated measures on the dependent variables were too proximal to each other (e.g., 15 min apart), thus raising the threat of testing measurement error (Scott et al., 1986). In contrast, some studies conducted their repeated measures of the dependent variables too distant from the CTX sessions when N, V, & R were likely to have occurred (LeBaron & Zeltzer, 1984; Zeltzer et al., 1983). Patients in one study were asked to recall their usual pattern of nausea and vomiting from previous CTX cycles (recall of at least 3 to 4 weeks required for this task) (Frank, 1985). The premeasures and postmeasures in another study were 6 months apart, with daily reporting on the parameters of vomiting (Zeltzer et al., 1983). The compliance rate of patients to their daily home diary recordings over a 6-month period was 50%. The investigators decided that these data introduced too much self-selection bias, and the data were not used in the study (Zeltzer et al., 1983).

The "blind" condition of the data collectors in these studies was present to a varying degree (Cotanch et al., 1985; Kolko & Rickard-Figueroa, 1985; Lyles et al., 1982) or was totally absent (Burish et al., 1987; Scott et al., 1986). For example, the nurse raters may not be blind to the patients' experimental condition, but they were blind to the patients' ratings of nausea and vomiting (Lyles et al., 1982).

The quality control of the behavioral technique intervention received varying amounts of attention by the investigators. In most (n = 14) studies the same therapist provided the intervention, so at the very least the intervention may have stayed constant. Two studies did not use the same therapists (Carey & Burish, 1987; Scott et al., 1986). The purpose of the first of these two studies was to compare different types of people and methods for administering the intervention (Carey & Burish, 1987). The types of people were professional therapists who included one licensed clinical psychologist, two doctoral candidates in clinical psychology, and one oncology nurse versus the paraprofessional therapists who were four community volunteers with no previous experience with PMRT and no postbaccalaureate training in psychology, nursing, or medicine. The paraprofessionals received extensive training requiring 8 to 12 hr of professional time (i.e., time for a professional therapist and a clinical psychologist to provide the training) and an additional 8 to 12 hr of self-study. The types of methods were professionally prepared audiotapes versus patient-therapist interaction sessions. Two clinical psychologists reviewed the patient-therapist session audiotapes, made by the professional and paraprofessional therapists, to determine the difference between the two groups. The review process was blind. Unfortunately, this review was conducted 2 weeks after the study was completed; thus, it was not possible to provide retraining to either group, if needed. Patients gave equivalent ratings to both types of therapists, but they were not exposed to both types. The clinical psychologists noted more skill in the professional therapist group. In the second study Scott and her associates (1986) provided a 2-week, 12-hr workshop in clinical relaxation. Nurses were supervised clinically and tested for their ability to carry out the experimental protocol. No ongoing reliability checks of the consistency of the intervention over time were reported by any of the studies in this series. In one study, a post hoc analysis was performed following the intervention period (Zeltzer et al., 1983). Patients in the hypnosis group were administered the Stanford Hypnotic Clinical Scale (Morgan & Hilgard, 1978/1979) to ensure that the patients' hypnotic susceptibility scores did not bias the therapists in their response to the children during the intervention (Zeltzer et al., 1983). Unfortunately, the results of this test were not presented in the report.

The adherence rate of the patients to the intervention was reported by only a few investigators (Cotanch, 1983; Cotanch & Strum, 1987; LeBaron & Zeltzer, 1984; Lyles et al., 1982; Zeltzer et al., 1983). The adherence rate was most appropriately determined when patients were to initiate the intervention in the absence of the therapist during follow-up CTX sessions, and when patients were to practice the intervention away from the clinic between CTX sessions. In Cotanch's study (1983) patients were given the PMRT audiotapes and a stamped addressed weekly schedule card to record their practice sessions. No adherence rate was reported. In another study, patients were to record the number of times they practiced the intervention at home (Lyles et al., 1982). The investigators reported the data as "very unreliable." In a study of adolescents, the investigators reported that the subjects did not practice any techniques at home despite being provided with audiotapes (LeBaron & Zeltzer, 1984). No adherence estimates were given for the intervention during follow-up sessions. In 11 of the 16 studies dependent variable measures were reported as improved or not, based on the assumption that patients performed the intervention during these sessions.

In two of the studies in the series of behavioral interventions to manage N, V, & R, a "placebo control" group was included in addition to a true control group (i.e., no intervention) (Cotanch & Strum, 1987; Lyles et al., 1982). The investigators provided the placebo control group with as much therapist attention as the experimental group. In one study, the placebo control group patients received support and encouragement from the therapist (Lyles et al., 1982). In the second study, the placebo control group patients listened to tapes of relaxing music in the presence of the therapist (Cotanch & Strum, 1987).

The findings from the behavioral intervention studies are consistent. All types of behavioral interventions yielded significant improvement in N, V, & R during the CTX sessions when the therapist was present and to a lesser extent during follow-up sessions when the therapist was absent. In studies where descriptive statistics were used the improvement in the N, V, & R scores appeared to be clinically important (Burish & Lyles, 1979; Burish et al., 1981). Only one study yielded a nonsignificant decrease in nausea and vomiting with PMRT with GI, and this was the study that tested different personnel as therapists as another of its study's aims. The investigators provided no insight into the lack of significant findings (Carey & Burish, 1987).

The behavioral techniques appear to be equivalent in their effectiveness

(Zeltzer et al., 1983). However, more than one intervention was administered to the experimental group. Thus, it is difficult to determine which intervention contributed to the improvement of the dependent variables (Scott et al., 1986; Shartner et al., 1985). One investigator offered the possible mechanisms of action to explain the interventions effectiveness (Cotanch & Strum, 1987); this was not a common practice.

The data analyses for these studies varied from descriptive to inferential and were appropriate for the type of data and study. The lack of significance of all dependent variable measures (N, V, & R) across all occasions/sessions may have been due to the small sample sizes in most of these studies. In one study, data were not presented on a dependent variable; nurses recorded observations and family and friends' subjective opinions regarding the nausea and vomiting the patient experienced (Cotanch, 1983).

Investigators were conservative in their statements of generalizability of their findings. Given the methodologic issues raised in this section, cautiousness was appropriate. Reported limitations included assessing the difficulty of a single group design, such as determining if the changes in the postintervention dependent variables were due to the intervention, testing, history, or maturation (Frank, 1985); and including the placebo control group for its possible dampening effect on the experimental intervention of PMRT with GI (Cotanch & Strum, 1987). For the problem of the confounded interventions, the investigators proposed a dismantling technique so biofeedback could be assessed independent of the PMRT with GI (Shartner et al., 1985). Other investigators commented on the inadequacy of the instruments (Kolko & Rickard-Figueroa, 1985), high dropout rates (Lyles et al., 1982), and the need for several baseline sessions owing to the variability of emesis over courses of CTX (Cotanch, 1983; Zeltzer et al., 1983).

There were five nonbehavioral intervention studies that had N, V, & R as their dependent or outcome variables. The interventions included patient-controlled infusion pumps (Edwards, Herman, Wallace, Pavy, & Harrison-Pavy, 1991; Wilder-Smith, Schuler, Osterwalder, Naji, & Senn, 1990), an exercise program (Winningham & MacVicar, 1988), hydration rates during CTX (Jordan, 1989), and time of CTX administration (Headley, 1987).

The first of the two patient-controlled infusion pump studies involved a two-group design; one group was the patient-controlled antiemetic therapy (PCAE) via an intravenous pump; the other group was a nurse-controlled antiemetic therapy via a nurse-administered mini-intravenous bags (Edwards et al., 1991). The second patient-controlled infusion pump study involved patients with the infusion pump filled with either one of two types of antiemetic drugs (metoclopramide or droperidol). The infusions were continuous with on-demand bolus of antiemetic drug that was administered on the patient pushing a button (Wilder-Smith et al., 1990). The primary emphasis of this study was the patients' behavior with the pump, not the two antiemetic drugs used in the study.

The third study in this series involved an exercise program using a cycle ergometer, aerobic-interval training protocol with a set of flexibility and stretching exercises (Winningham & MacVicar, 1988). The program involved exercising 3 times a week for 10 weeks. The last two studies in the series involved interventions where the investigators did *not* have control of the independent variables, that is, rate of hydration (Jordan, 1989) and time of CTX administration (Headley, 1987).

Three of the five nonbehavioral intervention studies measured all three side effects of N, V, & R (Edwards et al., 1991; Headley, 1987; Wilder-Smith et al., 1990); one study measured only nausea (Winningham & MacVicar, 1988); and another study measured only vomiting (Jordan, 1989). Other dependent variables measured in these studies were at a minimum in contrast to the variables measured in the previous section. The patient- versus the nurse-controlled antiemetic infusion pump study included measures of sedation level and other side effects of the antiemetic drugs (Edwards et al., 1991). The exercise program study included measures of symptoms other than N, V, & R; body weight; and height (Winningham & MacVicar, 1988). The other three studies did not include dependent variables in addition to N, V, & R (Headley, 1987; Jordan, 1989; Wilder-Smith et al., 1990).

The dependent variables other than N, V, & R were measured by standard methods for height and weight, established instruments, for example, Symptom Checklist 90 (Derogatis, 1977) and Rhodes Index of Nausea and Vomiting (Rhodes, Watson, & Johnson, 1986), or investigator-developed Likert scales (e.g., sedation level) (Edwards et al., 1991). The frameworks for these studies were provided by physiology, disability and rehabilitation, biologic rhythms and chronopharmacology, and perceived control.

All of the nonbehavioral intervention studies were conducted with adult patients. Patients in one of the infusion pump studies came to the study with a history of having not responded to high doses of an antiemetic in previous CTX sessions (Wilder-Smith et al., 1990). During the testing of the current interventions patients were receiving a high emetic potential drug, cis platinum (Headley, 1987; Jordan, 1989), or at least moderate emetic potential drugs (Edwards et al., 1991). Patients from three of the five studies had multiple types of cancer and consequently multiple CTX regimens (Edwards et al., 1991; Jordan, 1989; Wilder-Smith et al., 1990). There were notable exceptions to these heterogeneous samples. The exercise program study included only women with breast cancer who were receiving a selected type of CTX regimen (Winningham & MacVicar, 1988). The time of CTX administration study included only men with testicular or bladder cancer

(Headley, 1987). Furthermore, the exercise program study used some special sampling techniques to control for extraneous variables. The investigators matched patients on age and functional capacity (Winningham & MacVicar, 1988). One of the infusion pump studies recruited their sample as the patients were beginning their CTX (Edwards et al., 1991). The exercise program study required that patients had to have received three cycles of CTX before coming into the study (Winningham & MacVicar, 1988). Where the other studies' samples were in their course of CTX was not reported.

The exercise program study was the only true experimental study in this series, with the two infusion pump studies either lacking a control group (Edwards et al., 1991; Wilder-Smith et al., 1990) or some form of randomization (Wilder-Smith et al., 1990). The remaining two studies where the investigators had no control of the interventions were ex post facto designs (Headley, 1987; Jordan, 1989). Repeated measures of the dependent variables of N, V, & R varied across studies and occurred as frequently as hourly in one study (Headley, 1987), to every 2 hr in another study (Wilder-Smith et al., 1990), and at 12 hr in still another study (Edwards et al., 1991). In the exercise program study the dependent variables were measured "pre- and post-treatment"; it is unclear if "treatment" is CTX treatment or the exercise treatment. If it is the CTX treatment, the cycles for CTX administration are 3 to 4 weeks apart; if it is the exercise treatment, the dependent variables would have been measured 3 times a week for 10 weeks, which seems excessive considering some of the variables would not be expected to change in this time frame (e.g., body weight and height). In the hydration rate study, patients were to record the frequency of vomiting in 24 hr (Jordan, 1989). So in this study the repeated measures was ongoing during this period.

The instruments used to measure N, V, & R varied from self-report on a 100-mm visual analogue scale (Edwards et al., 1991) to nurses' observations of N, V, & R on Likert scales (Edwards et al., 1991; Wilder-Smith et al., 1990) to investigator-developed instruments (Headley, 1987) to established instruments (Headley, 1987; Winningham & MacVicar, 1988). The instrument to measure vomiting in the hydration rate study was not described (Jordan, 1989). In one study (Headley, 1987), family members asked the patient every hour for 12 hr if she or he had been nauseated and the number of times she or he had vomited in the last hour (Headley, 1987). There appeared to be a serious omission in one of the infusion pump studies, that is, patients did not provide any data on N, V, & R, but were only asked if they preferred the infusion pump. The nurses provided the N, V, & R data through observations (Wilder-Smith et al, 1990). Given the subjective nature of nausea, data from the patient are essential.

There were several design issues raised in this series of studies. The threat of testing measurement error occurred when patients were asked every hour their N, V, & R status (Headley, 1987). The timing of the exercise with the timing of the CTX administration was a question for the study by Winningham and MacVicar (1988). One clue was provided by the investigators who stated "it is best not to exercise until the day after CTX treatments" (p. 450). None of these five studies established a repeated measures baseline over several courses of CTX as had the behavioral intervention studies in the previous section. This was particularly of concern in the time of CTX administration study where patients were followed for only one cycle of CTX (Headley, 1987). Considerable time and effort were provided by the investigators in one of the infusion pump studies to establish and maintain the "double-blind" condition (Edwards et al., 1991). In the second infusion pump study (Wilder-Smith et al., 1990), why the blind condition was not established was not discussed in the report, and may rest with the primary purpose of this study not being the antiemetic drug effect but whether the patients preferred the pump.

The quality control of the nonbehavioral interventions received varying amounts of attention from the investigators. In the two infusion pump studies, either the pharmacist (Edwards et al., 1991) or the same physician (Wilder-Smith et al., 1990) handled the preparation of the pump solution and assignments. The difficulty reported in one of the pump studies (Edwards et al., 1991) was the reluctance of some patients to push the button to release the antiemetic when nausea occurred. In the exercise program study, the investigator provided all the interventions so that the technique would not have varied between other intervention personnel but may have varied during the 10-week exercise course. The patients' adherence to the exercise program was not an issue because the investigator was with these patients at each exercise session. The exercise program study was the only study in the five that included a "placebo control" as well as a true control group. The placebo control group patients received weekly stretching and flexing exercises provided by the investigator. This was extra attention, but it did not match the attention provided to the experimental group patients who exercised 3 times a week.

The findings from this series of five studies were more mixed than the findings from the behavioral interventions. Perhaps this was due to the wider range of interventions tested in this series. There were nonsignificant differences found between the patient- versus nurse-controlled antiemetic drug pumps for nausea. Because vomiting occurred so infrequently in both groups, differences could not be tested. However, the patient-controlled group used less antiemetic drugs during the course of the study (Edwards et al., 1991). It is important to note that the patients in this study received considerable dosages of antiemetics as premedication. In the other infusion study, eight of the nine patients preferred the pump, and both antiemetic drugs appeared to be effective in reducing N, V, & R (Wilder-Smith et al., 1990). The exercise program yielded a significant decrease in nausea (Winningham & MacVicar, 1988). In the two ex post facto studies, effects were obtained for different hydration rates for intravenous (more than 333 ml/hr) and for oral intake (between 400 and 1000 ml/day) for a significant decrease in vomiting (Jordan, 1989). Nonsignificant differences were obtained for the time of administration of CTX (Headley, 1987). In the hydration rate study, the 254 cis-platinum infusions were received by 60 patients, yet the investigator assumed incidents (infusions) were independent within patients for the purposes of the analyses. This may not be a safe assumption because the patient's own experiences with the infusions could be expected to be significantly related.

The investigators' discussions of their findings were within the confines of their data. Generalizability of the findings was limited to small samples: samples of only one gender (Headley, 1987; Wilder-Smith et al., 1990; Winningham & MacVicar, 1988) and type of cancer (Winningham & MacVicar, 1988; Headley, 1987). Investigator provided limitations centered on sampling and measurement issues. There was a sampling error in the exercise program study: 25% of the sample were recruited who were receiving CTX beyond the selected regimen (Winningham & MacVicar, 1988). The investigators in one of the infusion pump studies admitted that normal sleep may have confounded the measure of sedation, and the conclusions drawn from their study applied only to acute nausea and vomiting (Edwards et al., 1991). The question of feasibility was raised by the investigators in one of the pump studies (Wilder-Smith et al., 1990). They noted the high price of the pump, cassettes, and tubing extensions as a disadvantage of this intervention.

Studies of Anticipatory Nausea and Vomiting

Eight studies were found that used either behavioral (seven) or nonbehavioral (one) technique interventions. Interestingly, most of the studies targeted their intervention once AN & V had been experienced by patients, not to prevent AN & V from occurring.

The seven studies that used a behavioral intervention included hypnosis with direct muscle relaxation and GI (Redd, Andresen, & Minagawa, 1982); PMRT with GI (Burish & Lyles, 1981); two studies that used systematic desensitization (SD) (Morrow, 1986; Morrow & Morrell, 1982); two studies that used distraction, (video games) (Greene, Seime, & Smith, 1985; Redd et al., 1987); and a final behavioral study that included several techniques (Moore & Altmaier, 1981). Moore and Altmaier labeled their intervention "stress inoculation"; it involved teaching coping skills including cognitive- and behavior-based interventions.

The one study employing a nonbehavioral technique used an intervention that the investigators labeled as "stimulus manipulation" (Greene & Seime, 1987). A lemon solution was introduced to mask the taste sensation of CTX, thought to function as a conditioned stimulus eliciting anticipatory symptoms during CTX.

All of the interventions were provided by the investigators, with only one study hiring an additional therapist to provide the intervention (Redd et al., 1982). The interventions were administered over several sessions (cycles) of CTX.

Six of the studies identified AN & V as their outcome or dependent variables (Burish & Lyles, 1981; Greene et al., 1985; Moore & Altmaier, 1981; Morrow, 1986; Morrow & Morrell, 1982; Redd et al., 1982), and two studies identified only anticipatory nausea, not vomiting (Greene & Seime, 1987; Redd et al., 1987).

Other dependent variables measured were anxiety (Burish & Lyles, 1981; Greene & Seime, 1987; Moore & Altmaier, 1981; Morrow, 1986; Morrow & Morrell, 1982; Redd et al., 1987); depression and hostility (Burish & Lyles, 1981); control (Morrow & Morrell, 1982); physiologic stress (BP, P, R) (Burish & Lyles, 1981; Greene et al., 1985; Redd et al., 1982, 1987); inductive thought listing procedure to assess coping cognition (Moore & Altmaier, 1981); patients' expectations of results and credibility of the investigator/therapist and the intervention (Morrow, 1986); and patients' rating of credibility of the therapist alone (Morrow & Morrell, 1982). The instruments/techniques used to measure these dependent variables included patients' self-report (Greene & Seime, 1987; Redd et al., 1987), standard procedures for obtaining BP,P,R, investigator-developed instruments (Moore & Altmaier, 1981; Morrow, 1986; Morrow & Morrell, 1982), and established instruments, such as the Multiple Affect Adjective Checklist (Burish & Houston, 1979), State-Trait Anxiety Inventory (STAI) (Speilberger, 1970), and Health Locus of Control (Wallston, Wallston, & DeVellis, 1978) (Burish & Lyles, 1981; Greene & Seime, 1987; Moore & Altmaier, 1981; Morrow, 1986; Morrow & Morrell, 1982; Redd et al., 1987). Frameworks used in this series of studies were behavioral conditioning, cognitive and behavioral theory, and self-regulation models.

Adult cancer patients who were receiving multiple CTX protocols for their multiple types of cancer constituted all but one of the samples in this series of studies (Burish & Lyles, 1981; Greene et al., 1985; Green & Seime, 1987; Moore & Altmaier, 1981; Morrow, 1986; Morrow & Morrell, 1982, Redd et al., 1982). The one pediatric/adolescent report presented two studies: 26 patients were in the first study and then 15 of these patients were involved in the second study (Redd et al., 1987). The samples of most of the studies were comprised of patients who had experienced AN & V in prior and current

CTX despite receiving antiemetic medications (Burish & Lyles, 1981; Morrow, 1986; Morrow & Morrell, 1982; Redd et al., 1982, 1987). The two single case multiple sessions studies did not have this patient selection requirement (Greene et al., 1985; Greene & Seime, 1987). Special sampling techniques were used in two studies (Burish & Lyles, 1981; Moore & Altmaier, 1981). In the first study, patients were randomly assigned to the experimental conditions after equal numbers of patients with a given diagnosis and CTX protocol were included (Burish & Lyles, 1981). In the second study, the investigators designated patients as adjusting or failing to adjust based on the criteria of normal sleep, appetite pattern, correspondence between the patient's and the physician's description of the disease and the prognosis, and patient participation in decisions (Moore & Altmaier, 1981).

The predominant designs used in this series were experimental with repeated measures (Burish & Lyles, 1981; Morrow, 1986; Morrow & Morrell, 1982) and single case multiple sessions (Greene et al., 1985; Greene & Seime, 1987; Redd et al., 1982, 1987). The study that tested the "stress inoculation" intervention lacked randomization and a control group, but the very small sample size ($N = 9$) would have prohibited both (Moore & Altmaier, 1981). Another study involving the adolescent patients lacked randomization (Redd et al., 1987). The pattern of several baseline, intervention, and follow-up sessions was similar to that described in the previous section. Two of the experimental studies provided no follow-up sessions without the therapist (Moore & Altmaier, 1981; Redd et al., 1982). Therefore, the question of whether the patients could maintain the effects of the intervention could not be answered.

Instruments and techniques used to measure AN & V were either patients' self-report or the administration of an investigator-developed instrument. The methods used for the self-report were the patients' verbal complaint (Greene & Seime, 1987), Likert scales (Burish & Lyles, 1981), and visual analogue scales (Redd et al., 1987). Two studies by Morrow used his instrument, Morrow Assessment of Nausea and Emesis (Morrow, 1986; Morrow & Morrell, 1982). One study had the nurse and patient provide concurrent ratings of nausea and vomiting on a Likert scale (Burish & Lyles, 1981), and another had an observer record every 15 min if nausea, vomiting, or retching were present or absent (Greene & Seime, 1987). Anticipatory nausea is such a subjective phenomenon that the validity of the nurse's and observer's ratings are questioned. The agreement between the nurse's ratings and those of the patients was not reported (Burish & Lyles, 1981). Two studies failed to describe what methods were used to measure AN & V (Greene et al., 1985; Moore & Altmaier, 1981).

There were several design issues in the AN & V studies. In one study premeasures and postmeasures of nausea and anxiety occurred every 10 min for three periods (Burish & Lyles, 1981). Testing measurement error was a threat in that study. None of the studies attempted a "blind" design. As mentioned earlier, all the interventions were provided by the same investigator(s). How well the intervention protocol was maintained over the duration of the study was never addressed. One group of investigators hired a therapist to provide the intervention; the preparation and training of this therapist was not described (Redd et al., 1982). Patients in two of the studies were to practice their interventions at home (Burish & Lyles, 1981; Moore & Altmaier, 1981). The patient's adherence rates were never provided. Three of the studies had "placebo control" groups (Burish & Lyles, 1981; Morrow, 1986; Morrow & Morrell, 1982), and two of these studies had a true control group as well (Morrow, 1986; Morrow & Morrell, 1982). The investigator-provided attention to the placebo control group was counseling (Morrow, 1986; Morrow & Morrell, 1982), and the other type of attention was resting in a quiet place for the same length of time as the investigator/therapist spent with the experimental group patients (Burish & Lyles, 1981).

Behavioral and nonbehavioral interventions were effective in significantly reducing AN & V in frequency, intensity, and duration. These findings were obtained in the initial intervention sessions but in some studies were not maintained in the follow-up sessions. The hypnosis intervention with the single-subject multiple sessions was effective in decreasing nausea and vomiting during all CTX sessions with all patients (Redd et al., 1982). AN & V were totally eliminated when hypnosis was employed. Results were reversed (return of AN & V) when this intervention was not provided to three patients. The reversal design findings increased confidence that hypnosis was producing the effect on AN & V. The PMRT with GI intervention was effective in significantly reducing nausea but not vomiting as reported by both the nurses and the patients (Burish & Lyles, 1981). The PMRT with GI did yield a significant decrease in the experimental group's anxiety during the CTX sessions, and anxiety, depression, and anger at the post-CTX sessions. Systematic desensitization (SD) (Morrow, 1986; Morrow & Morrell, 1982) was found to decrease significantly the severity of anticipatory nausea and vomiting. In the first SD study (Morrow, 1986) (without the PMRT with GI) there was a significant decrease in state and trait anxiety. There were nonsignificant differences in either study variables of patients' expectations and their ratings of the credibility of the therapists (Morrow, 1986; Morrow & Morrell, 1982). Both distraction technique studies involved videos (Greene et al., 1985; Redd et al., 1987). In the first study, the video sessions showed initial decreases in AN & V, but this effect was not maintained (Greene et al., 1985). Instead, the later sessions with relaxation demonstrated initial and maintained effectiveness for decreasing AN & V. In the second distraction video study (Redd et al., 1987), a clear pattern was observed of significant decrease in nausea when the video sessions occurred and significant increase in nausea when the video was withdrawn. The stimulus manipulation study with lemon solution was effective for reducing nausea and retching, and this effect was observed even when the lemon solution was withdrawn (Greene & Seime, 1987). The lemon solution did not significantly reduce anxiety. Finally in the stress inoculation study (Moore & Altmaier, 1981), data on AN & V were not presented. The investigators did report that the three patients who had been designated as "failure to adjust" reported the intervention was beneficial in that they could attend clinic without previous anxiety-related responses. Perhaps these responses included AN & V.

In Morrow's later testing of SD (1986), he separated SD and PMRT. By separating the intervention into two parts he was able to determine SD's effectiveness in reducing the severity and duration of anticipatory nausea over simple relaxation, and thereby lend support to the classical conditioning model. Morrow warned that because he used different procedures to administer PMRT from those of other investigators (e.g., GI was not given, releaxation was not provided during CTX sessions, and patients were not told to use the relaxation technique during their CTX sessions), he appropriately cautioned against viewing this study as a direct comparison of SD and PMRT. However, the data suggested SD was more effective.

The two studies presented on the use of video games as a distractor demonstrated significant reductions in conditioned nausea. The effects were evident in a between-subjects comparison (first study) as well as in a within-subjects comparison of effects during a single CTX session (second study) (Redd et al., 1987).

All of the findings taken together would affirm the effectiveness of the tested interventions in decreasing AN & V in patients who were already experiencing difficulties with these symptoms. However, a major measurement issue with the AN & V studies was that it was to be anticipatory: nausea and vomiting needed to occur before the administration of CTX. To have dependent variable measures of nausea and vomiting during or after the CTX session was not by definition anticipatory nausea and vomiting that had its theoretic foundations in classical conditioning theory. Therefore, the premeasures of AN & V were appropriate, but the during and postmeasures were not. Once the CTX was administered, the emetic effects of the CTX drugs were responsible for the subsequent nausea and vomiting. This belief was founded in pathophysiologic theory.

Studies of Oral Mucositis

Mucositis or stomatitis is defined as an inflammation of the oral mucosa owing to local or systemic factors that may involve the buccal and labial mucosa, palate, tongue, floor of the mouth, and gingiva (Lindquist, Hickey, & Drane, 1978). Oral mucositis–producing agents are drugs that produce diminished mucosal thickness and keratinization, superficial sloughing, intense redness, and traumatic and atraumatic ulcerations of the oral mucosa. The frequency of CTX-induced oral mucositis ranges from 30% to 35% (National Institutes of Health, 1989).

Three studies were found where the primary aim was to prevent CTX-induced oral mucositis (Beck, 1979; Kenny, 1990; Mahood et al., 1991). Two studies tested specific protocols for oral care (Beck, 1979; Kenny, 1990). In the Beck (1979) study the protocols included rinsing with Cepacol (Merrill-Dow, Cincinnati, OH) four times a day if mild mucositis occurs; eating a bland diet; and performing oral hygiene every 1 to 2 hr with a solution of Cepacol (Merrill-Dow, Cincinnati, OH), hydrogen peroxide, and water. Beck outlined specific interventions for mild mucositis versus severe mucositis.

The protocol for the second oral care study consisted of four components: *Protocol A,* lip lubricant (nonocclusive preparation of lanolin and aloe vera); oral lubricant (sterile mint-flavored toothettes premoistened with aloe vera and chlorophyll); cleanser (sterile mint-flavored toothettes moistened with NaHCO3); mouthwash (NaHCO3 solution, 0.9%). *Protocol B* (control) included lip lubricant (vitamin A and B ointment in a lanolin petroleum base); oral lubricant (NaCl solution, 0.9%); cleanser (dry sterile mint-flavored toothettes) and mouthwash. Kenny (1990) tested two protocols that differed on the type of lip lubricant, oral lubricant, cleanser, and mouthwash. The third study to prevent oral mucositis tested cryotherapy (Mahood et al., 1991). The protocol involved patients putting ice chips in their mouths for 15 min prior to each dose of fluoracil.

The dependent variables in the first study included an Oral Exam Guide and a Physical Condition instrument (level of consciousness, breathing, habits, and self-care activities) that were completed by the investigator. A third instrument, the Oral Perception Guide, was completed by the patient. All three instruments were investigator-developed or adapted from others (Beck, 1979). The second study used an established instrument, the Oral Assessment Guide (OAG) (Eilers, Berger, & Peterson, 1988) to measure the dependent variables (Kenny, 1990). The study by Mahood and colleagues (1991) used two Likert 4-point scales with descriptors to measure the condition of the oral cavity (Mahood et al., 1991). The attending physician completed one scale and the patient the other scale.

The frameworks for this series of studies was based on theories of physiology, pathophysiology, pharmakinetics, and stress. All the samples were adults with different types of cancer and multiple CTX protocols. All were initiating their first CTX protocol.

The longitudinal design with repeated measures was used for both the oral protocol studies (Beck, 1979; Kenny, 1990). The Beck (1979) study used nonequivalent groups of patients. The oral care protocol study by Kenny (1990) included randomization to the experimental and control groups and repeated assessments of the oral cavity. The cryotherapy study included random assignment to an experimental or control group. Unfortunately the investigators conducted only a postmeasure of the oral cavity, that is, no baseline or repeated measures occurred in this study (Mahood et al., 1991).

There were several design and measurement issues raised in this series of studies. The threats to the internal validity of the findings are noteworthy in the nonequivalent groups study (Beck, 1979). Also in this same study, by not measuring the control group's oral care activities, data were not available on baseline or standard practice. The Kenny (1990) oral care protocol study used an established instrument, OAG (Eilers et al., 1988) to obtain dependent variable data (Kenny, 1990). The investigator also established interrater reliability among the four registered nurses who would be assessing the patients' mouths with the OAG. This extra effort was laudable. One of the major weaknesses of the cryotherapy study was the singular postmeasure conducted by the attending physician at a follow-up visit 1 month after CTX and by the patient 2 to 3 weeks after the CTX (Mahood et al., 1991). Why these assessments were done so distant from the administration of CTX and the possible occurrence of mucositis was not discussed. Baseline oral assessments were not obtained on these patients. A modification of a reverse design was seen in this study when 27 of the patients who returned for their second course of CTX were crossed over to the alternative protocol arm. Those patients who received cryotherapy showed improvement over the control patients, and this finding corroborates the findings during the first course of CTX (Mahood et al., 1991). None of the three studies were able to establish a blind condition. However the investigators in the cryotherapy study suggested that perhaps the attending physicians may have not known the group assignment because their assessments were distant from the cryotherapy intervention (Mahood et al., 1991).

The quality control of the intervention was most fully described by the two oral care protocol studies (Beck, 1979; Kenny, 1990). In the first study the investigator provided a 45-minute teaching session to all staff members. The content included: causes of stomatitis, assessment of the mouth, nursing interventions with stomatitis, explanation of protocol for oral care, patient teaching pamphlet, and an Oral Care Flow Sheet (Beck, 1979). The investigator in the second study gave each patient verbal and written instructions on self-care measures for oral care (Kenny, 1990). To maintain a consistent approach with each patient, the investigator reviewed each enumerated point contained in the written material, demonstrated the technique to be employed in oral care, and observed the patient demonstrating the correct technique for oral care. The investigator provided clarification and reinforcement of the instructions on self-care measures for oral care as needed during the study (Kenny, 1990). The important differences between these two oral care studies were: in the first study only one teaching session occurred, and the nurses provided the oral care and the investigator collected the dependent variable data. In the second study, the investigator provided both one time sessions with the patients but also reinforcement sessions as well, and the patients performed their own oral care while the nurses made the oral assessments. How well the oral protocol was implemented (i.e., quality) over time was not addressed in either study. The adherence of the nurses (Beck, 1979) and the patients (Kenny, 1990) to the intervention was discussed in the oral care protocol studies. In the first study where nurses completed the Oral Care Flow Sheet, the implementation of the oral protocol was documented on 82% of the flow sheets. However, the investigator commented that verbal feedback from both the patients and the staff indicated that more frequent oral care was provided than actually was recorded (Beck, 1979). A serendipitous finding was that reinforcement of oral care instructions and nurses' assessment of the oral cavity seemed to promote patient compliance with the oral regimen (Kenny, 1990).

Special attention was directed at the control group in the second oral care protocol study (Kenny, 1990). Indeed, the modified oral care protocol and mouth care guidelines that the control group received could explain the lack of significant differences between the experimental and control group patients.

The findings for the effectiveness of oral care protocols were mixed. In the Beck (1979) oral care study, the experimental group patients demonstrated a significant improvement in their oral status, and the level of infection was reduced by two thirds over the level of the control group in the control phase of the study. There were, however, nonsignificant differences in the patients' ratings of oral perceptions and the nurses' ratings of physical condition. The nonsignificant differences in the Kenny (1990) study perhaps were due to the similarities between the experimental and control groups' protocols. The cryotherapy significantly reduced mucositis as judged by both the attending physician and patients (Mahood et al., 1991).

The limitations in these three studies generally were recognized by the investigators. The problems inherent in nonequivalent groups were discussed by Beck (1979). The lack of independence of scores of the seven patients who were in both the control and experimental group (7 out of 22) warrants further comment by the investigator who decided each observation was to be treated independently. The lack of data on the patients' adherence to protocol is of concern, especially in the oral care studies where the intervention occurred over time. The nonsignificant differences seen in the second oral care study might be due in part to the lack of adherence to the protocol (Kenny, 1990).

DIRECTIONS FOR FUTURE RESEARCH

The intervention studies reviewed in this chapter for the side effects of CTX have several noteworthy characteristics. The interventions tested for N, V, & R and AN & V are by far where the most extensive work has occurred. The behavioral interventions for these side effects are effective and expensive (investigator's time). The *non*behavioral interventions for N, V, & R and AN & V have not demonstrated their effectiveness in as consistent a manner as the behavioral interventions, but they also suffer from being investigator intensive. There are several major concerns of these series of studies. First, there was a lack of attention provided by the investigators as to the study participants' adherence to the research protocol and the quality assurance of the intervention over time. Samples were too heterogeneous and small, although there were some matching and stratifying techniques used by a few of the investigators. Instruments to measure the studies' dependent variables were much too often developed by the investigators for the purposes of a specific study. Reliability and validity data on these instruments were scarce or missing altogether. Finally, the predominate design used was quasiexperimental often with no type of randomization or with no control group. These methodological issues has serious consequences for the validity of these studies' findings.

Future research should continue to test interventions to manage the side effects of cancer CTX. The issues raised in the summary of the studies reviewed provide the direction for designing subsequent studies in the area. There are more general issues or points that need further emphasis. For example, more attention should be placed on testing interventions with the pediatric and older cancer populations. There are many side effects of CTX that have received modest levels of attention or have received no attention from nurse researchers. Interventions need to be developed with cost effectiveness criteria in mind. Labor-intensive interventions are not in keeping with today's health care costs concerns. Well-conceived randomized clinical trials with large, more homogeneous samples will advance knowledge in the field rapidly. Selection of established instruments to measure the studies' dependent variables with their psychometric data are greatly preferred to the investigator-developed instruments. Serious attempts to at least single blind (e.g., intervention person is *not* also collecting the dependent variable data) the study design are needed. Investigators who elect to work in this area would do well to establish a program of research where one study builds on another.

REFERENCES

Beck, S. (1979). Impact of a systematic oral care protocol on stomatitis after chemotherapy. *Cancer Nursing, 2,* 185–199.

Borison, H. L. (1986). Anatomy and physiology of the chemoreceptor trigger zone and area postrema. In C. J. Davis, C. V. Lake-Bakaar, & D. G. Grahame Smith (Eds.), *Nausea and vomiting, mechanisms and treatment* (pp. 10–17). New York: Springer-Verlag.

Burish, T. G., Carey, M. P., Krozely, M. G., & Greco, F. A. (1987). Conditioned side effects induced by cancer chemotherapy: Prevention through behavioral treatment. *Journal of Consulting and Clinical Psychology, 55,* 42–48.

Burish, T. G., & Houston, B. K. (1979). Casual projection, similarity projection, and coping with threat to self-esteem. *Journal of Personality, 47,* 57–70.

Burish, T. G., & Lyles, J. N. (1979). Effectiveness of relaxation training in reducing the aversiveness of chemotherapy in the treatment of cancer. *Journal of Behavioral Therapists and Experimental Psychiatry, 10,* 357–361.

Burish, T. G., & Lyles, J. N. (1981). Effectiveness of relaxation training in reducing adverse reactions to cancer chemotherapy. *Journal of Behavioral Medicine, 4*(1), 65–78.

Burish, T. G., Shartner, C. D., & Lyles, J. N. (1981). Effectiveness of multiple muscle-site EMG biofeedback and relaxation training in reducing aversiveness of cancer chemotherapy. *Biofeedback and Self-Regulation, 6,* 523–535.

Carey, M. P., & Burish, T. G. (1985). Anxiety as a predictor of behavioral therapy outcome for cancer chemotherapy patients. *Journal of Consulting and Clinical Psychology, 53,* 860–865.

Carey, M. P., & Burish, T. G. (1987). Providing relaxation training to cancer chemotherapy patients: A comparison of three delivery techniques. *Journal of Consulting and Clinical Psychology, 55,* 732–737.

Cotanch, P. H. (1983). Relaxation training for control of nausea and vomiting in patients receiving chemotherapy. *Cancer Nursing, 6,* 277–283.

Cotanch, P. H., Hockenberry, M., & Herman, S. (1985). Self-hypnosis, an antiemetic therapy in children receiving chemotherapy. *Oncology Nursing Forum, 12*(4), 41–46.

Cotanch, P. H., & Strum, S. (1987). Progressive muscle relaxation as antiemetic therapy for cancer patients. *Oncology Nursing Forum, 14*(1), 33–37.

Derogatis, L. R. (1977). *SCL-90 R Manual I: Administration, scoring, and procedures manual for the revised version.* Baltimore, MD: Clinical Psychometrics Research Unit, Johns Hopkins University, School of Medicine.

Dodd, M. J. (1984). Measuring informational intervention for chemotherapy and self-care behavior. *Research in Nursing and Health, 7,* 43–50.

Dodd, M. J. (1988). Efficacy of proactive information on self-care in chemotherapy patients. *Patient Education and Counseling, 11,* 215–225.

Dodd, M. J. (1991). *Managing the side effects of chemotherapy and radiation.* New York: Prentice Hall Press.

Edwards, J. N., Herman, J., Wallace, B. K., Pavy, M. D., & Harrison-Pavy, J. (1991). Comparison of patient-controlled and nurse-controlled antiemetic therapy in patients receiving chemotherapy. *Research in Nursing and Health, 14,* 249–257.

Eilers, J., Berger, A. M., & Peterson, M. C. (1988). Development, testing and application of the Oral Assessment Guide. *Oncology Nursing Forum, 15,* 325–330.

Frank, J. M. (1985). The effects of music therapy and guided visual imagery on chemotherapy induced nausea and vomiting. *Oncology Nursing Forum, 12*(5), 47–52.

Gard, D., Edwards, P. W., Harris, J., & McCormack, G. (1988). Sensitizing effects of pretreatment measure on cancer chemotherapy nausea and vomiting. *Journal of Consulting and Clinical Psychology, 56*(1), 80–84.

Greene, P. G., & Seime, R. J. (1987). Stimulus control of anticipatory nausea in cancer chemotherapy. *Journal of Behavioral Therapists and Experimental Psychiatry, 18*(1), 61–64.

Greene, P. G., Seime, R. J., & Smith, M. E. (1985). *Distraction and relaxation training in the treatment of anticipatory nausea and vomiting: A single subject intervention.* Unpublished manuscript.

Guyton, A. (1980). *A textbook of medical physiology* (6th ed.). Philadelphia: Saunders.

Headley, J. A. (1987). The influence of administration time on chemotherapy-induced nausea and vomiting. *Oncology Nursing Forum, 14*(6), 14–47.

Hogan, C. M. (1990). Advances in the management of nausea and vomiting. *Nursing Clinics of North America, 25*(2), 475–497.

Jordan, L. N. (1989). Effects of fluid manipulation on the incidence of vomiting during outpatient cisplatin infusion. *Oncology Nursing Forum, 16,* 213–218.

Kenny, S. A. (1990). Effect of two oral-care protocols on the incidence of stomatitis in hematology patients. *Cancer Nursing, 13,* 345–353.

Kolko, D. J., & Rickard-Figueroa, J. L. (1985). Effects of video games on the adverse corollaries of chemotherapy in pediatric oncology patients: A single case analysis. *Journal of Consulting and Clinical Psychology, 53,* 223–228.

LeBaron, S., & Zeltzer, L. (1984). Behavioral intervention for reducing chemotherapy-related nausea and vomiting in adolescents with cancer. *Journal of Adolescent Health Care, 5,* 178–182.

Lindquist, S. F., Hickey, A. J., & Drane, J. B. (1978). Effect of oral hygiene on stomatitis in patients receiving cancer chemotherapy. *The Journal of Prosthetic Dentistry, 40*(3), 312–314.

Lyles, J. N., Burish, T. G., Krozely, M. G., & Oldham, R. K. (1982). Efficacy of relaxation training and guided imagery in reducing the aversiveness of cancer chemotherapy. *Journal of Clinical Oncology, 9,* 449–452.

Mahood, D. J., Dose, A. M., Loprinzi, C. L., Veeder, M. H., Athmann, L. M., Therneau, T. M., Sorensen, J. M., Gainey, D. K., Mailliard, J. A., Gusa, N. L., Finck, G. K., Johnson, C., & Goldberg, R. M. (1991). Fluorouracil induced stomatitis by oral cryotherapy. *Journal of Clinical Oncology, 9,* 449–452.

Moore, K., & Altmaier, E. M. (1981). Stress innoculation training with cancer patients. *Cancer Nursing, 4*(5), 389–393.

Morgan, A. H., & Hilgard, J. R. (1978/1979). The Stanford hypnotic clinical scale for children. *American Journal of Clinical Hypnosis, 21,* 148–169.

Morrow, G. R. (1986). Effect of the cognitive hierarchy in the systematic desensitization treatment of anticipatory nausea in cancer patients: A component comparison with relaxation only, counseling, and no treatment. *Cognitive Therapy and Research, 10*(4), 421–446.

Morrow, G. R., & Morrell, C. (1982). Behavioral treatment for the anticipatory nausea and vomiting induced by cancer chemotherapy. *The New England Journal of Medicine, 307,* 1476–1480.

National Institutes of Health (1989, April). Journal of N.I.H. *Consensus of development conference statement on oral complications of cancer therapies: Diagnosis, prevention, and treatment* (Monograph #9). Washington, DC: Author.

Needleman, R. (1987). Chemotherapy—an overview of nausea and vomiting in the cancer patient: Etiology and management of serious complications of chemotherapy. *American Association of Occupational Health Nursing Journal, 35,* 179–182.

Redd, W. H., Andresen, G. V., & Minagawa, R. Y. (1982). Hypnotic control of anticipatory emesis in patients receiving cancer chemotherapy. *Journal of Consulting and Clinical Psychology, 50,* 14–19.

Redd, W., & Hendler, C. (1984). Learned aversions to chemotherapy treatment. *Health Education Quarterly, 10*(Suppl.), 57–66.

Redd, W. H., Jacobsen, P. B., Die-Trill, M., Dermatis, H., McEvoy, M., & Holland, J. C. (1987). Cognitive/attentional distraction in the control of conditioned nausea in pediatric cancer patients receiving chemotherapy. *Journal of Consulting and Clinical Psychology, 55,* 391–395.

Rhodes, V. A. (1990). Nausea, vomiting, and retching. *Nursing Clinics of North America, 25,* 885–900.

Rhodes, V. A., Watson, P. M., & Johnson, M. H. (1986). Association of chemotherapy related nausea and vomiting with pretreatment and posttreatment anxiety. *Oncology Nursing Forum, 13*(1), 41–47.

Sallan, S. E., & Cronin, C. M. (1985). Nausea and vomiting. In V. T. DeVita, Jr., S. Hellman, & S. A. Rosenberg (Eds.), *Cancer: Principles and practice oncology* (2nd ed., pp. 2008–2013). Philadelphia: Lippincott.

Scott, D. W., Donahue, D. C., Mastrovito, R. C., & Hakes, T. B. (1986). Comparative trial of clinical relaxation and an antiemetic drug regimen in reducing chemotherapy related nausea and vomiting. *Cancer Nursing, 9,* 178–187.

Seigel, L. T., & Longo, D. L. (1981). The control of chemotherapy-induced emesis. *Annals of Internal Medicine, 95,* 352–359.

Shartner, C., Burish, T. G., & Carey, M. P. (1985). Effectiveness of biofeedback with progressive muscle relaxation training in reducing the aversiveness of cancer chemotherapy: A preliminary report. *Japanese Journal of Biofeedback Research, 12,* 33–40.

Speilberger, C. (1970). *The state-trait anxiety inventory test manual*. Palo Alto, CA: Consulting Psychologists Press.

Wallston, K. A., Wallston, B. S., & De Vellis, R. (1978). Development of the Multidimensional Health Locus of Control (MHLC) Scales. *Health Education Monographs, 6,* 160–170.

Wilder-Smith, C. H., Schuler, L., Osterwalder, B., Naji, P., & Senn, H.-J. (1990). Patient controlled antiemesis for cancer chemotherapy-induced nausea and vomiting. *Journal of Pain and Symptom Management, 5,* 375–378.

Winningham, M. L., & MacVicar, M. G. (1988). The effect of aerobic exercise on patient reports of nausea. *Oncology Nursing Forum, 15*, 447–450.

Zeltzer, L., Kellerman, L., Ellenberg, L., & Dash, J. (1983). Hypnosis for reduction of vomiting associated with chemotherapy and disease in adolescents with cancer. *Journal of Adolescent Health Care, 4*(2), 77–84.

Zeltzer, L., LeBaron, S., & Zeltzer, P. (1984). The effectiveness of behavioral intervention for reducing nausea and vomiting in children and adolescents receiving chemotherapy. *Journal of Clinical Oncology, 2*, 683–690.

Zuckerman, M., Lubin, B., Vogel, L., & Valerius, E. (1964). Measurement of experimentally induced affects. *Journal of Consulting Clinical Psychology, 28*, 418–425.

Chapter 5

Pain in Children

Nancy O. Hester
School of Nursing
University of Colorado Health Sciences Center

CONTENTS

Research on pain in children began in the early 1970s. The few studies on children's pain published in the 1970s primarily represented the efforts of nurses. Schultz (1971), Eland (1974, 1976, cited in Eland & Anderson, 1977), Hester (1979), and Savedra (1976) addressed issues related to children's pain: children's understanding and perceptions of pain, children's coping strategies during painful episodes, measurement of pain through self-report and behavioral observation, and postoperative analgesic use. These studies in addition to some unpublished work by nurses (e.g., Alyea, 1978; Hester, Davis, Hanson, & Hassanein, 1978; Loebach, 1979; Molsberry,

1979), formed the basis for the proliferation of research during the 1980s. During the 1980s researchers from other disciplines joined with nurse researchers in strengthening the knowledge base regarding pain in children.

This chapter presents an integrated review of nursing research related to children's pain, organized by prevalence of pain, children's perspective on pain, assessment of pain, and management of pain. A perspective on the state of the knowledge development and recommendations for the future is provided.

The nursing literature was selected using techniques described by Cooper (1982, 1989): (a) the invisible college approach, (b) professional meetings, (c) the ancestry approach, (d) abstracting services, and (e) on-line computer searches. The invisible college is an informal approach through which scientists working on similar problems exchange reprints. Proceedings of professional meetings were reviewed for abstracts on children's pain and authors contacted for status of publication. The ancestry approach involves tracking citations in publications. Reference lists and bibliographies in articles and the following books were reviewed for nursing citations: *Advances in Pain Research and Therapy, Vol. 15: Pediatric Pain* (Tyler & Krane, 1990); *Childhood Pain: Current Issues, Research, and Management* (Ross & Ross, 1988); *Key Aspects of Comfort: Management of Pain, Fatigue, and Nausea* (Funk, Tornquist, Champagne, Copp, & Wiese, 1989); *Pain: A Source Book for Nurses and Other Health Professionals* (Jacox, 1977); *Pain in Children and Adolescents* (McGrath & Unruh, 1987); and *Pain in Children: Nature, Assessment, and Treatment* (P. A. McGrath, 1990). In addition to Cooper's techniques, a list of studies on children's pain currently or previously funded through the National Institutes of Health was used to contact the investigators for the publication status of any papers or grant reports. Also the author participated on a federal panel to develop guidelines for pain management (Office of the Forum for Effectiveness and Quality of Health Care, Agency for Health Care Policy and Research) for which the National Library of Medicine retrieved pain references. The retrieval of unpublished papers was limited to those cited in published papers or presented at conferences.

Each article was screened to determine if (a) it was focused on pain or a related topic, (b) one of the authors was a nurse, (c) it reported a research study, and (d) the study sample involved infants, children, or adolescents (ages 0 through 19 years). Identification of the professional background(s) of the author(s) was difficult when the journal did not include author credentials or affiliations, so some articles appropriate for this review may be missing.

In 1977 Eland and Anderson reported that a review of articles from January 1970 to August 1975 yielded 1,380 pain articles. Of these, 33 were focused on pediatric pain: 19 on abdominal pain, 8 on headaches, and 6 on miscellaneous pain topics. All but one of the articles were medically oriented and not authored by nurses. The current retrieval yielded 142 studies conducted by nurses. Topics included (a) prevalence of pain, (b) children's perspectives on pain, (c) assessment of children's pain, and (d) management of children's pain.

Almost half (44%) of the studies used descriptive, correlational, and nonexperimental comparative designs. Twenty percent of the studies focused on developing instruments to measure children's pain and 18% examined the efficacy of interventions through experimental designs. Other designs such as survey, case study, meta-analysis, and qualitative approaches were used less frequently. A theoretic or conceptual framework guided 44% of the studies; common frameworks related to pain (e.g., the gate-control theory), development (e.g., Piaget's cognitive development theory), and stress arousal (e.g., physiological theory on stress arousal). Most studies were analyzed with inferential (44%) or descriptive (29%) statistics. Fewer studies employed nonparametric (18%) and content or qualitative (8%) analyses.

Most (98%) of the studies involved conveniently selected samples of children; random assignment to groups occurred in the experimental studies. In 65% of the samples, children were hospitalized. Most studies involved children; some, however, included parents and nurses. Preverbal children were studied less often than verbal children. For preverbal children, only 3% of the studies included premature infants; 11%, neonates; 13%, infants; and 12%, toddlers. In contrast, 51% of the studies included preschool children; 66%, school-age children; and 37%, adolescents. Sample sizes varied across the studies: 7% had fewer than 10 subjects; 29% included 10 to 29 subjects, the next 24% had 30 to 59 subjects, another 24% had 60 to 99 subjects, and the rest had more than 100 subjects.

These findings suggest a variety of problems regarding the validity of the studies comprising the state of the science. For example, the lack of random selection and small sample sizes limit the generalizability of the findings to the target populations while the use of descriptive and nonparametric analyses limit inferences to the target population. Further, the lack of theory specification limits theory testing and theory development. Substantively, gaps in the knowledge base are evident: Few studies have been conducted with preverbal children, and there is a dearth of work on the efficacy of interventions for children in pain.

PREVALENCE OF PAIN IN CHILDREN

The prevalence of pain in children lacks adequate documentation. Maunuksela, Saarinen, and Lahteenoja (1990), who measured prevalence of pain in children in the terminal stages by reviewing charts for pain treatment, reported that 41% had received treatment. Research using self-reported pain rather than treatment as a measure suggested the prevalence in hospitalized children is higher. Hester, Foster, and Kristensen (1990) measured self-reported pain in 72 hospitalized children (4 through 13 years). Measures taken 4 times during the day shift at mean time intervals of 1.5 to 2.0 hr revealed that 93% reported pain at least one time; 63%, all 4 times; and 7%, at no time. Johnston, Jeans, Abbott, Grey-Donald, and Edgar (1988) reported that 60% of hospitalized children interviewed recalled experiencing pain in the moderate to severe range for the previous 24 hr. These findings would indicate that most hospitalized children experienced pain, but documentation of the amount and intensity of pain for various conditions needs study.

CHILDREN'S PERSPECTIVE ON PAIN

A few researchers have studied children's perspective on pain through descriptive studies using either questionnaires or interviews.

Understanding of Pain

Eland (1974, 1983, 1988), Ward (1975), Hester et al. (1978), and Hester and Barcus (1986) addressed children's understanding of the word "pain." In each study researchers used convenient samples of hospitalized children (n = 25, 25, 100, & 28, respectively), 4 through 15 years, asking them to respond to the question: "What is pain?" Findings across studies were similar: Typically younger children (4 through 9) did not understand the word pain, whereas older children and adolescents (10 through 15) did. Molsberry (1978) asked mothers of 21 hospitalized children aged 4 through 7 whether the child had any special word(s) for pain. About two-thirds of the mothers reported hurt or "owie" as the words of choice.

Abu-Saad (1990), however, found that nonhospitalized Dutch children (n = 355) from 7 to 15 years responded adequately to the question: "What is pain?" The definitions were observed to be consistent with Piagetian theory: concrete for younger children and semiabstract/abstract for older children. Abu-Saad's findings were similar to those of psychologists Gaffney and Dunn (1986), and Ross and Ross (1988), who studied nonhospitalized Irish and American children.

Problems in the study designs do not permit interpretation of the apparent conflict in findings. None of the studies reported the process used to determine if a child's response to the question: "What is pain?" was adequate, and none reported interrater reliability for categorization of responses. Furthermore, the findings are restricted by the use of convenient, primarily white, and sometimes small samples. Despite these limitations, the findings indicated the importance of determining the language that is appropriate for discussing pain with children of specific age groups.

Experiences Associated with Pain

Research on children's experiences associated with pain showed that children from 5 through 17 years can describe the cause of their pain (Abu-Saad, 1984b, 1984c, 1984d; Jarrett, 1985; Savedra, Tesler, Ward, Wegner, & Gibbons, 1981; Savedra, Gibbons, Tesler, Ward, & Wegner, 1982; Savedra, Tesler, Ward, & Wegner, 1988). Typically, outpatient and hospitalized children identified causes such as surgery and medical procedures, whereas cohorts of well children listed falls and being hit (Savedra et al., 1981, 1982, 1988). Classification of causes as physical external, physical internal, and psychologic/miscellaneous revealed differences between hospitalized and nonhospitalized children: Hospitalized children reported physical internal causes, whereas nonhospitalized reported physical external (Savedra et al., 1981, 1982, 1988). Jarrett (1985), however, found that children using outpatient services also identified internal sources more frequently than external sources. These findings suggested that both illness and hospitalization accounted for differences in children's perceptions of causes.

Differences in the identification of causes as physical and psychological paralleled expectations of Piagetian theory: older children reported more psychologic causes than younger children did (Abu-Saad, 1984b; Savedra et al., 1982; Schultz, 1971). Abu-Saad (1984d), however, documented differences in causes according to culture. Although physical causes were identified more frequently for all three cultures, Latin American children identified physical causes almost exclusively, whereas approximately one-fourth of Asian-American and Arab-American also reported psychologic causes. Although gender was not a predominant factor in any of the studies pertaining to cause, Abu-Saad (1984c) found that older girls in the Asian-American culture reported more psychologic causes than older boys.

The most consistently reported cause of worst pain experiences for both hospitalized and nonhospitalized children was invasive procedures. Eland (1976), Eland and Anderson (1977), Hester et al. (1978), Jarrett (1985), and Loebach (1979) asked children about their worst pain experiences: shots or needles in the form of injections, lumbar punctures, and bone marrow aspirations accounted for 55%, 49%, 22%, 75%, and 15%, respectively. Other causes were more diverse but often included pain associated with surgery, illness, and medical treatment (Jarrett, 1985; Savedra et al., 1981, 1988). Children with cancer found most invasive procedures and treatments to be painful (Adams, 1990; Fowler-Kerry, 1990; Weekes & Savedra, 1988) and repeated invasive procedures as the most difficult to handle Ellerton, Caty, and Ritchie (1985) and (Fowler-Kerry, 1990). Menke (1981) validated the stressfulness of invasive procedures for children through play.

Fright or nervousness was present for most children undergoing painful procedures (Adams, 1990) or during pain experiences (Abu-Saad, 1984b, 1984c; Savedra et al., 1981, 1982). Other feelings children had during pain experiences included feel like crying and do, or feel like crying but don't (Abu-Saad, 1984b, 1984c, 1984d; Savedra et al., 1981, 1982; Schultz, 1971); sick to their stomach (Abu-Saad, 1984b, 1984c, 1984d; Savedra et al., 1981, 1982, and embarrassed (Abu-Saad, 1984b, 1984c; Savedra et al., 1982).

Abu-Saad (1984b, 1984c, 1984d) and Savedra et al. (1981, 1982, 1988) noted that children used sensory words primarily to describe their pain. Consistently, children selected red and sometimes black as the colors to represent pain (Abu-Saad, 1984c, 1984d; Eland, 1976; Hester et al. 1978; Jarrett, 1985; Jeans, 1983; Savedra et al., 1981, 1982, 1988). Interestingly, red and black are the most frequently used crayons generally, and research on children's drawings document extensive use of both colors. Thus, the conclusion that children equate pain with these colors is suspect.

ASSESSMENT OF CHILDREN'S PAIN

Research on assessment of children's pain has been focused on two perspectives: how nurses assess pain, and the developments and testing of tools to measure pain. Assessment is the comprehensive approach used to derive a clinical judgment of pain; measurement of pain is one aspect of assessment (McGrath & Unruh, 1987).

Approaches to Assessing Children's Pain

Research on assessment of pain has provided insight into the clinical criteria nurses use in determining presence and severity of pain. Primm (1971) developed criteria for assessment of children's pain when she discovered that a tool designed for assessing adult pain was inappropriate for use with children. Primm's criteria included the reason for the initiation of the assessment, who reported the child's discomfort, the severity of pain (none to severe), the importance of four indicators in decisions about severity of pain, a description of the child's behavior, and the nursing and medical care initiated as a result of the assessment. Severity was assessed according to the importance of four indicators: observation of the child's behavior, verbalization by the child, the child's emotional state, and the child's diagnosis and operative date. Behaviors described by nurses were categorized as to degree and description fo child's behavior, verbalization or vocalization by child, how the child was occupied, response to other people, judgment of child's emotional state, and physical signs. Lukens (1982) and Varchol (1983) used Primm's criteria in studies with small sample sizes (n = 13 and 26) of children aged 3 through 14 years experiencing acute and chronic pain. In both studies nurses rated observation of behavior as extremely important in assessing children's pain. Behaviors identified frequently by nurses were how the child was occupied, degree or description of body activity, and verbalization or vocal sounds. Response to other people, judgment of emotional state, and physical signs were used less frequently.

Atchison, Guercio, and Monaco (1986) surveyed 27 nurses in a burn care facility on assessing pain in children. Most nurses stated they ask children but also considered body language, changes in vital signs, emotional responses (e.g., crying, acting out) and a change in diet. For infants, almost all nurses reported crying as the most obvious cue. Other cues included diaphoresis, squirming, rigidity, agitation, irritability, and facial expression. Bradshaw and Zeanah (1986) conducted an open-ended survey on 99 pediatric nurses who cared for children (neonates through adolescents) with chronic and acute pain. Content analysis of responses revealed interrater agreement of .81 for the following criteria listed in order of frequency: oral expression, body language, affect, physiologic changes, verbal communication, facial expression, nurse's judgment, relief action, and parent's assessment. Pomietto (1988), using Bradshaw and Zeanah's criteria in a survey of 82 nurses, found frequency of use to be similar. Ritchie (1989) analyzed findings from a survey of 70 pediatric nurses and determined that age of the child affected the criteria nurses used. For example, oral expressions and responses to relief actions were ranked highly for infants, where verbal requests and body language were ranked highly for adolescents. One criterion, physiologic changes, was important across all age groups. Franck's (1987) survey of 76 nurses nationwide revealed that crying, activity, and physiologic parameters (e.g., heart rate, respiratory rate, blood pressure, transcutaneous oxygen/carbon dioxide, mean airway pressure, and skin color) were identified most frequently as criteria for neonates in intensive care units. In Powers' (1987) study, nurses expressed the importance of facial expression, holding or guarding the operative site, lack of ease in movements, and vocalizations in assessing pain in postoperative children.

Hester, Foster, Kristensen, and Bergstrom (1989) and Hester and Foster (1990) reported the cues used by 169 parents and 87 nurses to rate pain in 169 children, aged 4 through 13 years. Nurses and parents used the same types of cues: categories specific to pain (i.e., verbalization, vocalization, and body language) and categories not specific for pain (i.e., activity, appearance, interaction, physiology, and temperament). One of the most important findings of this study was the category named change. This refers to a change in the child's affect or behavior. Change was the primary process through which nurses and parents made judgments about children's pain.

Researchers reported similar criteria for assessing children's pain. The criteria differed according to the child's age or developmental level. Although physiologic changes were identified as criteria in all of the studies and verbalization was noted, measurement of pain through the formal self-report or behavioral/observational tools was not mentioned as a means for assessing pain.

Adequacy of Methods for Measuring Children's Pain

Researchers have emphasized the development and testing of methods for measuring children's pain. This emphasis began after Primm (1971) found that a tool for measuring pain in adults was unsatisfactory to measure children's pain. Three approaches dominate the research: self-report, observational/behavioral, and physiologic. Several self-report tools developed or tested by nurses measure one or more dimensions of pain: quantity, location, and quality. Nurse researchers have addressed four psychometric properties: reliability, generalizability, validity, and sensitivity.

The earliest and most predominant work was concentrated on the measurement of quantity. Quantification tools designed by nurses for use with children include Eland's Projective Tool (Eland, 1974, 1983, 1988), Eland's Color Tool (Eland, 1976, 1983, 1988), the Poker Chip Tool (PCT) (Hester, 1976, 1979), the Four Faces Tool (Alyea, 1978), Pain Thermometer (Molsberry, 1978) the Oucher (Beyer, 1984), Pain Ladder (Hay, 1984), the Faces Rating Scale (Wong & Baker, 1988), and the Adolescent Pediatric Pain Tool (Savedra, Tesler, Holzemer, & Ward, 1989; Savedra, Tesler, Holzemer, Wilkie, & Ward, 1989; Savedra, Holzemer, Tesler, & Wilkie, 1993). These tools are purported to measure only quantity except for Eland's Color Tool, which includes location, and the Adolescent Pain Tool, which includes location and quality. Some nurse researchers such as Adams (1990) have tested tools (i.e., the Children's Anxiety and Pain Scale [Kuttner & LePage, 1989] and the Faces Distress Scale [LeBaron & Zeltzer, 1984]) designed for children but developed by researchers from other disciplines. Versions of tools generally associated with measuring pain in adults also have been used: rating scales (Abu-Saad & Holzemer, 1981; Abu-Saad, 1984a, 1990; Fowler-Kerry & Lander, 1987; Fowler-Kerry & Ramsay-Lander, 1990; Lander, Fowler-Kerry, & Hargreaves, 1989; Tesler, Savedra, Holzemer, Wilkie, Ward, & Paul, 1990), diary (Richardson, McGrath, Cunningham, & Humphreys, 1983), word descriptor scales (Tesler et al., 1989), and visual analogue scales[1] (Aradine, Beyer, & Tompkins, 1988; Beyer & Aradine, 1987, 1988; Branson, McGrath, Craig, Rubin, & Vair, 1990; Moinpour, Donaldson, Wallace, Hiraga, & Joss, 1990; O'Hara, McGrath, D'Astrous, & Vair, 1987; Tesler et al., 1990).

Research on the psychometric properties of self-report measures is lacking for most tools. Researchers have studied convergent validity by using from two (e.g., Hester, 1979) to six tools (e.g., Wong & Baker, 1988) within the same study. Memory of an earlier rating may result in a misleading dependence between tools, threatening conclusions about validity. Findings from studies (e.g., Aradine et al., 1988; Beyer & Aradine, 1987, 1988; Dodd, 1988; Hester, 1979; Tesler et al., 1989; Wong & Baker, 1988) using multiple similar measures need further substantiation before accurate conclusions about validity can be drawn.

Three tools have undergone extensive testing and the research provides documentation of moderate to strong evidence for reliability/generalizability, validity, and sensitivity: the Oucher (Aradine et al., 1988; Beyer, 1984, 1988, 1989; Beyer & Aradine, 1986, 1987, 1988; Beyer, McGrath, & Berde, 1991; Datz, 1989; Jordan-Marsh, Brown, Watson, & Yoder, 1990), the Poker Chip Tool (Alyea, 1978; Aradine et al., 1988; Beyer, 1984, 1988; Beyer & Aradine, 1987, 1988; Datz, 1989; Foster & Hester, 1989a, 1989b, 1990; Hagedorn, 1990; Hay, 1984; Hester, 1976, 1979; Hester et al., 1978; Hester & Foster, 1990; Hester, Foster, & Kristensen, 1989b; Hester et al., 1990; Hester, Kristensen, & Foster, 1989; Hester, Foster, Kristensen, & Bergstrom, 1989; Jordan-Marsh et al., 1990; Molsberry, 1979; Wong & Baker, 1988) and the Adolescent Pediatric Pain Tool (Jordan-Marsh et al., 1990; Savedra et al., 1982; Savedra, Tesler, Holzemer, & Ward, 1989; Savedra, Tesler, Holzemer, Wilkie, & Ward, 1989, 1990; Tesler et al., 1990; Tesler, Savedra, Ward, Holzemer & Wilkie, 1988; Tesler, Savedra, Ward, Holzemer, & Wilkie, 1989; Tesler, Ward, Savedra, Wegner, & Gibbons, 1983; Wilkie, Holzemer, Tesler, Ward, Paul, & Savedra, 1990). Among the tools purported to measure

[1]In this chapter, visual analogue scale is recognized as a line of a specified length without markers other than a verbal or pictorial anchor on each end, indicating from the least to the greatest amount of the appropriate pain dimension. Scales such as the ones by Abu-Saad and Holzemer (1981) and Fowler-Kerry and Ramsay-Lander (1990) that were identified as visual analogue scales did not meet that definition; they were classified as rating scales because they included markers between the end points.

pain quantity, these tools emerge as the most well-developed with substantiated psychometric properties for use with children over four years. Of these three tools, the Poker Chip Tool is the only tool available in both English and Spanish (Jordan-Marsh et al., 1990).

Researchers have attempted to determine if child self-reports pertaining to quantification correspond to ratings by parents and nurses. Some researchers have used one tool for children and a different one for adult raters (Fradet, McGrath, Kay, Adams, & Luke, 1990), Lukens, 1982; Varchol, 1983; a situation that confounds measurement error. Other researchers have used the same tool for child and adult raters. Relationships between children and nurses (CN), children and parents (CP), and nurses and parents (NP) differ for three tools: visual analogue scale (VAS) (Abu-Saad, 1990; Powers, 1987), the Pain Ladder (PL) (Hester, Foster, & Kristensen, 1989; Hester, Foster, Kristensen, & Bergstrom, 1989), and the PCT (Hester, Foster, & Kristensen, 1989; Hester, Foster, Kristensen, & Bergstrom, 1989). Correlation coefficients for the VAS were low to moderate (.14 to .48) for CN, and moderate (.44) for CP and NP; for the PL ranged from low to moderate (.21 to .63) for CN and low to moderate (.39 to .66) for CP, but moderate to high (.42 to .74) for NP; and for the PCT were from moderate to high (.59 to .81) for CN, high (.74 to .80) for CP, and moderate to high (.46 to .78) for NP. Hester, Foster, Kristensen, and Bergstrom (1989) speculated that the PCT may have performed better across raters because of its simplicity and limited range of five points rather than 11 points (PL) and infinite points (VAS).

Two nurse-originated tools include pain maps to measure the location of pain. Eland's Color Tool (1976, 1983, 1988; Eland & Anderson, 1977) uses clothed, gender-linked body outlines, and the Adolescent Pediatric Pain Tool (Savedra, Tesler, Holzemer, & Ward, 1989; Savedra, Tesler, Holzemer, Wilkie, & Ward 1989; Savedra, Holzemer et al., 1993) includes unclothed, nongender-linked body outlines. Studies by Eland and Savedra and colleagues on these tools indicated that reported location on the body outline corresponded to actual body location of pain and to location predicted by pathology or surgery. In using Eland's body outline, Hester et al. (1978) identified some problems: (a) the lack of the three-dimensional aspects of specific body parts such as the foot, (b) the occlusion of certain body parts by the clothing on the body outline, (c) the distraction of the clothing to the location of pain (i.e., some children colored the shirt instead of locating the pain), and (d) left-right reversals. These issues primarily affected the location of pain by younger children except for the dimensionality issue.

Tools to assess the qualitative dimension of pain included lists of words. The earliest and most extensive work on word lists has been accomplished by Savedra, Tesler, and colleagues (Savedra et al., 1982, 1988; Savedra, Tesler, Holzemer, & Ward, 1989; Savedra et al., 1990; Tesler et al., 1983, 1988,

1989; Wilkie et al., 1990). Others who have studied the use of words to measure children's pain include Abu-Saad (1984a, 1984b, 1984c, 1990), Branson et al. (1990), and Jarrett and Evans (1986). Word choices differed according to type of clinical conditions and whether the child was hospitalized. Research on the use of words as a qualitative measure of pain is in its infancy and has not yet provided information on how to use the selection of words as a measure of pain.

Tools for measuring behavior are few but include both unidimensional and multidimensional perspectives: Neonatal Facial Coding System (Grunau & Craig, 1987, 1990; Grunau, Johnston, & Craig, 1990), Maximally Discriminative Facial Movement Coding System (Izard, 1979; Johnston & Strada, 1986), cry spectrograph (Fuller, 1984; Fuller & Horii, 1986, 1988; Fuller, Conner, & Horii, 1990; Fuller, Horii, & Conner, 1989; Grunau & Craig, 1987; Grunau et al., 1990; Johnston & O'Shaungnessy, 1988; Johnston & Strada, 1986), photogrammetry (Franck, 1986), Behavioral Observation Tool (Hester, 1976, 1979), Child Behavior Observation Rating Scale (adapted, Broome, 1985), and Behavioral Checklist (Abu-Saad & Holzemer, 1981). Observations without the aid of specific tools occurred frequently (e.g., Dale, 1986, 1989; Davis & Calhoon, 1989; Mills, 1989a, 1989b; Taylor, 1983). Reported levels of interrater agreement were generally adequate whether or not a specific tool was used. Subjects in most of these studies were children undergoing medical and nursing procedures or were infants. The emphasis was on vocal (primarily crying), facial expression, and motor behaviors with little attention given to verbal behavior.

Crying behavior has been studied from two perspectives: observation of crying behaviors and the measurement of acoustic attributes (e.g., pitch, jitter, shimmer). Davis and Calhoon (1989), Wiliamson and Williamson (1983), Franck (1986), and Dale (1986, 1989) observed crying associated with painful care (e.g., chest physiotherapy, removal and restart of intravenous lines, and dressing changes) in preterm infants, with circumcisions and heelsticks in newborns, and with diphtheria injections in infants 2 to 4.5 months of age, respectively. Although cries sometimes occurred before the start of the painful procedure, crying responses were strongly associated with skin penetration or immediately following. Characteristics of cries such as number, duration, loudness, and breath-holding episodes varied across infants within these studies. Grunau et al. (1990) found that infants who had cried previously exhibited higher pitch and intensity after the injection, suggesting that some infants are more sensitive or expressive. Cry may also be related to type of pain. Cote (1987), through ethologic analysis, concluded that crying occurred infrequently in newborns with postoperative pain. Studies on the acoustical attributes of cries using a cry spectrograph (Fuller, 1984; Fuller et al., 1990; Fuller & Horii, 1986, 1988; Fuller et al.,

1989; Grunau & Craig, 1987; Grunau et al., 1990; Johnston & O'Shaughnessy, 1988; Johnston & Strada, 1986) have yet to document whether a cry is related to pain or something else. Few studies have been focused on the influence of infant behavioral states, gender, and age on crying behavior associated with painful events. Latency to cry but not number of cry cycles or duration differed according to behavioral states (Grunau & Craig, 1987). The effect of gender on cries associated with pain has shown differences in number of cry cycles and for latency to cry (Grunau & Craig, 1987) but no differences in tenseness (Fuller & Horii, 1988).

Age per se has been explored minimally, but the influence of age on pain-related crying behavior can be inferred by examining findings across studies. Previously cited studies documented the occurrence of crying in infants undergoing procedures. Observations of infants and toddlers experiencing acute pain showed a decrease in crying behavior as verbal facility increased (Mills, 1989a, 1989b), and observations on preschool and school-age children undergoing bone marrow aspirations and lumbar punctures revealed a decrease in crying for older children (Foster, 1981). Other researchers (Abu-Saad, 1984a; Abu-Saad & Holzemer, 1981; Beyer, McGrath, & Berde, 1991; Hester, 1979; Hester & Foster, 1990) reported the absence of crying behavior during postoperative periods or during painful procedures for a majority of children as young as 3 years. Absence of crying, however, did not indicate the absence of pain even though the occurrence of crying was related to higher levels of pain (Hester, 1976, 1979).

Mills (1989a, 1989b) noted a decrease in crying as verbal facility increased. This finding should not be construed to mean that as verbal facility increases, verbal expression of pain increases; in fact, research shows otherwise. Although the findings reported by Dauz-Williams (1973) suggested that 60% of pain response behaviors in the postoperative period were verbal, only 40 verbal behaviors occurred during 4 days of observations on seven preadolescents. Evidence from Hester (1979) and Beyer et al. (1991) also would not substantiate that verbal expression about pain increases with verbal facility, even though verbal expression has been associated with higher levels of pain (Hester, 1976, 1979).

Facial expression is a potential behavioral expression of pain, particularly in infants. Dale (1986, 1989), Johnston and Strada (1986), Grunau and Craig (1987), Johnston and O'Shaughnessy (1988), and Grunau et al. (1990) documented, for infants undergoing painful procedures, specific facial parameters that form an expression of pain. The facial expression, a cry face, is comprised of brow bulge, eye squeeze, nasolabial furrow, open lips, lip purse, stretch mouth, taut tongue, and chin quiver. For newborns, facial activity was greatest with the shortest reaction time to an injection and least with slowest reaction time to the umbilical procedures (Grunau et al., 1990).

Tongue protrusion was greatest for noninvasive procedures while taut tongue was greatest with the invasive procedure. Co-occurrence of brow action, eye squeeze, nasolabial furrow, and open lips for most of the infants was observed during the injections but not during noninvasive procedures. Facial expression in newborns may be related to behavioral state (Grunau & Craig, 1987) and to type of pain (Cote, 1987).

The influence of age on facial expression can be inferred from studies on children from preterm through 15 years. For children from birth through 3 years of age experiencing acute pain, relevant facial parameters change with age. The cry face evident in early months of age is replaced with behaviors such as anger, vigilance, and pouting (Mills, 1989a, 1989b). Findings from Abu-Saad (1984a), Abu-Saad and Holzemer (1981), Beyer et al. (1991), and Hester (1979) suggested an absence of any particular facial expression in the majority of children from 3 through 15 years experiencing acute pain and procedural pain. Interestingly, facial expressions with closed eyes, wrinkled forehead, and clenched jaw have been related significantly to lower levels of pain; Hester (1976, 1979) suggested that facial expression may be a coping mechanism for pain.

Research on body movements associated with pain in inconclusive. According to Dale (1986), Franck (1986) and Johnston and Strada (1986), infants expressed variable and nonspecific behaviors during heelsticks and injections. Froese-Fretz (1986) documented the increase of body movement with arterial blood draws, through analogues generated from the Infant Activity Mattress (Keefe, 1984) in infants up to 5 months of age hospitalized in a neonatal intensive care unit. The photogrammetric techniques used by Franck (1986) suggested that velocity of leg movements, number of leg movements, and number of movements directed toward the stimuli might be valuable measures for infants undergoing heelsticks. Mills's (1989a, 1989b) observation of infants and toddlers in acute pain showed that body movements became more controlled and purposeful across time; some of the behaviors were protective or self-consoling. Motor behaviors in older children are diminished or inhibited (Abu-Saad, 1984a; Abu-Saad & Holzemer, 1981; Beyer er al., 1991; Hester, 1979). In fact, only 34% of the pain response behaviors in preadolescents were documented as motor (Dauz-Williams, 1973). This finding is not surprising considering that many adults try to remain calm and to not appear in pain (Jacox, 1979). As did Mills, Abu-Saad and Holzemer (1981) described body movements as purposeless, protective, or consoling. The occurrence of exaggerated body movements has been associated with lower pain scores, suggesting that movements may function as a way to reduce pain from injections (Hester, 1976, 1979). This finding is substantiated by Taylor (1983), who observed more than 4,000 pain-related movements and vocalizations during the first 3 hr after surgery in 20 postoperative children aged 18 months to 4 years. Typical movements, somewhat different from those generally studied included restlessness, guarding site, touching or contacting operative site, and grimacing; vocalizations consisted of crying, groaning, whining, and verbal statements of pain. Movements often exacerbated pain. Taylor observed that children used movement as means of coping with the pain experience (e.g., supporting and protecting painful area).

Stress arousal alters physiologic responses; if pain is a stress arousal, then physiologic responses would be expected to change with its presence. To that end researchers have focused on determining whether physiologic responses can be used as indicators of pain. Physiologic parameters that have been studied in relationship to pain include temperature (Abu-Saad, 1984a; Abu-Saad & Holzemer, 1981); pulse/heart rate (Abu-Saad, 1984a; Abu-Saad & Holzemer, 1981; Dale, 1986; Froese-Fretz, 1986; Johnston & Strada, 1986; Mills, 1989a, 1989b; Wiliamson & Williamson, 1983); respiratory rate (Abu-Saad, 1984a; Abu-Saad & Holzemer, 1981; Mills, 1989a, 1989b); blood pressure (Abu-Saad, 1984a; Abu-Saad & Holzemer, 1981); transcutaneous po_2 ($TCpO_2$) (Froese-Fretz, 1986; Norris, Campbell, & Brenkert, 1982; Wiliamson & Williamson, 1983); skin color (Mills, 1989a, 1989b); diaphoresis (Mills, 1989a, 1989b); and cortisol levels (Williamson & Evans, 1986).

Findings regarding physiologic parameters differ according to type of pain (i.e., acute pain from trauma or surgery and induced pain from diagnostic or therapeutic procedures). Abu-Saad (1984a), Abu-Saad and Holzemer (1981), and Mills (1989a, 1989b) studied commonly assessed vital signs (temperature, pulse, respiratory rate, and blood pressure) in relationship to observed or self-report of pain from children in the postsurgical period. For infants and toddlers experiencing acute pain from trauma or surgery, heart and respiratory rates (excluding those during cry episodes) were sometimes elevated but within normative ranges (Mills, 1989a, 1989b). No episodes of diaphoresis (apparently discerned through observation rather than skin conductance) occurred. Reports on the occurrence of skin pallor in two reports of the same study by Mills are discrepant: one instance (in 75 observations) of pallor was reported in Mills (1989a), and five infants and three toddlers with pallor in Mills (1989b). For school-age children, Abu-Saad and Holzemer (1981) implied that pain scale scores were correlated with physiologic parameters but this finding was not substantiated with statistical testing. In a subsequent report of the same study, Abu-Saad (1984a) noted the lack of a relationship between these four physiologic parameters and self-report of pain.

Studies of pain induced by procedures were conducted more rigorously than those on acute pain. In most studies of procedures, heart and respiratory rates were measured by electrocardiometers. Dale (1986), Froese-Fretz (1986), and Johnston and Strada (1986) documented a variable response to injections/venipunctures in infants, with some heart rates increasing, some decreasing, and others remaining stable. Froese-Fretz (1986), Johnston and Strada (1986) and Wiliamson and Williamson (1983), found different dominant response patterns: increasing heart rates with venipunctures and with dissection during circumcision versus decreasing heart rates with injections and following the application of the circumcision clamp. Respiratory rates, measured by electrocardiometers, varied considerably in response to venipunctures and circumcisions; no discernible pattern evolved (Froese-Fretz, 1986; Wiliamson & Williamson, 1983).

Findings regarding $TCpO_2$ are inconsistent. Norris et al. (1982) studied $TCpO_2$ under three circumstances: suctioning, repositioning, and heelsticks. Despite drops in $TCpO_2$ for all three circumstances, changes from the preprocedure to postprocedure time were statistically significant for suctioning and repositioning but not for heelsticks. Mean $TCpO_2$ levels also dropped in response to the injection and dissection phases in the circumcision procedure (Wiliamson & Williamson, 1983) but increased for arterial punctures (Froese-Fretz, 1986). However, no one pattern of response was confirmed.

Williamson and Evans (1986) provided the only information on hormonal response to invasive procedures by examining cortisol response during circumcision. The cortisol level increased from baseline for all infants.

The use of physiologic parameters for measuring pain is not substantiated by the research in this area. Findings are inconsistent, demonstrating a great amount of variability across individuals. Further, the findings suggested that physiologic responses differ depending on type of pain. Changes in physiologic parameters may have occurred with other stress-arousing events limiting physiologic parameters as measures of pain.

Salient Factors for Assessing Children's Pain

Researchers suggested similarities but also discrepancies between findings on how to measure pain most appropriately and how nurses actually assess pain. Nurses use verbalizations about pain in their assessments, documenting the importance of self-reports, yet they do not include validated self-report tools in their assessments. Nurses rely on physiologic indicators, particularly vital signs, in assessing pain but research has yet to show their value in measuring pain. Nurses report behavioral observations in their assessments, but these observations are not consistent with the content of tools designed to measure pain. Although some behavioral and physiologic responses may be similar across children, a common pain response has yet to be documented. Review of the extensive body of research on assessment of pain revealed that cues nurses use to assess pain are often vague and nonspecific for pain. The matrix of cues relevant for a diagnosis of pain has yet to be documented.

This review suggested that the most salient factor for assessing pain is measuring the quantity of pain through a valid self-report tool for children greater than 4 years of age. Facial expression is promising as a measure for young infants experiencing acute and procedural pain. Existing research does not provide an adequate and practical method for measuring pain in older infants, toddlers, and young preschoolers.

MANAGEMENT OF CHILDREN'S PAIN

Two models of pain management are nurse management and child management. Nurse management of pain consists of pharmacologic and nonpharmacologic strategies. Child management refers to those strategies that the child prefers and initiates.

Nurse management of pain is dependent on knowledge of a patient's pain. Children not unlike adults may be reluctant to discuss their pain with others. Atchison et al. (1986) found that a majority of nurses believed that children may try to conceal pain, yet children may assume that nurses or their parents know they are in pain and will automatically do something to relieve it (Eland, 1983, 1988; Jacox, 1979; Taylor, 1983).

Studies on nurse management revealed that the goal of pain relief for most nurses is to relieve as much pain as possible rather than complete pain relief (Burokas, 1985; Gadish, Gonzalez, & Hayes, 1988; Page & Halvorson, 1991). The determination of pain may result in no nursing action, the use of nonpharmacologic interventions, and administration of analgesics (Atchison et al., 1986; Burokas, 1986; Franck, 1987; Gadish et al., 1988; Gonzalez & Gadish, 1990; Lukens, 1982; Pomietto, 1988; Ritchie, 1989; Varchol, 1983). Nurses taking no action has been documented primarily through observations. For example, Lukens (1982) and Varchol (1983) reported that as many as 39% and 50%, respectively, of the nurses did nothing following an assessment of pain in children postoperatively and that 72% initiated verbal interactions as the only invervention (Varchol, 1983).

Through meta-analysis of interdisciplinary literature, Broome, Lillis, and Smith (1989) determined the effectiveness of pain management interventions on behavioral distress, self-reports of pain, and physiologic responses. Nonpharmacologic interventions predominated in the 27 studies (Broome & Lillis, 1989). Effect sizes for the interventions were significant, with the greatest change in behavioral distress and the least in physiologic responses. These findings suggested that, in general, pain management interventions are successful in altering pain-related responses.

Pharmacologic management, according to nurses, is dependent on evaluation of vital signs, type of surgery, severity of pain, body language, age of child, time lapse since last analgesic, response to previous analgesic, nonverbal behavior, and nurse's experience (Atchison et al., 1986; Burokas, 1985; Davis, 1990; Gonzalez & Gadish, 1990; Gadish et al., 1988; Powers, 1987). For infants, type of pain and the effectiveness of nonpharmacologic interventions took precedence over infant's condition and clinical indicators (Franck, 1987).

Pharmacologic management of pain has been examined from several perspectives by researchers. Paramount issues are whether analgesics were ordered and administered. Findings about the percentage of hospitalized children with orders vary across studies, ranging from 77% to 98% (Abu-Saad, 1984a; Abu-Saad & Holzemer, 1981; Beyer, Ashley, Russell, & DeGood, 1984; Beyer, DeGood, Ashley, & Russell, 1983; Eland, 1974; Foster & Hester, 1989a, 1989b, 1990a, 1990b; Lukens, 1982). However, analgesic orders differed by age: older children had more analgesics ordered (Beyer et al., 1983, 1984; Burke & Jarrett, 1989; Schnurrer, Marvin, & Heimbach, 1985). Of those who had analgesics ordered, 57% had both narcotics and nonnarcotics ordered (Eland, 1974). Foster and Hester (1989a) reported that 33% of children on the postoperative day had orders for all three of the following analgesics: morphine sulfate, acetaminophen with codeine, and acetaminophen.

Doses for ordered analgesics have been examined to determine whether they are within the recommended therapeutic ranges (generally calculated by drug-specific dose per kilogram).[2] Beyer et al. (1983, 1984) and Schnurrer et al. (1985) reported 50% and 69% within the recommended ranges, 27% and 13% below (38% in Burokas, 1985), and 23% and 17% above, respectively. Gadish et al. (1988) reported ranges for narcotics versus acetaminophen: within recommended ranges, 55% versus 20%; below, 31% versus 47%; and above, 14% versus 33%. Foster and Hester (1989a, 1989b) identified the extremes of dosages ordered for three commonly used analgesics: morphine sulfate, 7% to 200%; acetaminophen with codeine, 31% to 224%; and acetaminophen, 39% to 180%. Older children tended to have more analgesic per kilogram ordered (Schnurrer et al., 1985). When children and adults were matched on diagnoses, fewer and less potent analgesics were ordered for children (Beyer et al., 1983, 1984; Eland & Anderson, 1977).

[2]The therapeutic dose ranges may have been calculated differently depending on the standard used. The author did not attempt to reinterpret the findings according to one standard.

Analgesic administration varied across studies with 39% to 60% of children with orders receiving analgesics (Eland, 1974; Foster & Hester, 1989a, 1990b; Lukens, 1982). According to Foster and Hester (1990a, 1990b), nurses administered 38% to 131% of the maximum dose range for morphine sulfate, 31% to 209% for acetaminophen with codeine, and 39% to 180% for acetaminophen. Generally, narcotics were reserved for major surgeries such as open heart and spinal fusion (Ritchie, 1989) and for the terminally ill, but were used less frequently for younger children (Burokas, 1985; Gonzales & Gadish, 1990). A general trend was evident for analgesic use: infants and toddlers received smaller (as adjusted per kilogram) doses or no analgesics compared with older school-age children and adolescents (Beyer et al., 1983, 1984; Schnurrer et al., 1985). Infants were medicated after major surgery but rarely before or after procedures (Caire & Erickson, 1986; Franck, 1987; Hockenberry & Bologna-Vaughan, 1985). Wallace (1989) found that children who were high on the intensity dimension of temperament received significantly more analgesics for pain. Children with high intensity exhibited more overt reactions to pain than those with lower intensity.

On the first postoperative day, children who had analgesics ordered and whose nurses identified them as having pain received analgesics only 33% of the times they were eligible for them (Foster & Hester, 1990b). Typically, postoperative analgesics were administered most often in the first 24 hr following surgery (Beyer et al., 1983, 1984; Datz, 1989; Foster, 1990; Ritchie, 1989). Analgesics were discouraged as patients were healing and preparing to go home (Atchison et al., 1986). When adults and children were matched for diagnosis, children rated poorly: Fewer and less potent analgesics were administered to children (Beyer et al., 1983, 1984; Eland & Anderson, 1977).

Researchers have identified reasons for pharmacologic undertreatment of children's pain; nurses may not be confident in their assessment of pain (Foster, 1990); the unit culture may not emphasize pain and its treatment as a priority (Foster, 1990); and nurses may lack knowledge about analgesics and their uses. Potential knowledge deficits include analgesic effects of medications, the unique qualities of analgesics (dosage ranges, route, rates for administration, and side effects), equianalgesics, and drug tolerance (Franck, 1987; Gadish et al., 1988; Pomietto, 1988). Additionally, fear of addiction may preclude the administration of analgesics although results from studies are conflicting (Foster, 1990; Gadish et al., 1988, Pomietto, 1988). Fear of respiratory depression may be a deterrent to administering narcotic analgesics (Foster, 1990; Pomietto, 1988) and nurses may be reluctant to administer analgesics ordered on a *pro re nata* basis (Eland & Anderson, 1977).

Recognition of the undertreatment problem led O'Brien and Konsler (1988) to institute an ongoing educational program on pediatric pain management for staff nurses. Although results showed that the use of intravenous narcotics increased by 48% and the use of intramuscular narcotics decreased by 9%, these findings should be viewed tentatively because the study design was weak and lacked significance testing.

The efficacy of pharmacologic approaches in reducing pain has received minimal attention. Few nursing studies have been focused on efficacy of analgesics. Findings in measurement studies on the Oucher and the Poker Chip Tool revealed that pain levels after analgesic administration decreased (Aradine et al., 1988; Datz, 1989; Hester, Foster, Kristensen, & Bergstrom, 1989).

The efficacy of two clinical regimens, oral morphine every 4 hr and injected meperidine every 3 to 4 hr *pro re nata,* was examined by O'Hara et al. (1987) through a randomized controlled trial. Although the researchers demonstrated that the resolution of pain was better with oral morphine, the results must be viewed tentatively. Embedded in the alternative treatment were three variables, that is, analgesic (morphine vs. meperidine), route (oral vs. intramuscular), and administration protocol (routine vs. *pro re nata*). Any combination of these variables may have been responsible for the study results.

The use of patient-controlled analgesia with children is relatively new and issues of concern include degree of pain control, safety, satisfaction, incidence of respiratory depression, and child's level of consciousness. The degree of pain control was reported to be satisfactory; however, mean pain scores were 4.01 on a 0 to 10 visual analogue (Rodgers, Webb, Stergios, & Newman, 1988; Webb, Stergios, & Rodgers, 1989a, 1989b) and 2.8 on a 1 to 5 behavioral rating scale (Rauen & Ho, 1989). Younger children tended to use less morphine sulfate (Rauen & Ho, 1989). Interpreting these levels of pain as satisfactory is questionable; comparative data with other modes of administration through randomized controlled trials are needed. Although some problems in the mechanical device occurred, risk to the safety of the child was minimal (Rodgers et al., 1988; Webb et al., 1989a, 1989b). Satisfaction with patient-controlled analgesia was rated high by nurses and physicians (Rauen & Ho, 1989), and by children and parents (Rodgers et al., 1988; Webb et al., 1989a, 1989b). Respiratory depression did not occur and level of consciousness was acceptable (Rauen & Ho, 1989).

Examination of the effectiveness of specific anesthetic agents has been demonstrated in studies on thoracotomies, circumcisions, and injections. Fleming and Sarafian (1977) studied the use of intercostal blocks with bupivacaine for the ligation of patent ductus arteriosus through a thoracotomy. Children with the block received statistically fewer doses of analgesics and spent fewer days in the hospital postoperatively. Wiliamson and Williamson (1983) showed that dorsal penile nerve block reduced the stress of circumcisions. Although crying time was significantly longer for the experimental group during the anesthetic injection, crying time was significantly less during the dissection period for the experimental group. Additionally, the drop of $TCpO_2$ was significantly less and the heart rate was significantly lower. If crying time, $TCpO_2$, and heart rate are valid indicators of pain, then the dorsal penile block was effective in reducing pain. The resolution of pain using a penile block is paradoxic in that to reduce the pain of the circumcision a pain-inducing procedure (anesthetizing injection) had to occur.

The efficacy of anesthetic agents for relief of pain associated with injections has been shown by Eland (1981) and Hagedorn (1990). In a two-by-two factorial design, Eland examined the effect of a topical coolant versus an aerosol air spray with and without cognitive information on injection pain. The only significant finding was a main effect: The topical coolant significantly reduced pain. Similarly, Hagedorn demonstrated significant differences between another topical coolant, ethyl chloride, and the standard preparation using alcohol. In these well-controlled studies researchers strongly suggested the efficacy of topical coolants in reducing injection pain.

The pharmacologic approach to managing children's pain is efficacious in treating pain but is underused, thus causing children to suffer needlessly. Resolution of the undertreatment problem has not been adequately addressed through research.

Information on the nurse's application of nonpharmacologic measures is difficult to obtain because it is generally not documented in patient records. Research using observation, vignettes/simulated patient situations, and nurse recall has identified several nonpharmacologic measures: reassurance, positioning, music, diversion/distraction, deep breathing, comfort measures, relaxation, imagery, therapeutic touch, massage, presence of others, minimization of environmental stimulation (Atchison et al., 1986; Burke & Jarrett, 1989; Gadish et al., 1988; Gonzalez & Gadish, 1990; Lukens, 1982; Pomietto, 1988; Ritchie, 1989; Varchol, 1983). Franck (1987) discovered that nurses preferred nonpharmacologic interventions for infants: pacifier, position change, swaddle, minimization of stimulation, holding/rocking, tactile stimulation, and music/voice. Studies addressing nonpharmacologic strategies include one meta-analysis (Olson, Heater, & Becker, 1990). Although only 11 studies comprised the sample, the findings suggested that nonpharmacologic interventions benefited the subjects by 81% over the standard or routine care.

Studies of nonpharmacologic strategies are organized using the framework for nursing interventions developed by Bulechek and McCloskey (1985). When a study was focused on more than one type of intervention, the study is discussed under the intervention that was most prominent. Studies in this section all involved potentially painful events; however, some of the studies did not use pain level as an outcome measure. Instead mood, anxiety, fear, upset, and physiologic parameters were frequently reported. Inclusion of such studies in this review is based on the assumption that pain is manifested in patient outcomes other than subjective or observed pain.

Relaxation techniques are strategies directed toward preventing or reducing the psychologic and physiologic effects of stress. Examples of strategies for relief of pain in children include progressive muscular relaxation, biofeedback, hypnosis, and meditation (Scandrett & Uecker, 1985). No research studies focused on the application of relaxation techniques to prevent or reduce pain. However, Hockenberry and Bologna-Vaughan (1985) surveyed 29 pediatric oncology institutions on their use of relaxation and hypnosis for bone marrow aspirations, lumbar punctures, radiation, and radiographic testing. Relaxation techniques were used sometimes in most of the institutions for bone marrow aspirations and lumbar punctures but seldom for radiation therapy and radiographic testing. Hypnosis was used rarely with any of the procedures. Hockenberry and Bologna-Vaughan concluded that use of these strategies could benefit children with minimal risk, but research is needed to substantiate the efficacy of their use.

Music therapy is "the use of music in the accomplishment of therapeutic aims" (National Association for Music Therapy, 1977, p. 2, cited in Buckwalter, Hartsock, & Gaffney, 1985). The therapeutic aim is to prevent or reduce pain. In a descriptive study, Caire and Erickson (1986) examined the use of child/parent-selected taped music or taped relaxation suggestions with soothing music for 28 infants and children undergoing cardiac catherizations. Self-report and staff observations suggested that most of the children, particularly those 7 to 12 years of age, benefited, but the outcome measures were unclear. In a more rigorous experimental study, Fowler-Kerry and Lander (1987) and Fowler-Kerry and Ramsay (1990) tested the effect of music with and without suggestion. Music but not suggestion was statistically effective in reducing self-reported pain. Although Ryan's small (n = 14) sample (1989) potentially precluded statistical significance, Ryan also found clinical significance in that hospitalized children who listened to taped music reported less pain during venipunctures. These studies, although few in number, suggested that taped music may be a practical and inexpensive therapeutic intervention for pain.

Preparatory sensory information is an intervention that is focused on the description of the subjective and objective aspects of an experience (Christman & Kirchhoff, 1985). Johnson, Kirchhoff, and Endress (1975) studied the use of preparatory sensory information with 84 children during the removal of orthopedic casts. Distress in the sensory information group was significantly less than in either control group. Pulse rates increased significantly in the control groups but not the sensory information group. Fear was not altered but possibly the stick figure scale used to measure fear was not reliable and valid. Sturner, Rothbaum, Visintainer, and Wolfer (1980) examined the effects of preparatory information (including sensory expectations) with and without venipunctures on human figure drawings by children hospitalized for surgery. Emotional indicators were significantly lower in the group who received venipunctures with preparation. Preparation, however, did not alter pulse rates or coping behaviors. Schreiber (1982) found that distress and resistance associated with injections were not less for children who received a preparatory program that included expected body sensations.

Preprocedural/preoperative preparation includes supportive and educational actions the nurse takes to assist children scheduled for procedures or surgery in alleviating their pain (adapted from Felton, 1985). No significant differences between preparation techniques (including verbal and visual-verbal) were evident for self-reported injection pain (Alyea, 1978; Gadaly-Duff, 1987) or for mood, behavior, and sweat (Gadaly-Duff, 1987). Similarly, Sinacore (1984) found that type of preparation (group, individual, and standard preoperative preparation) did not make a difference on heart rate, mood, and time until first postoperative voiding, and posthospitalization behavior.

Play is an appropriate strategy for use with children. Ellerton et al. (1985) found that 10 children with extensive hospitalizations expressed concerns about intrusive procedures during play interviews. Three intrusive procedures dominated the play: blood draws, intramuscular injections, and intravenous injections. The authors concluded that play helped the children to master difficult experiences. Haycraft (1983) used verbal explanation and doll play with 40 children experiencing laceration repair; the experimental group exhibited significantly lower pulse and respiratory rates and had diminished signs and symptoms of emotional distress.

Wolfer and Visintainer (1975) found that psychologic preparation and supportive care effectively diminished emotional distress and improved post-operative recovery in 89 children undergoing minor surgical procedures. A subsequent study (Visintainer & Wolfer, 1975) was focused on four types of preparation (stress-point preparation, single-session preparation, consistent supportive care, and control conditions) for 84 children scheduled for ear, nose, and throat surgery. Findings demonstrated the efficacy of the stress-point and single-session types of preparation in increasing child cooperation, decreasing upset behavior, and improving posthospital behavior. The final study in this series (Wolfer & Visintainer, 1979) has focused on combinations of home preparation with different types of inhospital preparation and supportive care. In this study researchers replicated the findings of the previous studies: home and inhospital preparations were efficacious in decreasing child upset and resistance and increasing cooperation.

Presence is being there for the purpose of meeting the needs of the child in pain (adapted from Gardner, 1985, p. 317). Presence is operationalized cognitively as verbal communication of empathy or understanding of the child's experience; affectively as a generation of positive regard, trust, and genuineness evidence by interpersonal rapport; and physically by being physically available as a helper (Gardner, 1985, pp. 320–321). Parental presence is important to children during pain experiences. Researchers addressed parental presence in only four studies. Atchison et al. (1986) explored 27 nurse's perceptions of parental presence. Nurses who worked in acute care burn units reported that parents increased children's anxiety and that children cried more during their presence, whereas nurses in the reconstructive care burn units felt parents helped to console their child, decreased the child's anxiety, and helped the child to cope with pain. Johnston, Bevan, Haig, Kirnon, and Tousignant (1988) examined parental presence during anesthesia induction. Children accompanied by highly anxious parents were more anxious than those children accompanied by nonanxious parents, and those children not accompanied by either anxious or nonanxious parents. Broome and Endsley (1989) found that mother's anxiety during her child's immunization was significantly and positively correlated with the child's anxiety. The 83 mothers in this study were restricted to an area 3 ft away from the child; potentially the separation produced anxiety in some mother-child pairs. Eland (1983, 1988) categorized parental presence as not present, infrequently present, present during child's awake time and present for 24 hr per day. She found an inverse relationship between parental presence and use of analgesics: increased parental presence was associated with receipt of fewer analgesics. Plausible explanations for this finding include that nurses relinquished their role regarding pain management to the parent(s) or the presence of parents was therapeutic, alleviating the child's pain. This research suggested the importance of examining the effect of parental presence on children's pain. The findings from Johnston et al. (1988) and Broome and Endsley (1989) suggested that to enhance the efficacy of parental presence, strategies to decrease parental anxiety need to be developed and tested.

Triplett and Arneson (1979) examined the deliberate use of verbal or tactile comfort to reduce the distress (i.e., crying) of 63 young hospitalized children. Most interventions were considered successful with the combination of verbal and tactile the most effective. Another study (n = 8) on tactile stimulation (Beaver, 1987) showed that stroking the medial side of the leg during heelsticks corresponded with an increase of heart rate and blood pressure and a decrease in $TCpO_2$. These physiologic responses are consistent with stress arousal and suggest that the pain experienced by the infant was not alleviated.

Cutaneous stimulation is "stimulating the skin for the purpose of relieving pain" (McCaffery & Beebe, 1989, p. 130). The only cutaneous stimulation that has been studied is transcutaneous electrical nerve stimulation (TENS). In a double-blind study, Froese-Fretz (1986) studied the effectiveness of the TENS in reducing pain associated with radial arterial punctures in infants. No differences were found in heart or respiratory rates, $TCpO_2$ levels, and body movement. Through presentation of cases, Eland (1989) described the efficacy of the TENS in reducing pain in children with cancer.

Advocacy, a philosophical ideal, has yet to be operationalized for clinical practice. As Donahue (1985) noted, strategies of advocacy must be identified and tested. A clinically tested strategy of advocacy related to children's pain is providing children with more involvement during potentially painful events by increasing children's sense of predictability and control. Kavanagh (1983a, 1983b) tested the effect of providing nine children on a burn unit with predictability and control. Children were taught to focus on the aversive event rather than being distracted from it; they were given sensation and event information before and during each phase of dressing change. Through controllability, children as young as 18 months took active roles in dressing changes and were encouraged to do as much burn care as safely possible under the nurse's supervision. Children in the experimental group experienced fewer maladaptive behaviors during the first 2 weeks of hospitalization and less depression at discharge. They used fewer analgesics before dressing changes but more between dressing changes. The use of more may suggest that children who took more active roles in their care during dressing changes also took more active roles between dressing changes (i.e., being unwilling to suffer needlessly). Lasoff and McEttrick (1986), in replicating Kavanagh's work, found that although nurses initially had difficulty in allowing children more control and predictability, they adopted this strategy as part of their nursing practice with burned children.

Some of the nonpharmacologic interventions successfully altered the degree of pain, mood, behavior, and other pain-related outcomes. Too little research has been done in this area to state conclusively that nonpharmacologic interventions are efficacious.

Child Management of Pain

Children attempt to manage their pain whether or not health care providers do. Through interviews, questionnaires, and observations, researchers have elicited child-preferred or child-initiated strategies; these strategies are focused on preventing pain or alleviating it.

Several studies have focused on children's perceptions of what helps when they have pain. The two most consistently reported strategies preferred by children from 5 through 17 years were medication and parental presence (especially mother's presence) (Abu-Saad, 1984b, 1984c, 1984d; Adams, 1990; Branson et al., 1990; Hester, 1987, 1989; Hester & Ray, 1987; Savedra et al., 1982, 1988; Tesler, Wegner, Savedra, Gibbons, & Ward, 1981). Unfortunately, these preferred strategies often are not under the child's control. Children in four studies (Adams, 1990; Fowler-Kerry, 1990; Jarrett, 1985; Weekes & Savedra, 1988) mentioned parental presence but not medication. Children in these studies had undergone procedures related to the diagnosis of cancer. Because analgesics are typically not used for children undergoing these procedures (Adams, 1990), children may not have realized that analgesia was a plausible alternative.

In addition to medication and parental presence, Abu-Saad (1984b, 1984c, 1984d), Adams (1990), Branson et al. (1990), Hester (1987, 1989), Hester and Ray (1987), Savedra et al. (1982, 1988), Tesler et al. (1981) documented numerous child-initiated strategies as helpful: holding someone's hand, using distraction, sleeping/resting, relaxing, holding a stuffed toy or favorite blanket, seeking information, using imagery, and positioning. Hester (1987) discovered that girls from 7 through 12 years often reported "Don't show it" (i.e., pain) as a strategy.

Children also try to avert inevitable painful situations such as described by Savedra (1976). Observations of children with burns reveal they attempted to avoid painful dressing changes by telling others not to hurt them, postponing the dressing change, asking nurses to pretend to do it, keeping nurses at a distance through physical absence at the time of the dressing change, or by kicking to keep the nurse away, using distraction, and sleeping.

A strategy that has received little attention is the use of humor for pain relief. Wessell (1975) reported a case study of an immobilized adolescent girl who used humor as a defense against anxiety, as an outlet for aggression, and as a social device. The use of humor, however, was not exhibited at times of pain or intense emotion.

Painful situations may elicit responses from children that may indicate either severity of pain or a child-initiated relief strategy. For example, Foster (1981) described children's responses to lumbar punctures and bone marrow aspirations as cognitive (e.g., avoiding/resisting verbally, seeking comfort or information verbally), emotional (e.g., crying, forced breath sounds, statements of feelings), and motor (initiating actions nonverbally, resisting nonverbally). Potentially, responses such as these may be indicating severity of pain or may be alleviating pain, thus suggesting a paradox for interpreting behavioral responses. This paradox may provide insight into the problems associated with observational/behavioral measurement of pain.

Two studies (Fowler-Kerry, 1990; Hester & Ray, 1987) provided information on the importance of the relationship between caregiver and child. Adolescents in the Fowler-Kerry study (1990) described procedures as being easier if caregivers were known and trusted. They did not want to be handled in a rough manner nor be rushed for a procedure. Similarly, Hester and Ray (1987) found that children and adolescents want others to be caring when they are in pain. Child-identified caring behaviors were consistent with the types of ideal caring described by Watson (1985) and with the intervention presence (Gardner, 1985). Environmental factors can serve to make the pain worse. Children with cancer undergoing procedures reported cold room temperature, crowded rooms, and delayed appointments made the pain worse (Fowler-Kerry, 1990). Children hospitalized for a variety of reasons noted that quiet, dark rooms were helpful for relieving pain (Hester, 1989; Hester & Barcus, 1986). One adolescent specifically mentioned that the noise from "beepers" on the machines made her pain worse.

Salient Factors for Managing Pain

The management literature documents the efficacy of analgesic and anesthetic agents for pain relief. A repertoire of nonpharmacologic strategies has been examined, but each strategy has been the focus of only a few studies and, in some cases, the results are conflicting. Although many of the nonpharmacologic strategies are promising, the evidence for their efficacy in relieving pain is insufficient.

Several of the preprocedural preparation interventions did not significantly reduce pain. Potentially, the experimental intervention was not potent enough to alter pain below the levels attained by the interventions already incorporated in the standard care procedures.

None of the studies on nurse management of pain addressed child preference and studies on child management described only strategies documented through interview, questionnaire, or observation. Efficacy of the child-initiated strategies has yet to be tested. Potentially, success of interventions in relieving children's pain will, in part, depend on the appropriateness of the intervention for a particular child. Criteria for selecting appropriate interventions have not been addressed.

STATE OF KNOWLEDGE DEVELOPMENT AND RECOMMENDATIONS

In the past 20 years, research on pain in children has increased remarkably. Measurement of pain has been and continues to be the primary emphasis.

Researchers have perpetuated the development of self-report quantification tools without adequately substantiating their psychometric properties. Too often tools lacking reliability and validity estimates are used prematurely in testing the efficacy of interventions. Although less research has been focused on behavioral and physiologic measures of pain, research indicates that these responses may differ with type of pain experienced (i.e., procedural, acute, and chronic pain). Thus, the generalizability of the findings from one type of pain to another is limited.

Research has demonstrated discrepancy between clinical assessment of pain by nurses and the approaches used in research to measure pain, particularly regarding behavioral manifestations and the use of physiologic indicators. The gap between assessment and measurement can be minimized by strengthening the clinician-researcher partnership to determine valid indicators of pain.

Underrepresented in this body of measurement literature is an emphasis on measuring acute and chronic pain in the preverbal population of infants, toddlers, and young preschoolers and in the nonverbal, cognitively impaired, or multiply handicapped population of children from infants through adolescents. Approaches to self-report, behavioral, and physiologic measures of pain must be validated with these special-need populations.

Research on the management of pain is less well developed than the assessment research. The undertreatment of pain from a pharmacologic perspective has been well documented. Although the efficacy of analgesic and anesthetic agents is minimally substantiated, the issue of therapeutic dose ranges is not addressed other than from a description. A consensus panel said studies should be focused on what factors in children might influence drug action (National Institutes of Health, 1986) and thereby affect the dose range regarding safety and therapeutic effect.

Nonpharmacologic strategies need more thorough examination. Research such as that by Visintainer and Wolfer (1975) and by Kavanagh (1983) and Lasoff and McEttrick (1986) attests to the importance of building a program of research across time to refine and substantiate the intervention strategies.

None of the researchers addressed the use of analgesia in conjunction with nonpharmacologic approaches or with child-initiated strategies. Questions for future research should be focused on the combined effect on pain relief and the effect of strategies such as relaxation or preoperative preparation on amount of analgesia needed for pain relief.

Potentially, improving knowledge and clinical judgment skills of nurses regarding pain would alleviate the problem. Other potential strategies include the adoption of policies or practice guidelines for the assessment and treatment of pain, and the prioritization of pain management through quality assurance. The effectiveness of such strategies in resolving the undertreatment of pain needs to be documented through research.

Research by nurse scientists has contributed greatly to the breadth and depth of the knowledge about children's pain. Although addressing gaps in knowledge is paramount, research must be focused also on minimizing the disparity between knowledge development and clinical practice. The incorporation of scientifically based pain assessment and management strategies into practice logically follows the development of knowledge. Without clinical implementation, knowledge development is for naught, and the problem of undertreatment of children's pain will remain unresolved.

REFERENCES

Abu-Saad, H. (1984a). Assessing children's responses to pain. *Pain, 19,* 163–171.

Abu-Saad, H. (1984b). Cultural components of pain: The Arab-American child. *Issues in Comprehensive Pediatric Nursing, 7,* 91–99.

Abu-Saad, H. (1984c). Cultural components of pain: The Asian-American child. *Children's Health Care, 13*(1), 11–14.

Abu-Saad, H. (1984d). Cultural group indicators of pain in children. *Maternal-Child Nursing Journal, 13,* 187–196.

Abu-Saad, H. H. (1990). Toward the development of an instrument to assess pain in children: Dutch study. In D. C. Tyler & E. J. Krane (Eds.), *Advances in pain research and therapy: Vol. 15. Pediatric pain* (pp. 101–106). New York: Raven Press.

Abu-Saad, H., & Holzemer, W. L. (1981). Measuring children's self-assessment of pain. *Issues in Comprehensive Pediatric Nursing, 5,* 337–349.

Adams, J. (1990). A methodological study of pain assessment in Anglo and Hispanic children with cancer. In D. C. Tyler & E. J. Krane (Eds.), *Advances in pain research and therapy: Vol. 15. Pediatric pain* (pp. 43–52). New York: Raven Press.

Alyea, B. (1978). *Child pain rating after injection preparation.* Unpublished master's thesis, University of Missouri, Columbia, MO.

Aradine, C. R., Beyer, J. E., and Tompkins, J. M. (1988). Children's pain perception before and after analgesia: A study of instrument construct validity and related issues. *Journal of Pediatric Nursing, 3,* 11–23.

Atchison, N., Guercio, P., & Monaco, C. (1986). Pain in the pediatric burn patient: Nursing assessment and perception. *Issues in Comprehensive Pediatric Nursing, 9,* 399–409.

Beaver, P. K. (1987). Premature infants' response to touch and pain: Can nurses make a difference? *Neonatal Network, 6*(3), 13–17.

Beyer, J. E. (1984). *The Oucher: A user's manual and technical report.* Charlottesville, VA: University of Virginia Alumni Patent Foundation.

Beyer, J. E. (1988). The Oucher: A pain intensity scale for children. In S. G. Funk, E. M. Tornquist, M. T. Champagne, L. A. Copp, & R. A. Wiese (Eds.), *Key aspects of comfort: Management of pain, fatigue, and nausea* (pp. 65–71). New York: Springer Publishing Co.

Beyer, J. E. (1988). *The Oucher: A user's manual and technical report*. Denver: University of Colorado Health Sciences Center, Unpublished Instrument.

Beyer, J. E., & Aradine, C. R. (1986). Content validity of an instrument to measure young children's perceptions of the intensity of their pain. *Journal of Pediatric Nursing, 1,* 386–395.

Beyer, J. E., & Aradine, C. R. (1987). Patterns of pediatric pain intensity: A methodological investigation of a self-report scale. *The Clinical Journal of Pain, 3,* 130–141.

Beyer, J. E., & Aradine, C. R. (1988). Convergent and disciminant validity of a self-report measure of pain intensity for children. *Children's Health Care, 16*(4), 274–282.

Beyer, J. E., Ashley, L. C., Russell, G. A., & DeGood, D. E. (1984). Pediatric pain after cardiac surgery: Pharmacologic management. *Dimensions of Critical Care Nursing, 3,* 326–334.

Beyer, J. E., DeGood, D. E., Ashley, L. C., & Russell, G. A. (1983). Patterns of postoperative analgesic use with adults and children following cardiac surgery. *Pain, 17,* 71–81.

Beyer, J. E., McGrath, P. J., & Berde, C. C. (1991). Discordance between self-report and behavioral measures in 3–7 year old children following surgery. *Journal of Pain and Symptom Management, 5,* 350–356.

Bradshaw, C., & Zeanah, P. D. (1986). Pediatric nurses' assessments of pain in children. *Journal of Pediatric Nursing, 1,* 314–322.

Branson, S. M., McGrath, P. J., Craig, K. D., Rubin, S. Z., & Vair, C. (1990). Spontaneous strategies for coping with pain and their origins in adolescents who undergo surgery. In D. C. Tyler & E. J. Krane (Eds.), *Advances in pain research and therapy: Vol. 15. Pediatric pain* (pp. 237–246). New York: Raven Press.

Broome, M. E. (1986). The relationship between children's fears and behavior during a painful event. *Children's Health Care, 14,* 142–145.

Broome, M. E., & Endsley, R. C. (1987). Group preparation of young children for painful stimulus. *Western Journal of Nursing Research, 9,* 484–497.

Broome, M. E., & Lillis, P. P. (1989). A descriptive analysis of the pediatric pain management research. *Applied Nursing Research, 2,* 74–81.

Broome, M. E., Lillis, P. P., & Smith, M. C. (May–June 1989). Pain interventions with children: A meta-analysis of research. *Nursing Research, 38,* 154–157.

Buckwalter, K., Hartsock, J., & Gaffney, J. (1985). Music therapy. In G. M. Bulechek & J. C. McCloskey (Eds.), *Nursing intervention: Treatments for nursing interventions* (pp. 68–74). Philadelphia: W. B. Saunders.

Bulechek, G. M., & McCloskey, J. C. (1985). *Nursing intervention: Treatments for nursing interventions*. Philadelphia: W. B. Saunders.

Burke, S. O., & Jerrett, M. (1989). Pain management across age groups. *Western Journal of Nursing Research, 11,* 164–180.

Burokas, L. (1985). Factors affecting nurses' decisions to medicate pediatric patients after surgery. *Heart & Lung, 14,* 373–379.

Caire, J. B., & Erickson, S. (1986). Reducing distress in pediatric patients undergoing cardiac catheterization. *Children's Health Care, 14,* 146–152.

Christman, N., & Kirchoff, K. T. (1985). Preparatory sensory information. In G. M. Bulechek & J. C. McCloskey (Eds.), *Nursing intervention: Treatments for nursing intervention* (pp. 259–276). Philadelphia: W. B. Saunders.

Cooper, H. M. (1982). Scientific guidelines for conducting integrative research reviews. *Review of Educational Research, 52*(2), 291–302.

Cooper, H. M. (1989). *Integrating research: A guide for literature reviews* (2nd ed). Newbury Park: Sage.

Cote, J. (1987, May). *A description of the pain response of the postoperative newborn.* Paper presented at Nursing Research Conference, Edmonton, Alberta, Canada.

Dale, J. C. (1986). A multidimensional study of infants' responses to painful stimuli. *Pediatric Nursing, 12,* 37–31.

Dale, J. C. (1989). A multidimensional study of infants' behaviors associated with assumed painful stimuli: Phase II. *Journal of Pediatric Health Care, 3,* 34–38.

Datz, L. (1989). *Comparison of mother's and children's rating of children's tonsillectomy pain intensity.* Unpublished master's thesis, University of California, Los Angeles, CA.

Dauz-Williams, P. (1973). Reactions of preadolescent boys and girls to post-operative pain. *The ANPHI Papers,* 8–12.

Davis, D. H., & Calhoon, M. (1989). Do preterm infants show behavioral responses to painful procedures? In S. G. Funk, E. M., Tornquist, M. T. Champagne, L. A. Copp, & R. A. Wiese (Eds.), *Key aspects of comfort: Management of pain, fatigue, and nausea* (pp. 35–45). New York: Springer Publishing Co.

Davis, K. L. (1990). Postoperative pain in toddlers. In D. C. Tyler & E. J. Krane (Eds.), *Advances in pain research and therapy: Vol. 15. Pediatric pain* (pp. 53–61). New York: Raven Press.

Dodd, J. (1988). The efficacy of nursing management of pain in post-operative paediatric patients. *Nursing Praxis in New Zealand, 4*(1), 4–7.

Donahue, P. (1985). Advocacy. G. M. Bulechek & J. C. McCloskey (Eds.), *Nursing intervention: Treatments for nursing intervention* (pp. 338–351). Philadelphia: W. B. Saunders.

Eland, J. M. (1974). *Children's communication of pain.* Unpublished master's thesis, University of Iowa, Iowa City.

Eland, J. M. (1976). *Children's experience of pain: A descriptive study.* Unpublished manuscript, University of Iowa, Iowa City.

Eland, J. M. (1981). Minimizing pain associated with prekindergarten intramuscular injections. *Issues in Comprehensive Pediatric Nursing, 5,* 361–372.

Eland, J. M. (1983). Children's pain: Developmentally appropriate efforts to improve identification of source, intensity, and relevant intervening variables. G. Felton & M. Albert (Eds.), *Nursing research: A monograph for non-nurse researchers* (pp. 64–79). Iowa City: University of Iowa Press.

Eland, J. M. (1988). Persistence in pediatric pain research: One nurse researcher's efforts. *Recent Advances in Nursing, 21,* 43–62.

Eland, J. M. (1989). The effectiveness of transcutaneous electrical nerve stimulation (TENS) with children experiencing cancer pain. In S. G. Funk, E. M. Tornquist, M. T. Champagne, L. A. Copp, & R. A. Wiese (Eds.), *Key aspects of comfort: Management of pain, fatigue, and nausea* (pp. 87–100). New York: Springer Publishing Co.

Eland, J. M., & Anderson, J. E. (1977). The experience of pain in children. In A. K. Jacox (Ed.), *Pain: A sourcebook for nurses and other health professionals* (pp. 453–473). Boston: Little, Brown.

Ellerton, M.-L., Caty, S., & Ritchie, J. A. (1985). Helping young children master intrusive procedures through play. *Children's Health Care, 13,* 167–173.

Felton, G. (1985). Preoperative teaching. In G. M. Bulechek & J. C. McCloskey (Eds.), *Nursing intervention: Treatments for nursing interventions* (pp. 288–300). Philadelphia: Saunders.

Fleming, W. H., & Sarafian, L. B. (1977). Kindness pays dividends: The medical benefits of intercostal nerve block following thoractomy. *The Journal of Thoracic and Cardiovascular Surgery, 74*(2), 273–274.

Foster, R. (1981). *Coping strategies of the child with leukemia: The stress of invasive procedures*. Unpublished master's thesis, University of Colorado Health Sciences Center, Denver, CO.

Foster, R. L. (1990). *A multi-method approach to the description of factors influencing nurses' pharmacologic management of children's pain*. Unpublished doctoral dissertation, University of Colorado Health Sciences Center, Denver.

Foster, R., & Hester, N. (1989). The relationship between assessment and pharmacologic intervention for pain in children. In S. G. Funk, E. M. Tornquist, M. T. Champagne, L. A. Copp, & R. A. Wiese (Eds.), *Key aspects of comfort: Management of pain, fatigue, and nausea* (pp. 72–79). New York: Springer Publishing Co.

Foster, R., & Hester, N. (1989). Pain relief for children on the first postoperative day. *Journal of Pain and Symptom Management, 4*(4), 57.

Foster, R., & Hester, N. (1989). The relationship between assessment and pharmacologic intervention for pain in children. In S. G. Funk, E. M. Tornquist, M. T. Champagne, L. A. Copp, & R. A. Wiese (Eds.), *Key aspects of comfort: Management of pain, fatigue, and nausea* (pp. 72–79). New York: Springer Publishing Co.

Foster, R. L., & Hester, N. O. (1990). The relationship between pain ratings and pharmacologic interventions for children in pain. In D. C. Tyler, & E. J. Krane (Eds.), *Advances in pain research and therapy: Vol. 15. Pediatric pain* (pp. 31–36). New York: Raven Press.

Foster, R. L., & Hester, N. O. (1990). Administration of analgesics for children's pain. *Pain, 5* (Suppl.), S31.

Fowler-Kerry, S. (1990). Adolescent oncology survivors' recollection of pain. In D. C. Tyler & E. J. Krane (Eds.), *Advances in pain research and therapy: Vol. 15. Pediatric pain* (pp. 365–371). New York: Raven Press.

Fowler-Kerry, S., & Lander, J. R. (1987). Management of injection pain in children. *Pain, 30,* 169–175.

Fowler-Kerry, S., & Ramsay-Lander, J. (1990). Utilizing cognitive strategies to relieve pain in young children. In D. C. Tyler & E. J. Krane (Eds.), *Advances in pain research and therapy: Vol. 15. Pediatric pain* (pp. 247–254). New York: Raven Press.

Fradet, C., McGrath, P. J., Kay, J., Adams, S., & Luke, B. (1990). A prospective survey of reactions to blood tests by children and adolescents. *Pain, 40,* 53–60.

Franck, L. S. (1986). A new method to quantitatively describe pain behavior in infants. *Nursing Research, 35,* 28–31.

Franck, L. S. (1987). A national survey of the assessment and treatment of pain and agitation in the neonatal intensive care unit. *Journal of Obstetric, Gynecologic, and Neonatal Nursing, 16,* 387–393.

Froese-Fretz, A. (1986). *The use of transcutaneous electrical nerve stimulators (TENS) during radial arterial blood sampling in newborn infants*. Unpublished master's thesis, University of Colorado Health Sciences Center, Denver.

Fuller, B. (1984). Signals in infant vocalizations. *Cry, 6,* 5–10.

Fuller, B. F., Connor, D., & Horii, Y. (1990). Potential acoustic measures of infant pain and arousal. In D. C. Tyler, & E. J. Krane (Eds.), *Advances in pain research and therapy: Vol. 15. Pediatric pain* (pp. 137–146). New York: Raven Press.

Fuller, B. F., & Horii, Y. (1986). Differences in fundamental frequency, jitter, and shimmer among four types of infant vocalizations. *Journal of Communication Disorders, 19,* 111–117.

Fuller, B. F., & Horii, Y. (1988). Spectral energy distribution in four types of infant vocalizations. *Journal of Communication Disorders, 21,* 251–261.

Fuller, B., Horii, Y., & Connor, D. (1989). Vocal measures of infant pain. In S. G. Funk, E. M. Tornquist, L. A. Copp, M. T., Champagne, & R. A. Weise (Eds.), *Key aspects of comfort: Management of pain, fatigue, and nausea* (pp. 46–51). New York: Springer Publishing Co.

Funk, S. G., Tornquist, E. M., Champagne, M. T., Copp, L. A., & Wiese, R. A. (1989). *Key aspects of comfort: Management of pain, fatigue, and nausea.* New York: Springer Publishing Co.

Gadaly-Duff, V. (1987). Preparing young children for painful procedures. *Journal of Pediatric Nursing, 3,* 169–179.

Gadish, H. S., Gonzalez, J. L., & Hayes, J. S. (1988). Factors affecting nurses' decisions to administer pediatric pain medication postoperatively. *Journal of Pediatric Nursing, 3,* 383–389.

Gaffney, A., & Dunne, E. A. (1986). Developmental aspects of children's definitions of pain. *Pain, 26,* 105–117.

Gardner, D. (1985). Presence. In G. M. Bulechek & J. C. McCloskey (Eds.), *Nursing intervention: Treatments for nursing interventions* (pp. 316–324). Philadelphia: W. B. Saunders.

Gonzalez, J. L., & Gadish, H. (1990). Nurses' decisions in medicating children postoperatively. In D. C. Tyler, & E. J. Krane (Eds.), *Advances in pain research and therapy: Vol. 15. Pediatric pain* (pp. 37–42). New York: Raven Press.

Grunau, R. V. E., & Craig, K. D. (1987). Pain expression in neonates: Facial action and cry. *Pain, 28,* 395–410.

Grunau, R. V. E., & Craig, K. D. (1990). Facial activity as a measure of neonatal pain expression. In D. C. Tyler & E. J. Krane (Eds.), *Advances in pain research and therapy: Vol. 15. Pediatric pain* (pp. 147–156). New York: Raven Press.

Grunau, R. V. E., Johnston, C. C., & Craig, K. D. (1990). Neonatal facial and cry responses to invasive and non-invasive procedures. *Pain, 42,* 295–305.

Hagedorn, M. (1990). *Does a topical skin cooling agent alter a child's pain perception during a D. P. T. injection?* Unpublished master's thesis, University of Colorado Health Sciences Center, Denver.

Hay, H. (1984). *The measurement of pain intensity in children and adults—A methodological approach.* Unpublished master's research report, McGill University, Montreal, Canada.

Haycraft, L. (1983). *Caring for young children who sustain lacerations that require sutures: A study of two methods of preparation.* Unpublished master's thesis, St. Louis University, St. Louis, MO.

Hester, N. O. (1976). *The preoperational child's reaction to immunizations.* Unpublished master's thesis, University of Kansas Medical Center, Kansas City.

Hester, N. (1987, March). *Child participation in the pain experience.* Paper presented at the Second International Conference on Research and Maternal Child Nursing, Montreal, Quebec, Canada.

Hester, N. O. (1989). Comforting the child in pain. In S. G. Funk, E. M. Tornquist, M. T. Champagne, L. A. Copp, & R. A. Weise (Eds.), *Key aspects of comfort: Management of pain, fatigue, and nausea* (pp. 290–298). New York: Springer Publishing Co.

Hester, N. O., & Barcus, C. S. (1986). The human experience of pain in hospitalized children. *Proceedings: New Frontiers in Nursing Research* (p. 172). Edmonton, Alberta, Canada: Faculty of Nursing, University of Alberta.

Hester, N. O., Davis, R. C., Hanson, S. H., & Hassanein, R. S. (1978, June). *The hospitalized child's subjective rating of painful experiences*. Paper presented at the Association of Care of Children in Hospitals, Washington, DC.

Hester, N. O., & Foster, R. L. (1990). Cues nurses and parents use in making judgments about children's pain. *Pain, 5*(Suppl.), S31.

Hester, N. O., Foster, R. L., & Kristensen, K. (1989, March). *Sensitivity, convergent and discriminant validity of the Pain Ladder and the Poker Chip Tool*. Paper presented at the Third International Nursing Research Symposium, Clinical Care of the Child and Family, Montreal, CAN.

Hester, N. O., Foster, R. L., & Kristensen, K. (1989). Do nurses' and parents' ratings of children's pain correspond with children's ratings? *Journal of Pain and Symptom Management, 4*(4), S6.

Hester, N. O., Foster, R. L., & Kristensen, K. (1990). Measurement of pain in children: Generalizability and validity of the Pain Ladder and Poker Chip Tool. In D. C. Tyler & E. J. Krane (Eds.), *Advances in pain research and therapy: Vol. 15. Pediatric pain* (pp. 79–84). New York: Raven Press.

Hester, N. O., Foster, R. L., Kristensen, K., & Bergstrom, L. (1989). *Measurement of children's pain by children, parents and nurses: Psychometric and clinical issues related to the poker chip tool and pain ladder. Generalizability of procedures assessing pain in children: Final report*. Research funded by NIH, National Center for Nursing Research under Grant Number R23NR01382.

Hester, N. O., Kristensen, K., & Foster, R. (1989). Measuring children's pain: The convergent and discriminant validity of the pain ladder and poker chip tool. *Journal of Pain and Symptom Management, 4*(4), S6.

Hester, N. K. & Olson. (1979). The preoperational child's reaction to immunization. *Nursing Research, 28*, 250–254.

Hester, N. O., & Ray, M. A. (1987). Assessment of Watson's carative factors: A qualitative research study. *Clinical Excellence in Nursing International Networking* (pp. 91–92), Edinburgh, Scotland: The Department of Nursing Studies, University of Edinburgh, the Royal College of Nursing, and Sigma Theta Tau.

Hockenberry, M. J., & Bologna-Vaughan, S. (1985). Preparation for intrusive procedures using noninvasive techniques in children with cancer: State of the art vs. new trends. *Cancer Nursing, 8*(2), 97–102.

Izard, C. E. (1979). *The Maximally Discriminative Facial Movement Coding System (MAX)*. Neared, DE: University of Delaware Instructional Resources Center.

Jacox, A. K. (1977). *Pain: A source book for nurses and other health professionals*. Boston: Little, Brown.

Jacox, A. (1979). Assessing pain. *American Journal of Nursing, 79*, 895–900.

Jeans, M. ED. (1983). Pain in children: A neglected area. In P. Firestone, P. J. McGrath, & W. Feldman (Eds.), *Advances in behavioral medicine for children and adolescents* (pp. 23–27). Hillsdale, NJ: Erlbaum.

Jerrett, M. D. (1985). Children and their pain experience. *Children's Health Care, 14,* 83–89.

Jerrett, M., & Evans, K. (1986). Children's pain vocabulary. *Journal of Advanced Nursing, 11,* 403–408.

Johnson, J. E., Kirchhoff, K. T., & Endress, M. P. (November–December 1975). Altering children's distress behavior during orthopedic cast removal. *Nursing Research, 24,* 404–410.

Johnston, C. C., Bevan, J. C., Haig, M. J., Kirnon, V., & Tousignant, G. (1988). Parental presence during anesthesia induction. *AORN Journal, 47,* 187–194.

Johnston, C. C., Jeans, M. E., Abbott, F. V., Grey-Donald, K., & Edgar, L. (1988, July). *A survey of pain in hospitalized children: Preliminary results.* Poster presented at the 1st International Symposium on Pediatric Pain, Seattle, WA.

Johnston, C. C., & O'Shaughnessy, D. (1988). Acoustical attributes of infant pain cries: Discriminating features. In R. Dubner, G. F. Gebhart, & M. R. Bond (Eds.), *Proceedings of the VIth World Congress on Pain: Pain research and clinical management* (Vol. 3, pp. 336–340). Amsterdam: Elsevier.

Johnston, C. C., & Strada, M. E. (1986). Acute pain response in infants: A multidimensional description. *Pain, 24,* 373–382.

Jordan-Marsh, M., Brown, R., Watson, R., & Yoder, L. (1990, October). *Pediatric pain assessment research: Application challenges in a multicultural acute care setting.* Paper presented at the American Pain Society, St. Louis, MO.

Kavanagh, C. (November 1983a). A new approach to dressing change in the severely burned child and its effect on burn-related psychopathology. *Heart and Lung, 12,* 612–619.

Kavanagh, C. (1983b). Psychological interventions with the severely burned child: Report of an experimental comparison of two approaches and their effects of psychological sequelae. *American Academy of Child Psychiatry, 22,* 145–156.

Keefe, M. (1984). *The effect of the hospital environment of infant state behavior and maternal sleep.* Unpublished doctoral dissertation, University of Colorado, Denver.

Kuttner, L., & LePage, T. (1989). Faces scales for assessment of pediatric pain: A critical review. *Canadian Journal of Behavioral Science, 21*(2), 198–209.

Lander, J., Fowler-Kerry, S., & Hargreaves, A. (1989). Gender effects in pain perception. *Perceptual and Motor Skills, 68,* 1088–1090.

Lasoff, E. M., & McEttrick, M. A. (1986). Participation versus diversion during dressing change: Can nurses' attitudes change? *Issues in Comprehensive Pediatric Nursing, 9,* 391–398.

LeBaron, S., & Zeltzer, L. (1984). Assessment of acute pain and anxiety in children and adolescents by self-reports, observer reports, and a behavior checklist. *Journal of Consulting and Clinical Psychology, 52,* 729–738.

Loebach, S. (1979). *The use of color to facilitate communication of pain in children.* Unpublished master's thesis. University of Washington, Seattle, WA.

Lukens, M. (1982). *The identification of criteria used by nurses in the assessment of pain in children.* Unpublished master's thesis, University of Cincinnati, Cincinnati, OH.

Maunuksela, E.-L., Saarinen, U. M., & Lahteenoja, K.-M. (1990). Prevalence and management of terminal pain in children with cancer: Five-year experience in Helsinki, Finland. In D. C. Tyler, & E. J. Krane (Eds.), *Advances in pain research and therapy: Vol. 15. Pediatric pain* (pp. 383–390). New York: Raven Press.

McCaffery, M., & Beebe, A. (1989). *Pain: Clinical manual for nursing practice*. St. Louis: C. V. Mosby.

McGrath, P. A. (1990). *Pain in children: Nature, assessment, & treatment*. New York: Guilford.

McGrath, P. J., & Unruh, A. M. (1987). *Pain in children and adolescents*. Amsterdam: Elsevier.

Menke, E. M. (1981). School-aged children's perception of stress in the hospital. *Children's Health Care, 9,* 80–86.

Mills, N. (1989). Acute pain behavior in infants and toddlers. In S. Funk, E. Tornquist, M. Champagne, L. Copp, & R. Wiese (Eds.), *Key aspects of comfort: Management of pain, fatigue, and nausea* (pp. 52–59). New York: Springer Publishing Co.

Mills, N. M. (1989). Pain behaviors in infants and toddlers. *Journal of Pain and Symptom Management, 4,* 184–190.

Moinpour, C. M., Donaldson, G., Wallace, K., Hiraga, Y., & Joss, B. (1990). Parent/child agreement in rating child mouth pain. In D. C. Tyler, & E. J. Krane (Eds.), *Advances in pain research and therapy: Vol. 15. Pediatric pain* (pp. 69–78). New York: Raven Press.

Molsberry, D. (1979). *Young children's subjective quantifications of pain following surgery*. Unpublished master's thesis, University of Iowa, Iowa City.

National Institutes of Health (1986). The integrataed approach to the management of pain. *National Institutes of Health Consensus Development Conference Statement 6*(3), 1–8.

Norris, S., Campbell, L. A., & Brenkert, S. (1982). Nursing procedures and alterations in transcutaneous oxygen tension in premature infants. *Nursing Research 31,* 300–336.

O'Brien, S. W., & Konsler, G. K. (1988). Alleviating children's postoperative pain. *American Journal of Maternal-Child Nursing, 13,* 183–186.

O'Hara, M., McGrath, P. J., D'Astous, J., & Vair, C. A. (1987). Oral morphine versus injected meperidine (demerol) for pain relief in children after orthopedic surgery. *Journal of Pediatric Orthopedics, 7,* 78–82.

Olson, R. K., Heater, B. S., & Becker, A. M. (1990). A meta-analysis of the effects of nursing interventions on children and parents. *American Journal of Maternal-Child Nursing, 15,* 104–108.

Page, G. G., & Halvorson, M. (1991). Pediatric nurses: The assessment and control of pain in preverbal infants. *Journal of Pediatric Nursing, 6,* 99–106.

Pomietto, M. (1988). Pain management at children's hospital: Results of 1987 survey. *Express 88, 3*(1), 1, 8.

Powers, D. M. (1987). Ratings of pain from postoperative children and their nurses. *Nursing Papers, 19*(4), 49–58.

Primm, P. (1971). *Identification of criteria used by nurses in the assessment of pain in children*. Unpublished master's thesis, University of Iowa, Ames.

Rauen, K. K., & Ho, M. (1989). Children's use of patient-controlled analgesia after spine surgery. *Pediatric Nursing, 15,* 589–593.

Richardson, G. M., McGrath, P. J., Cunningham, S. J., & Humphreys, P. (1983). Validity of the headache diary for children. *Headache, 23,* 184–187.

Ritchie, J. (1989, May). *Nurses' assessments and management strategies for children's pain*. Paper presented at the Association of the Care of Children's Health, Anaheim, CA.

Rodgers, B. M., Webb, C. J., Stergios, D., & Newman, B. M. (1988). Patient-controlled analgesia in pediatric surgery. *Journal of Pediatric Surgery, 23*(3), 259–262.

Ross, D. M., & Ross, S. A. (1988). *Childhood pain: Current issues, research, and management.* Baltimore: Urban & Schwarzenberg.

Ryan, E. (1989). The effect of musical distraction on pain in hospitalized school-aged children. In S. Funk, E. Tornquist, M. Champagne, L. Copp, & R. Wiese (Eds.), *Key aspects of comfort: Management of pain, fatigue, and nausea* (pp. 101–104). New York: Springer Publishing Co.

Savedra, M. (1976). Coping with pain: Strategies of severely burned children. *Maternal-Child Nursing Journal, 5,* 197–203.

Savedra, M., Gibbons, P., Tesler, M., Ward, J., & Wegner, C. (1982). How do children describe pain? A tentative assessment. *Pain, 14,* 95–104.

Savedra, M., Holzemer, W., Tesler, M., & Wilkie, D. (1993). Assessment of postoperative pain in children and adolescents using the Adolescent Pediatric Pain Tool. *Nursing Research, 42,* 5–9.

Savedra, M. C., Tesler, M. D., Holzemer, W. L., & Ward, J. A. (1989). *Adolescent pediatric pain tool (APPT) preliminary user's manual.* San Francisco: University of California.

Savedra, M. C., Tesler, M. D., Holzemer, W. L., Wilkie, D. J., & Ward, J. A. (1989). Pain location: Validity and reliability of body outline markings by hospitalized children and adolescents. *Research in Nursing and Health, 12,* 307–314.

Savedra, M. C., Tesler, M. D., Holzemer, W. L., Wilkie, D. J., & Ward, J. A. (1990). Testing a tool to assess postoperative pediatric and adolescent pain. In D. C. Tyler, & E. J. Krane (Eds.), *Advances in pain research and therapy: Vol. 15. Pediatric pain* (pp. 85–94). New York: Raven.

Savedra, M., Tesler, M., Ward, J., Wegner, C., & Gibbons, P. (1981). Description of the pain experience: A study of school-age children. *Issues in Comprehensive Pediatric Nursing, 5,* 373–380.

Savedra, M. C., Tesler, M. D., Ward, J. D., & Wegner, C. (1988). How adolescents describe pain. *Journal of Adolescent Health Care, 9,* 315–320.

Scandrett, S., & Uecker, S. (1985). Relaxation training. In G. M. Bulechek & J. C. McCloskey (Eds.), *Nursing intervention: Treatments for nursing interventions* (pp. 22–48). Philadelphia: W. B. Saunders.

Schnurrer, J. A., Marvin, J. A., & Heimbach, D. M. (1985). Evaluation of pediatric pain medications. *Journal of Burn Care and Rehabilitation, 6*(2), 105–107.

Schreiber, M. (1982). *Verbal interaction: A preparatory method to decrease distress of four and five year-olds during immunizations.* Unpublished master's thesis, University of Michigan, Ann Arbor.

Schultz, N. V. (1971). How children perceive pain. *Nursing Outlook, 19,* 670–673.

Sinacore, M. L. (1984). *A comparison of group and individual preparation of young children for surgery.* Unpublished master's thesis, St. Louis University, St. Louis, MO.

Sturner, R. A., Rothbaum, F., Visintainer, M., & Wolfer, J. (1980). The effects of stress on children's human figure drawings. *Journal of Clinical Psychology, 36*(1), 324–331.

Taylor, P. L. (1983). Post-operative pain in toddler and pre-school age children. *Maternal-Child Nursing Journal, 12,* 35–50.

Tesler, M., Savedra, M., Ward, J. A., Holzemer, W. L., & Wilkie, D. (1988).

Children's language of pain. In R. Dubner, D. F. Gebhart, & M. R. Bond (Eds.), *Proceedings of the Fifth World Congress on Pain* (pp. 348–352). Amsterdam: Elsevier Science.

Tesler, M. D., Savedra, M. C., Ward, J. A., Holzemer, W. L., & Wilkie, D. J. (1989). Children's words for pain. In S. G. Funk, E. M. Tornquist, M. T. Champagne, L. A. Copp, & R. A. Wiese (Eds.), *Key aspects of comfort: Management of pain, fatigue, and nausea* (pp. 60–65). New York: Springer Publishing Co.

Tesler, M., Ward, J., Savedra, M., Wegner, C. B., & Gibbons, P. (1983). Developing an instrument for eliciting children's description of pain. *Perceptual and Motor Skills, 56,* 315–321.

Tesler, M. D., Wegner, C., Savedra, M., Gibbons, P. T., & Ward, J. A. (1981). Coping strategies of children in pain. *Issues in Comprehensive Pediatric Nursing, 5,* 351–359.

Triplett, J. L., & Arneson, S. W. (1979). The use of verbal and tactile comfort to alleviate distress in young hospitalized children. *Research in Nursing and Health, 2,* 17–23.

Tyler, D. C., & Krane, E. J. (1990). *Advances in pain research and therapy: Vol. 15. Pediatric pain.* New York: Raven Press.

Varchol, D. (1983). *The relationship between nurses's and children's perceptions of pain in the acute and chronic pain experiences of children.* Unpublished master's thesis, University of Cincinnati, Cincinnati, OH.

Visintainer, M, A., & Wolfer, J. A. (August 1975). Psychological preparation for surgical pediatric patients: The effect on children's and parents' stress responses and adjustment. *Pediatrics, 56,* 187–202.

Wallace, M. R. (1989). Temperament: A variable in children's pain management. *Pediatric Nursing, 15,* 118–121.

Ward, B. (1975). *Externally observed pain—Associated behavior and internally perceived pain intensity in the four through eight year old child.* Unpublished master's thesis, University of Kansas Medical Center, Kansas.

Watson, J. (1985). *Nursing: The philosophy and science of caring.* Boston: Little, Brown.

Webb, C. J., Stergios, D. A., & Rodgers, B. M. (1989a). Patient-controlled analgesia as postoperative pain treatment for children. *Journal of Pediatric Nursing, 4,* 162–171.

Webb, C. A., Stergios, D. A., & Rodgers, B. M. (1989b). Use of patient-controlled analgesic by children. In S. G. Funk, E. M. Tornquist, M. T., Champagne, L. A. Copp, & R. A. Wiese (Eds.), *Key aspects of comfort: Management of pain, fatigue, and nausea* (pp. 80–86). New York: Springer Publishing Co.

Weekes, D. P., & Savedra, M. C. (1988). Adolescent cancer: Coping with treatment-related pain. *Journal of Pediatric Nursing, 3,* 318–328.

Wessell, M. L. (1975). Use of humor by an immobilized adolescent girl during hospitalization. *Maternal-Child Nursing Journal, 4,* 35–48.

Wiliamson, P. S., & Williamson, M. L. (1983). Physiologic stress reduction by a local anesthetic during newborn circumcision. *Pediatrics, 71,* 36–40.

Wilkie, D. J., Holzemer, W. L., Tesler, M. D., Ward, J. A., Paul, S. M., & Savedra, M. C. (1990). Measuring pain quality: Validity and reliability of children's and adolescents' pain language. *Pain, 41,* 151–159.

Williamson, P. S., & Evans, N. D. (1986). Neonatal cortisol response to circumcision with anesthesia. *Clinical Pediatrics, 25*(8), 412–415.

Wolfer, J. A., & Visintainer, M. A. (July–August 1975). Pediatric surgical patients' and parents' stress responses and adjustment. *Nursing Research, 24,* 244–255.

Wolfer, J. A., & Visintainer, M. A. (November 1979). Prehospital psychological preparation for tonsillectomy patients: Effects on children and parents' adjustment. *Pediatrics, 64,* 646–655.

Wong, D. L., & Baker, C. M. (1988). Concerns expressed on pain article. *Pediatric Nursing, 14,* 320–331.

PART II

Research on Nursing Care Delivery

Chapter 6

Patient Care Outcomes Related to Management of Symptoms

SUE T. HEGYVARY
SCHOOL OF NURSING
UNIVERSITY OF WASHINGTON

CONTENTS

The provision of health care services has the general objective of promoting health. The search for positive outcomes of care and treatment is implicit in volumes of research in all the health professional literature. Yet the systematic investigation and documentation of the results of care and treatment are recent and limited.

In 1988 the National Center for Nursing Research defined the national nursing research agenda that included a high priority on outcomes of symptom management. This chapter assesses the status of research about the outcomes of care related to managing patient symptoms. What is the state of the science in regard to managing patients' symptoms effectively? This review does not attempt to present a comprehensive analysis of the literature about any specific symptoms. Instead, it addresses the question of the development of the knowledge base of the discipline in this aspect of nursing practice. The review and assessment includes the problem and its significance, methods of data collection and evaluation, presentation and interpretation of findings, and the conclusions and recommendations.

PROBLEM AND ITS SIGNIFICANCE

Deviations from or threats to a state of health are manifest by signs and symptoms. Signs generally are regarded as the objective measures of abnormal functioning, such as a cardiac arrhythmia, that are observable and measurable by clinicians. Symptoms are the perceived indicators of change in normal functioning as experienced by patients, though clinicians also attempt to measure symptoms.

Although the distinction between signs and symptoms at times becomes artificial, this chapter focuses on research related to symptoms that may be managed by nursing interventions. This area of research is important for several reasons. First, symptom management is part of comprehensive health care that aims to treat both disease and the manifestations of illness. Second, research can uncover the conditions under which various interventions are or are not successful. To what extent can clinicians generalize in regard to predicting results from the treatment of symptoms? How does symptom management relate not only to the disease under treatment and the clinical interventions, but simultaneously to other conditions, such as physiologic, mental, social, and cultural variables? Are the desired outcomes of treatment merely the absence of symptoms, or do the outcomes of symptom management go beyond the cure or reduction of symptoms?

Addressing these questions requires that research consider the overall context of health. Research about clinical outcomes of symptom management must be combined with related research toward theoretic development to guide clinicians. Such theories to guide care and treatment require precision in the definition of symptoms and outcomes, and evaluation of the implicit assumption in the use of the term *outcomes* that causal linkages are present.

Symptoms are the red flags of threats to health and are an essential focus of health care. Verbrugge and Ascione (1987) called symptoms "the iceberg of mortality." They observed that symptoms seldom are studied, because they are regarded as indicators for treatment of disease and for research into the underlying mechanisms of disease. Further, successful reduction in symptoms is, often appropriately, regarded as effective treatment of the underlying disease process. Research directed only toward the management of symptoms and not at their underlying causes would be inadequate and incomplete. Yet a sole focus on disease processes ignores an essential component of human experience and health care services.

Outcomes research usually focuses on disease and morbidity and mortality associated with disease states and medical procedures. Numerous efforts have been directed toward relating medical practices to outcomes, but definitions and measures of outcomes generally lack consistency (Welch & Grover, 1991). The very necessary research into mechanisms of disease and methods of treatment dwarfs attention to the management of symptoms, as if assuming that diagnosis and treatment of disease cures the symptoms. Fortunately, such is often the case.

For two reasons, however, *research into management of symptoms is an essential adjunct to research about disease and treatment.* First, symptoms usually are manifestations of disease processes. People have to live with the symptoms before and during successful treatment. Management of symptoms during that time is important to individuals, families, and practitioners. Second, naming and treating the disease may not cure the symptoms, as some become chronic even when the disease process is under control. This common occurrence adds emphasis to the need to research to define and measure patient symptoms, and to develop and test effective approaches to the management of symptoms.

Research into *outcomes* of care and treatment confronts even greater problems of definition and measurement (Marek, 1989; Nadzam, 1991). Complex variables and constructs must be measured and isolated, and ambiguous, abstract notions must be reduced to concrete, behavioral indicators (Waltz, Strickland, & Lenz, 1991). Conceptually, outcomes are the end results of care and treatment. In practice, however, such definition is not straightforward. Lohr (1988) indicated that "the desirability of one outcome rather than another in any given clinical situation . . . may differ markedly according to the values and preferences of patients" (p. 38). Those conceptual differences are reflected in the wide range of measures of outcomes, varying according to definitions, values, approaches to research and practice, and human experience.

The conduct of research about the processes and outcomes of managing symptoms requires consideration of five issues: definition, timing, level of analysis, attribution, and data base (Hegyvary, 1991). How are the phenomena, both symptoms and outcomes, defined and measured? What methodologic issues must be addressed when symptoms are both the indicator for and the outcome of treatment? In situations in which cure of symptoms is not possible, do other outcomes indicate effectiveness of interventions? Over what period does a measure constitute a result of a particular action? Does the research focus on individuals, groups, or populations—and with what characteristics? How do we know that *Z*, that is, an outcome measure, is attributable to *Y*, an intervention, for the treatment of *X* symptom? What data at what levels of analysis, from individual to large population, are necessary to document the relationships among symptoms, clinical interventions, and outcomes, and thereby enhance theoretic development?

The subjective nature of symptoms, the difficulties in defining and measuring both symptoms and outcomes, and the assumption of causal linkages between interventions and outcomes pose serious threats to the validity of outcomes research. This review considers such threats in individual studies and also in assessment of the overall status of outcomes research in relation to management of patient symptoms.

METHODS OF DATA COLLECTION AND EVALUATION

This review and analysis takes a developmental approach to determine the status of outcomes research regarding symptom management. Questions for investigation include what symptoms are cited as phenomena for investigation? What outcomes are studied, and do they pertain to changes in presenting symptoms? What levels of theory are generated as guides for practice?

Defining the database for this analysis required some limitations to keep the survey manageable. The review includes health professional literature in the 5-year period between 1987 and 1991, though several meta-analyses published during this time included studies conducted before 1987. A MEDLINE search was conducted, using the following key words: outcomes, patient care outcomes, and symptom management. In addition, manual screening of contents during this time produced additional reports from these journals: *Nursing Research, Medical Care,* the *Journal of Nursing Quality Assurance,* the *Western Journal of Nursing Research,* and *Research in Nursing and Health.* Because of the lack of comprehensive studies identified in these screens, further manual search was done in the *Cumulative Index to Nursing and Allied Health Literature* for the following selected common symptoms: constipation, dyspnea, fatigue, insomnia, nausea, pain, and premenstrual syndrome.

No a priori list of symptoms guided this review. The scope for inclusion became more targeted during the literature reviews. Ultimately, however, the choice was the author's interpretation of symptoms and research especially pertinent to nursing. Therefore, it is not an exhaustive review of research related to outcomes of symptom management.

Studies were included in this review if they (a) were published in English between 1987 and 1991, (b) focused on the management of patient symptoms, and (c) included assessment of outcomes. Studies that reported outcomes of disease processes or of specific medical procedures and treatments were excluded (e.g., reduction in pain following surgical or pharmacologic intervention). Similarly, reports limited to outcomes screening in quality assurance programs were excluded unless they met the overall criteria as research projects.

Initially, the criteria for inclusion were aimed at studies that were adequately comprehensive to yield predictive- or prescriptive-level theory. A complete analysis of outcomes would require documentation of causal relationships, and thus these higher levels of theory. Because of the paucity of such studies in this emerging field of research, this review instead surveys studies of symptom management and outcomes at four levels of theory development (Dickoff & James, 1968): factor isolating, factor relating, predictive, and prescriptive levels.

These four levels of theory illustrate increasing complexity, culminating in guides to practice. Factor-isolating theory defines a conceptual entity, factor, or phenomenon. Factor-relating theory depicts situations in which factors are associated with each other, but the analysis stops short of determining causal relationships. Predictive theory relates not only factors but conditions in which factors are related. These three levels build to the fourth level of situation-producing or prescriptive theory. Dickoff and James (1968) contended that "a theory for a profession or practice discipline must provide for more than mere understanding or 'describing,' or even predicting reality, and must provide conceptualization specifically intended to guide the shaping of reality to that profession's purpose" (p. 199).

Selection of this framework for review of research is arbitrary. Although the levels of theory sound linear, few would regard the development of knowledge as linear. Further, the distinction between categories sometimes is blurred, for example, the use of experimental designs to yield only factor-relating theory. Yet the implicit assumption of causality and prediction in the word "outcomes" suggests the heuristic value of the Dickoff and James typology. Thus, the following review is organized according to that typology. The conclusions examine both the state of the science and the utility and limitations of this somewhat linear view of theory development in this area of research and practice.

Factor-Isolating Studies of Symptoms and Outcomes

The most frequent type of research related to symptoms and outcomes focuses on defining, describing, and measuring symptoms. Review of 39 research reports is described in this category. This section illustrates the developing nature of this area of research, the importance of such studies in documenting validity and reliability of measures, and the nature of descriptive research as a basis for predictive and prescriptive theoretic development.

The difficulty in assessing and managing symptoms is the lack of precision, as they are, in large part, private, subjective experiences. Further, their expression reflects that they are not unitary but are multidimensional constructs. Leidy (1990) found that symptoms experienced by a sample of 109 patients with chronic obstructive lung disease varied in relation to their psychosocial resources, gender, and perceived stress. That and other studies reported in this review indicate that alleviating symptom discomfort requires (a) an understanding of the experience, (b) skills to assess its characteristics, and (c) tools to reduce it effectively (Jacox, 1989).

Funk, Tornquist, Champagne, Copp, and Wiese (1989) identified pain, fatigue, and nausea as three of the problems that cause the most human suffering. Lists of symptoms for clinical management vary widely including incontinence, alteration in skin integrity, patient knowledge levels, confusion, nutrition, sleep, and discomfort (Lang & Marek, 1991), and nursing diagnostic elements in the nursing minimum data set (Werley & Lang, 1988).

Jacox (1989) asserted that descriptive studies of phenomena that cause discomfort are essential. Using the example of pain, she recommended the conduct of epidemiologic studies on the incidence and prevalence of pain to find out what constitutes the average course of pain for patients experiencing different conditions and treatments, what are the peak periods of pain, how pain is expressed, and how it can be measured in clinical research.

The example of pain is a prototype for factor-isolating research about patient symptoms. Champagne and Wiese (1989) concluded that pain is a complex experience with at least four components: (a) nociception, (b) sensation, (c) suffering or distress, and (d) behavior. The multidimensionality of pain is taken into account in measuring tools such as the McGill Pain Questionnaire (Melzack, 1975), which consists of verbal descriptors of pain in 20 categories, each reflecting a distinct quality of the pain experience. Subscales reflect sensory, affective, and evaluative components (Hand & Reading, 1986). Extensive research has been done to test its validity and reliability and its use in cross-cultural research (Hand & Reading, 1986; Kiss, Muller, & Abel, 1987; Radvila, Adler, Galeazzi, & Vorkauf 1987; Vanderiet, Adriaensen, & Carton, 1987; Wilkie, 1990).

The extent and rigor of testing of this instrument is unusual. Researchers in several countries have built on previous studies to test this measure of pain. Validity of the German version, for example, was documented by expert panels, pilot testing in different groups with pairwise comparisons, and double-blind, crossover designs. Similar studies were done to test the Italian and Dutch versions (Maiani & Sanavio, 1985; Vanderiet et al., 1987).

Davis (1988) studied the adequacy of the McGill Pain Questionnaire (Melzack, 1975) for assessing patients with a nursing diagnosis of alteration in comfort, that is chronic pain. The sample was composed of 30 patients with a nursing diagnosis of chronic pain. The second sample group was selected from patients admitted to the hospital for general surgery. These 30 patients had the potential for acute pain and met the same demographic criteria as patients in the group with chronic pain. Descriptive statistics showed that the McGill Pain Questionnaire measured and differentiated chronic and acute pain (Melzack, 1975). Davis suggested further evaluation of construct validity, for example the possible relationship of chronic pain to depression, which was observed informally but was not measured.

Wilkie, Savedra, Holzemer, Tesler, and Paul (1990) conducted a meta-analysis of 51 studies of the McGill Pain Questionnaire (Melzack, 1975) to measure pain in 3,624 subjects with seven painful conditions. Their conclusions were limited because use of the tool was not standardized across studies; analyses were inconsistently reported; and studies did not adequately test for differences by age, gender, or ethnicity. They recommended consistent, standardized measurement and reporting as a basis for describing a common language of pain.

Such meticulous measurement of symptoms is an essential base for the conduct of outcome studies. Piper (1989) urged such extensive work in relation to other symptoms, such as fatigue. She portrayed the multidimensionality of fatigue in four components: subjective, physiologic, biochemical, and behavioral. Before proceeding with intervention studies, clarity and validity of the construct is essential. Thus, Piper asserted, it is necessary to conduct research about the assessment and measurement of fatigue including the differentiation of concepts of tiredness, weakness, fatigue, and exertion.

Although not as extensive as the testing of measures of pain, the literature reflects efforts to define and measure fatigue. Piper, Lindsey, Ferketich, Paul, and Weller (1989) developed a self-report scale with dimensions. They labeled as temporal, severity, emotional, sensory, evaluative, associated symptoms, and relief. Schaefer (1990) reported a qualitative assessment of the experience of fatigue according to Levine's model of conservation of energy. These tests included limited samples and demonstrated the need for further work, such as testing for use with older patients.

A series of studies attempted to measure the presence and experience of fatigue in different patient populations, such as cardiac surgical patients (Gregersen, 1988), patients with advanced cancer (Aistars, 1987; Bruera & MacDonald, 1988; Piper, Lindsey, & Dodd, 1987), patients with multiple sclerosis compared with a control group of healthy adults (Krupp, Alvarez, LaRocca, & Scheinberg, 1988), patients with chronic pain (Williams, 1988), and cancer patients with pain and nausea (McMillan, 1989). These descriptive studies contributed to development and validation of the construct; however, the use of different tools in single studies with small, selected samples precluded a cumulative advancement to higher levels of theory development regarding the management of fatigue.

Voith, Frank, and Pegg (1989) defined fatigue for adoption as a nursing diagnosis by the North American Nursing Diagnosis Association (NANDA). A sample of 173 nurses identified and described the fatigued individual as (a) verbalizes fatigue, (b) is unable to maintain usual activity level, (c) has poor task performance, (d) has impaired ability to concentrate, (e) feels irritable, and (f) expresses increased physical complaints. On the basis of these factor-isolating studies, NANDA defined fatigue as "an overwhelming, sustained sense of exhaustion and decreased capacity for physical and mental work" (Carroll-Johnson, 1989).

Similar research has targeted definition and measurement of other patient symptoms, for example, nausea (Cotanch, 1989; Dilorio, 1988; Hogan, 1990; McMillan, 1989); dyspnea (Gift, 1989; Renfroe, 1988); premenstrual syndrome (Kirkpatrick, Brewer, & Stocks, 1990; Woods, 1987); constipation (McMillan & Williams, 1989; Ross, 1990); comfort/discomfort (Kolcaba, 1991); and depression (Franks & Faux, 1990).

Factor-isolating, descriptive studies of the outcomes of management of patient symptoms implicitly regard measures of symptoms as both phenomena and outcome. Clinical interventions focus on reducing distress, thus a change between two or more times of measurement. Methodologic issues in this approach are discussed in a later section.

Factor-Relating Studies of Symptoms and Outcomes

Volumes of studies related to patient care outcomes link various interventions to outcomes. These studies tend to rely on correlation of intervention and outcome and thus fall short of documenting a causal relationship, even if an experimental or quasi-experimental design is used. This section surveys reports that relate outcomes to methods of managing patient symptoms. It does not include large numbers of studies that may imply attention to managing symptoms but actually focus the research on disease or treatment, for example, nursing care of patients with various pathologic conditions or undergoing specific medical procedures.

A total of five meta-analyses and 22 individual research reports constituted the database for review of factor-relating studies of symptoms and outcomes. The Heater, Becker, and Olson (1988) meta-analysis was directed toward nursing interventions and patient outcomes. They reviewed 84 studies, including 4,146 subjects, in nursing literature over the previous 8-year period.

Patient outcomes were defined as effects of interventions by nurses that led to measurable responses in relation to identified criteria. Outcomes were categorized as behavioral, knowledge, physiologic, or psychosocial. Studies in this analysis compared patient outcomes of two types of nursing care: systematic, research-based care and routine, procedural nursing care. The analysis concluded that patients who receive research-based interventions can expect 28% better outcomes than patients who receive standard nursing care.

This meta-analysis detected consistencies and similarities in the conclusions of nursing studies of patient care outcomes. Nearly all interventions under study were significantly associated with desired outcomes, and the results of the meta-analysis in a general way supported its implicit aim: the contention that scientifically based care is superior to "routine" care that is based less on data and reason than on established procedure. However, lack of conceptual and methodologic distinction between and within the two types of nursing care, possible Hawthorne effects, and issues of validity and reliability in individual studies complicated the meta-analysis. Nursing interventions require greater methodologic rigor than was present in several studies to establish causal linkages with patient outcomes.

Broome, Lillis, and Smith (1989) conducted a meta-analysis of pain interventions with children. The review included 27 studies of pain management interventions over 2 decades of literature from five disciplines. They reported small but significant relationships between pain management interventions and children's responses in behavioral, self-report, and physiologic measures. This analysis pointed out the need for greater methodologic and theoretic development to enable causal analysis of interventions and outcomes.

Brown's (1988) meta-analysis of educational interventions in diabetes care included 47 studies of the effects of patient teaching on knowledge, self-care behaviors, and metabolic control. The conclusion was that patient teaching has positive outcomes in care of adults with diabetes. This analysis, like those cited earlier, makes a significant contribution to the literature. However, the lack of specific definition of measures of knowledge deficit, educational interventions, and patient outcomes impedes theoretic development as a basis for practice. These meta-analyses show that "something is going on" that requires study, yet the studies are limited to illustrating linkages of variables in small-scale, parallel studies.

Malone and Strube (1988) conducted a meta-analysis of nonmedical management of pain. The 109 studies showed short-term efficacy for most types of pain. They wrote: "Results suggest that outcomes may be attributable not to the differences between treatments, but to the features they have in common" (p. 231). They speculated that pain management may lie in reducing fear and depression associated with pain, more than in relieving pain directly. Limited samples, however, prohibited analysis of differences with combinations of variables.

In a meta-analysis of critical outcomes of nonnutritive sucking in preterm infants, Schwartz, Moody, Yaraneti, and Anderson (1987) reviewed five studies. The number was limited because few studies included the same independent and dependent variables, a criterion for the meta-analysis. They found that the magnitude and consistency of benefits from nonnutritive sucking were small; there was a positive relationship between care related to nonnutritive sucking and two outcome variables, time to first bottle, and days of hospitalization.

Wells et al. (1989) studied function and well-being in 1,242 depressed, chronically ill adults in three cities. The study was carefully constructed and coordinated to assess outcomes related to physical, social, role functioning, and perceptions of health. Analysis of covariance and multiple regression analysis indicated that function and well-being varied according to age, sex, education of the clinician, and comorbidity. However, specific clinical interventions that were associated with variations were not delineated. This study's attention to factor isolation and to some factor-relating analysis provides a basis for further study.

Most of the factor-relating studies focused on pain including postoperative pain (McQuay, Carroll, & Moore, 1988); use of TENS (transcutaneous electrical nerve stimulation) for relief of pain (Eland, 1989; Hargreaves & Lander, 1989; Nelson & Planchock, 1989); pain and related factors in children undergoing tonsillectomy (Rauen & Holman, 1989); use of guided imagery for pain reduction (Geden, Lower, Beattie, & Beck, 1989; Moran, 1989); changes in pain associated with relaxation techniques (Dulski & Newman, 1989; Laframboise, 1989; Levin, Malloy, & Hyman, 1987); biofeedback to reduce pain (Duchene, 1989); treatment of acute and chronic low-back pain (Tollison, Kriegel, & Satterthwaite, 1989); and relationship of low-back pain to disability (Lanier & Stockton, 1988). This set of studies varied from case analysis (Eland, 1989) to two-group comparative design (Duchene, 1989; Dulski & Newman, 1989; Moran, 1989). The studies described "effects" within limited samples and recommended more precise measurement and intervention in the study of outcomes. They are regarded in this review as factor-relating because, despite the use of designs commonly assumed to yield prediction, the limitations of studies prevented theoretic development at the level of prediction.

Additional factor-relating studies included Holtzclaw's (1990) study of drug-induced shivering and the use of extremity wraps to reduce shivering; Kolanowski's (1990) analysis of artificial lighting to reduce restlessness in the elderly; the Becker, Grunwald, Moorman, and Stuhr (1991) test of altered nursing care to improve respiratory and feeding status, behavioral organization, and level of morbidity in LBW infants; the Fowler et al. (1988) study of symptom status and quality of life after prostatectomy; and acupressure therapy for morning sickness (Hyde, 1989).

McCorkle, Benoliel, and Georgiadou (1989) and McCorkle, Benoliel, Donaldson, et al. (1989) reported study of symptom distress including pain, mood disturbances, nausea, appetite, fatigue, bowel patterns, insomnia, and dyspnea in cancer patients. They randomly assigned 166 patients to either oncology home care, standard home care, or office care groups. After 6 months, they concluded that home care was associated with less symptom distress and greater independence than care only in office visits, but patients in the office care group perceived that their health status was better, despite clinical indicators to the contrary. This study moved close to prediction, yet was compromised by 66% attrition of the sample, and lack of precise measurement of the large numbers of symptoms and interventions, especially in the routine care groups. The investigators recommended larger, controlled studies with more refined methods to assess and monitor symptoms.

Dickoff and James (1968) would suggest that these factor-relating studies provide an important basis for further theory development. They document associations among symptoms, interventions, and outcomes, and thus are preliminary as guides to practice. Establishing reliability, validity, and prediction requires precise measures of symptoms, interventions, and outcomes, and controlled studies with large samples to determine that clinical interventions effect changes in symptoms and related outcomes.

Predicting Outcomes of Symptom Management

Outcomes research implies documenting prediction. Jacox (1989) recommended that descriptive, factor-isolating, and factor-relating studies lead to experimental studies to test the effects of interventions. Wall (1988) urged progress beyond simply relating variables toward analyzing multiple dimensions of factors and intervening conditions that lead to outcomes. Developing predictive theory related to symptom management is enhanced, but not assured, through clinical trials using experimental designs. Nursing literature is extremely limited in this type of study, and clinical trials reported in the medical literature generally refer to testing of pharmacologic agents and treatment of disease. Some of the factor-relating studies cited previously used the complex techniques of clinical trials: random group assignment, and cross-over designs. Yet the findings were judged to be factor relating and not predictive because of very limited sample sizes, failure to meet the assumptions of statistical tests, one-time testing without follow-up or replication, or lack of attention to the context and potential intervening variables.

The road to predictive theory is a long one, extending beyond a single study. A program of study, however, may culminate in a single report that illustrates the development of predictive theory. Achieving predictive theory regarding symptom management results, not simply from the choice of methods (i.e., experimental design in clinical trials), but by the overall questions being addressed, the conceptual and methodological rigor of investigation, and the analysis of symptom, intervention, and outcome in a larger context.

The studies of Barnard et al. (1988) illustrate detailed, longitudinal efforts toward predictive theory. They evaluated two intervention strategies focused on preventing parenting alterations in women with low social support. The two interventions, the mental health model and the information-resource model, were derived from previous work that showed these interventions to be more effective than routine, usual care, yet raised the question of need for differential application with clients. Both interventions targeted outcomes to prevent socioemotional disturbances and developmental delay in children, used home visits for delivery of services, and were organized with written protocols. Pregnant women meeting the criteria for study were randomly assigned to the two groups, 68 to the mental health group and 79 to the information-resource group. Multiple tested methods of data collection measured a large set of variables related to subject characteristics, living conditions, interventions, maternal responses and outcomes, and child behaviors and outcomes at intervals over a 3-year period.

The results showed that less socially competent mothers had better outcomes in the mental health group, and more competent mothers had better outcomes in the information-resource group. Women in the mental health group attained more treatment goals and had less depression on repeated measures. The study suggested areas for further research and testing in clinical practice including further analysis of the importance of cultural variations in the sample. Thus, some predictive theory was presented, yet the need for further refinement and prescription was addressed.

A series of studies of children exhibiting conduct disorders was reported by Webster-Stratton and Fjone (1989). These problems were regarded as symptoms of underlying dysfunction or pathology in the family and social environment. They compared parent-child interactions in two groups: children and parents referred from a clinic for conduct problems, and a control group without known conduct problems. Those comparisons led to extensive descriptions of differences in characteristics and interactive patterns between groups, particularly the cycle of aversive interactions. Parents, especially mothers, confronted by conduct-problem children, exhibited more criticism, threats, negative gestures, and expressions. On the basis of documented patterns of behavior, the researchers designed and tested interventions, with careful attention to reliability of measures. The results with a limited sample were predictive of more positive outcomes in the presence of the defined interventions. Wider-scale testing was recommended with more diverse populations to test methods of breaking the cycle of aversive interactions and measuring behavioral outcomes.

Two studies of urinary incontinence illustrate building toward predictive theory to guide practice. Schnelle et al. (1989) studied prompted voiding treatment of 126 incontinent, severely impaired patients in six nursing homes. Subjects were randomly divided into immediate or delayed treatment groups after baseline observation. Experimental treatment of prompted voiding, first every hour, then progressing to every 2 hours, was shown to correlate highly with reduced incontinence, in both the immediate and delayed treatment groups. They recommended expanded study of a wider range of patients. Attention also should be focused on variations by site.

Burns, Pranikoff, Nochajski, Desotelle, and Harwood (1990) studied treatment of stress incontinence with pelvic floor exercises and biofeedback, based on methods and findings in previous studies. The randomized clinical trial assigned the 135 female subjects to three groups: (a) the Kegal exercise group, (b) the biofeedback plus Kegal exercise group, and (c) the control group. Outcomes were episodes of urinary loss, pelvic muscle activity recorded on electromyograph, and maximal urethral closure pressures as determined during urethral profilometry. Careful attention was given to reliability and prevention of research bias. Results showed reduced incontinence in both experimental groups, with even greater reduction with biofeedback. The investigators cautioned that the sample was homogeneous, and that continued research is necessary for further testing of these methods in practice.

These nursing research programs combined elements of clinical trials and field study to yield prediction of some outcomes. They tested for and documented some predictive theory. However, recognizing the frequent limitations of such studies, including samples limited by size and homogeneity, and the inability to account for large numbers of contextual variables, they recommended directions to progress toward prescriptive theory—the basis for generalizations that can guide practice.

Yet the possibility of conclusive, situation-producing or prescriptive theory in such complex situations is debated in the literature. Rettig (1991) suggested that randomized clinical trials may not be the answer for the study of complex situations. In reviewing the medical effectiveness initiatives of the Institute of Medicine, researchers concluded "that only a few very specific questions can be asked in a controlled trial. A lot of money will be spent, it will take a long time, and the selection of participants will exclude everyone over 65. . . . The emphasis on effectiveness made it necessary to move beyond clinical trials and to use large administrative data bases and other primary data" (Rettig, 1991, pp. 15–16).

These reports and observations suggest the possibility of moving directly to the level of prescriptive theory in patient outcomes research. Or is it the case that data from clinical trials constitute a major element of the data set embedded in broader analyses of large databases? Review of prescriptive theoretic development in relation to outcomes of managing patient symptoms provides data about progress in that direction.

Prescriptive Theory of Outcomes of Symptom Management

Prescriptive or situation-producing theory is necessary to guide actions of practitioners (Dickoff & James, 1968). Such theory focuses on goals or intended outcomes of clinical activities and the conditions under which these causal linkages pertain. Such extensive field testing is complex, expensive research, and it requires assessment of structures, processes, and outcomes simultaneously in multiple, defined contexts.

No prescriptive theories related to outcomes of symptom management were found in nursing or medical literature. Donovan (1989) questioned whether such conclusive theory is possible. She argued for "successive approximation" in therapy in relation to management of pain: "If what we already know about pain is true at all, it's that we will never have the perfect answer to such a complex phenomenon" (Champagne & Wiese, 1989, p. 177). Yet work toward prescriptive theory can document under what conditions the interventions of clinicians can be expected to produce desired outcomes.

The emphasis on effectiveness requires complex field studies (Berwick, 1989; Jacox, 1989; Roper, Winkenwerder, Hackbarth, & Krakauer, 1988; Stewart et al., 1989). Tarlov et al. (1989) reported a current series of studies of clinical outcomes that have promise of producing prescriptive-level theory about the effectiveness of health care services. The four categories of outcomes in their studies are (a) clinical end points including signs and symptoms, laboratory values, and mortality; (b) functional status: physical, mental, social, and role; (c) general well-being: health perceptions, energy, fatigue, pain, life satisfaction; and (d) satisfaction with care including access, convenience, financial coverage, quality, and general satisfaction. Their studies include 22,462 patients being treated by 523 clinicians in Boston, Chicago, and Los Angeles. The series of studies attempted to link outcomes with differences in systems of care, specialty of clinicians, the clinicians' technologic and interpersonal styles, and various other structural and process measures in the delivery of health care services. The design was present to move toward prescriptive theory. Yet the authors emphasized the need for further work to develop tools to monitor outcomes—again illustrating the constant need for precision in factor isolation, and refuting a linear view of theory development.

The conceptual framework for the study by Tarlov et al. (1989) indicated the necessary but overwhelming complexity of studies designed to produce prescriptive theory to guide practice. Validity of studies requires careful attention to definition and measurement of all relevant variables, wide-scale testing under field conditions, and analysis of very large databases. Even with such a complex design, some variables are omitted including careful measurement of aspects of the psychosocial environment and the varied care-related activities of multiple practitioners.

Werley and Lang (1988) argued for development and validation of a nursing minimum data set that would account for the nursing component of patient care in such comprehensive analyses. Components of the minimum data set include (a) nursing care elements: nursing diagnosis, interventions, outcomes, and intensity of nursing care; (b) patient or client demographic elements; and (c) service elements. Work continues on the construction of the nursing minimum data set as a potential element in the development of prescriptive theory to guide clinical practice.

DISCUSSION AND INTERPRETATION

This review indicates progress in the emerging field of symptom management, but reveals many conceptual and methodologic issues. Studies show wide-scale efforts in factor-isolating and factor-relating investigations of outcomes of symptom management. The symptom most commonly addressed is pain, though a variety of additional patient symptoms are the focus of research. Although the stage is set for predictive and prescriptive levels of theories (i.e., generalizations that serve as guides to practice), few studies were judged to be at those levels. Why?

Studies at more complex theoretic levels build on years of effort in research programs, not just individual projects. Because the emphasis on outcomes research is relatively recent, nursing research is young, and the dominant research tradition and socialization focuses on description, perhaps the field simply has not had time and concerted efforts to evolve. It also is possible that predictive studies are intimidating because of the requisite time, expense, and rigor, but also because they are perceived as artificial situations. A repeated theme in the literature, though, is the need for predictive and prescriptive level theories to guide practice. Simply producing more studies at the same level, that is, factor relating, does not help the field to advance to a higher level. A shift in both thinking and design is necessary to progress to predictive and prescriptive levels.

Studies of outcomes of symptom management reflect many conceptual and methodological issues. Conceptually there still is a struggle with the definition of outcomes, particularly in relation to patient symptoms. Is the outcome of symptom management simply the reduction in distress from the symptom, or are there other variables that also constitute outcomes of those interventions? Who defines the desired outcomes—the patient, the practitioner, or both? Similarly, there is difficulty with the definition of symptoms and the overlap of signs and symptoms. Those difficulties are portrayed in the review, particularly the inclusion of both subjective and objective measures of symptoms.

Tilden, Nelson, and May (1990) observed that content validity is the generally achieved level of validity in the measurement of research variables in nursing. Murphy (1989) urged greater assurance of validity through multiple triangulation including diverse procedures related to data, investigator, and methods. Reliability and validity in each measure, combined with simultaneous analysis, adds rigor and perspective to investigation. Gioia and Pitre (1990) urged both methodologic and theoretic triangulation to assure that multiple perspectives are taken into account in the interpretation of differences in findings.

The measurement of symptoms and outcomes raises the issue of standardization. The widely tested McGill Pain Questionnaire comes close to being a standard measure through its extensive testing and use. Other measures of pain also were included in the studies reported in this review. The question of a standard, or at least commonly triangulated measures, is basic to comparison of results and the conduct of analytic techniques such as meta-analysis. Documenting an adequate level of reliability and validity to regard a measure as a standard, however, requires extensive testing and application under widely ranging field conditions, and runs the risk of obscuring valid alternative measures. The inevitable dilemma is the desirability of highly reliable and valid tools, but the difficulties in establishing such conclusive standards in the measurement of either symptoms or outcomes.

Another methodologic issue in measuring outcomes is the use of change or difference scores. Repeated application of the same tool assumes that outcomes are documented by changes in scores. Bindman, Keane, and Lurie (1990) cautioned that change scores may be deceiving. Using repeated measures of perceived health status, patients reported improvements in their health, despite clinical indicators to the contrary. The inconsistency may have reflected lack of reliability or changes in patients' definitions of health as they lived with chronic conditions. Hinds (1989) further pointed out that measures may lack reliability over time, and that change is neither unidimensional nor unidirectional. Assessing the conceptual and methodological questions about change scores, Norman (1989) concluded that difference scores can be appropriately derived to measure change or may be used as adjuncts to other statistical measures.

Kazis, Anderson, and Meenan (1989) assessed the importance of effect sizes for interpreting changes in health status. They defined effect sizes as the mean change found in a variable divided by the standard deviation of that variable. Effect size, then, is a standard unit of measurement for changes in a single group. Data were drawn from (a) a 21-week double-blind, multi-centered drug trial of 97 patients with active rheumatoid arthritis, (b) a clinical trial with 135 rheumatoid arthritis subjects in a 12-week double-blind treatment, and (c) a descriptive study of 299 patients with rheumatoid arthritis over a 5-year period. They concluded that effect sizes supplement standard statistical testing in interpreting the results of clinical trials.

A major conceptual and methodological issue is establishing causal linkages between interventions and outcomes. The word "effects" frequently is used in titles of research reports that indicate correlations between intervention and outcome in limited studies. Establishing effects requires documentation of causality. There is no agreement in the statistical and methodological literature that establishing causality actually is possible. The general view is that it always remains controversial and tentative. There is agreement that causal relations are more than mere correlations that show two factors varying in relation to each other. Causality means that the presence of *A* actually determines the presence of *B* (Heise, 1975; Polit & Hungler, 1983).

Lazersfeld (1955) gave a classic definition of the three criteria for causality: (a) temporal, that is, the cause precedes the effect; (b) a demonstrated empiric relationship between the presumed cause and presumed effect; and (c) the relationship cannot be explained as being due to a third variable. This third criterion makes experimental design with randomization a strong approach for testing causal relations. Experimental designs, however, set up artificial situations that preclude measuring all potentially influential variables. Heise (1975) contended that "few phenomena of interest depend on just a single cause and effect" (p. 27). He advocated research of causal systems in which there are networks of multiple causes, multiple effects, and mutual causation, that is, a prescription for prescriptive theory.

In this review of research related to outcomes of symptom management, almost all studies reported significant relationships between interventions and outcomes. It appeared that nearly any activity, no matter how well or how poorly defined and measured, was related positively to desired outcomes. Three nonmutually exclusive interpretations of this finding are possible. First, researchers may be reporting and publishing only those studies that show positive findings. Reporting studies that show negative findings could be very useful. Second, limited studies may simply be producing Hawthorne effects.

A third interpretation is suggested in the findings of Wells et al. (1989), Cherkin (1988), and Burns and Wholey (1991) that outcomes were related to characteristics of the practitioners performing the interventions. This possibility commands further study. Numerous reports noted that symptoms are multidimensional, highly subjective, complex phenomena. They are not signs of illness that are readily and objectively measured and treated by the clinician. It is possible that factors in the clinician-patient interaction, instead of or in addition to the precise intervention itself, cause a change in distress from symptoms. The methods that work in alleviating (or intensifying) symptom distress may depend as much on the characteristics of the practitioners as on the methods themselves, as well as many intervening variables.

The quality of the practitioner-patient relationship is not a new theme, and may be considered a "soft" aspect of outcomes research. Yet the composite view of studies in this analysis requires that researchers give it a closer look. Professional socialization emphasizes the microlevel one-to-one relationship between practitioner and patient. Comprehensive analysis of patient care outcomes centers on that microlevel core, but extends to include multiple interacting layers of variables to combine microanalysis and macroanalysis.

RECOMMENDATIONS FOR FUTURE RESEARCH

Outcomes research related to symptom management is an essential adjunct to outcomes research related to mechanisms and treatment of disease. This field of research is in the early stages of development. Indeed, the recency of emphasis on outcomes research in general would suggest that factor-isolating and factor-relating research still would predominate in the literature. However, the long-standing assumption of health care practitioners that their services produce desired effects is challenged by the paucity of research studies that can guide clinical practice.

The framework for theory development presented by Dickoff and James (1968) served as a heuristic guide for this review and categorization of studies. This framework invites a developmental approach to analysis because of the view of successive stages of building theory, that is, factor-isolating, factor-relating, predictive, and then prescriptive or situation-producing theory. This review does not treat the levels as necessarily linear.

The issue of linearity is significant, however, in the tendency to regard controlled, randomized trials as a prerequisite to wide-scale field testing. Not all clinical trials yield prediction, and new technologies in information systems may allow more rapid progression to analysis of large data sets. Conceptually one could argue that determining efficacy under controlled conditions gives the level of clarity and evidence to suggest wider-scale study with large databases in natural conditions. Research into medical effectiveness currently in progress, however, challenges this linear view, as the wide-scale testing is not as dependent on clinical trials as on information systems to analyze very large sets of data that include contextual variables. In either case, the literature suggests that some basic themes in the conduct of research remain central at any level of theory development: conceptual clarity, methodologic rigor, and reliability and validity of measures.

The findings of this review suggest four conclusions:

First, factor-isolating research is essential to define and measure symptoms, interventions, and outcomes. This need is ongoing to assure reliability and validity in any studies and will recur even in studies targeting higher levels of theory.

Second, measurement must take into account that this field of research pertains to measuring change in subjective, multidimensional phenomena and events. The necessity of multiple methods produces complex research designs and requires advanced analyses.

Third, doing more and more of the same type of research does not advance the field to higher levels, nor do singular, small-scale intervention studies without adequate controls yield prediction. Findings from such studies may even be misleading when a wide range of variables associated with outcomes is not taken into account, or when studies go unreplicated or untested in progressively developing research programs.

Finally, developing predictive and prescriptive theory to guide practice requires rigorous, complex intervention studies and causal analysis, built on solid factor-isolating and factor-relating research. It also requires shifts in thinking, beyond the simple microlevel of the practitioner-patient dyad to complex macrodesigns, and beyond description to intervention and results. Field studies with large, longitudinal data sets are essential for prescriptive theory to guide practice. An area of research cannot begin at the level of predictive or prescriptive theory. Research programs over time, not just parallel projects, provide the basis for progress to more difficult and complex, but essential levels of theory.

Efforts of practitioners, over centuries of health care, have aimed to relieve suffering and improve the state of health. Further development of the field of outcomes research in relation to symptom management will provide a necessary scientific basis to guide clinicians toward better health of society.

REFERENCES

Aistars, J. (1987). Fatigue in the cancer patient: A conceptual approach to a clinical problem. *Oncology Nursing Forum, 14,* 25–30.

Barnard, K. E., Mgyary, D., Sumner, G., Booth, C. L., Mitchell, S. K., & Spieker, S. (1988). Prevention of parenting alterations for women with low social support. *Psychiatry, 51,* 248–253.

Becker, P. T., Grunwald, P. C., Moorman, J., & Stuhr, S. (1991). Outcomes of developmentally supportive nursing care for very low birth weight infants. *Nursing Research, 40,* 150–155.

Berwick, D. M. (1989). Health services research and quality of care: Assignments for the 1990s. *Medical Care, 27,* 763–771.

Bindman, A. B., Keane, D., & Lurie, N. (1990). Measuring health changes among severely ill patients: The floor phenomenon. *Medical Care, 28,* 1142–1152.

Broome, M. E., Lillis, P. P., & Smith, M. C. (1989). Pain interventions with children: A meta-analysis of research. *Nursing Research, 38,* 334–344.

Brown, S. A. (1998). Effects of educational interventions in diabetes care: A meta-analysis of findings. *Nursing Research, 37,* 223–230.

Bruera, E., & MacDonald, R. N. (1988). Overwhelming fatigue in advanced cancer. *American Journal of Nursing, 88,* 99–100.

Burns, L. R., & Wholey, D. R. (1991). The effects of patient, hospital and physician characteristics on length of stay and mortality. *Medical Care, 29,* 251–271.

Burns, P. A., Pranikoff, K., Nochajski, K., Desotelle, P., & Harwood, M. K. (1990). Treatment of stress incontinence with pelvic floor exercises and biofeedback. *Journal of the American Geriatrics Society, 38,* 341–344.

Carroll-Johnson, R. M. (1989). *Classification of nursing diagnosis: Proceedings of the eighth conference*. Philadelphia: Lippincott.

Champagne, M. T., & Wiese, R. A. (1989). Intervening with adults in pain: A discussion. In S. G. Funk, E. Tornquist, M. T. Champagne, L. A. Copp & R. Wiese (Eds.), *Key aspects of comfort* (pp. 173–178). New York: Springer Publishing Co.

Cherkin, D. C. (1988). Commentary. *Journal of Family Practice, 27,* 488–489.

Cotanch, P. H. (1989). Management of nausea: Current bases for practice. In S. G. Funk, E. Tornquist, M. T. Champagne, L. A. Copp, & R. Wiese (Eds.), *Key aspects of comfort* (pp. 243–247). New York: Springer Publishing Co.

Davis, G. C. (1988). Measuring the clinical outcomes of the patient with chronic pain. In C. F. Waltz & O. L. Strickland (Eds.), *Measurement of nursing outcomes: Vol. 1. Measuring client outcomes* (pp. 160–184). New York: Springer Publishing Co.

Dickoff, J., & James, P. (1968). A theory of theories: A position paper. *Nursing Research, 17,* 197–203.

Dilorio, C. (1988). The management of nausea and vomiting in pregnancy. *Nurse Practitioner, 13*(5), 23–28.

Donovan, M. I. (1989). Relieving pain: The current basis for practice. In. S. G. Funk, E. Tornquist, M. T. Champagne, L. A. Copp, & R. A. Wiese (Eds.) *Key aspects of comfort* (pp. 25–31). New York: Springer Publishing Co.

Duchene, P. (1989). The effectiveness of biofeedback in relieving childbirth pain. In S. G. Funk, E. Tornquist, M. T. Champagne, L. A. Copp, & R. A. Wiese (Eds.), *Key aspects of comfort* (pp. 145–149). New York: Springer Publishing Co.

Dulski, T. P., & Newman, A. M. (1989). The effectiveness of relaxation in relieving pain of women with rheumatoid arthritis. In S. G. Funk, E. Tornquist, M. T. Champagne, L. A. Copp, & R. A. Wiese (Eds.), *Key aspects of comfort* (pp. 150–154). New York: Springer Publishing Co.

Eland, J. M. (1989). The effectiveness of transcutaneous electrical nerve stimulation (TENS) with children experiencing cancer pain. In S. G. Funk, E. Tornquist, M. T. Champagne, L. A. Copp, & R. A. Wiese (Eds.), *Key aspects of comfort* (pp. 87–100). New York: Springer Publishing Co.

Fowler, F. J., Wennberg, J. E., Timothy, R. P., Barry, M. J., Mulley, A. G., & Hanley, D. (1988). Symptom status and quality of life. *Journal of the American Medical Association, 259,* 3018–3024.

Franks, F., & Faux, S. A. (1990). Depression, stress, mastery and social resources in four ethnocultural women's groups. *Research in Nursing and Health, 13,* 282–292.

Funk, S. G., Tornquist, E., Champagne, M. T., Copp, L. A., & Wiese, R. A. (1989). *Key aspects of comfort: Management of pain, fatigue and nausea*. New York: Springer Publishing Co.

Geden, E. A., Lower, M., Beattie, S., & Beck, N. (1989). Effects of music and imagery on physiological and self-report analogued labor pain. *Nursing Research, 38,* 37–41.

Gift, A. G. (1989). Validation of a vertical visual analogue scale as a measure of clinical dyspnea. *Rehabilitation Nursing, 14,* 323–325.

Gioia, D. A., & Pitre, E. (1990). Multiparadigm perspectives on theory building. *Academy of Management Review, 14,* 584–602.

Gregersen, R. A. (1988). Fatigue in the cardiac surgical patient. *Progress in Cardiovascular Nursing, 3*(4), 106–111.

Hand, D. J., & Reading, A. E. (1986). Discriminant function analysis of the McGill Pain Questionnaire. *Psychological Reports, 59,* 763–770.

Hargreaves, A., & Lander, J. (1989). Use of TENS for postoperative pain. *Nursing Research, 38,* 159–161.

Heater, B. S., Becker, A. M., & Olson, R. K. (1988). Nursing interventions and patient outcomes: A meta-analysis of studies. *Nursing Research, 37,* 303–307.

Hegyvary, S. T. (1991). Issues in outcomes research. *Journal of Nursing Quality Assurance, 5*(2), 7–12.

Heise, D. R. (1975). *Causal analysis*. New York: Wiley.

Hinds, P. S. (1989). Method triangulation to index change in clinical phenomena. *Western Journal of Nursing Research, 11,* 440–447.

Hogan, C. M. (1990). Advances in the management of nausea and vomiting. *Nursing Clinics of North America, 25,* 475–497.

Holtzclaw, B. J. (1990). Effects of extremity wraps to control drug-induced shivering: A pilot study. *Nursing Research, 39,* 280–283.

Hyde, E. (1989). Acupressure therapy for morning sickness: A controlled clinical trial. *Journal of Nurse-Midwifery, 34,* 171–178.

Jacox, A. K. (1989). Key aspects of comfort. In S. G. Funk, E. Tornquist, M. T. Champagne, L. A. Copp, & R. A. Wiese (Eds.), *Key aspects of comfort*. New York: Springer Publishing Co.

Kazis, L. E., Anderson, J. J., & Meenan, R. F. (1989). Effect sizes for interpreting changes in health status. *Medical Care, 27,* S178–S189.

Kirkpatrick, M. D., Brewer, J. A., & Stocks, B. (1990). Efficacy of self-care measures for peri-menstrual syndrome. *Journal of Advanced Nursing, 15,* 183–188.

Kiss, I., Muller, H., & Abel, M. (1987). The McGill Pain Questionnaire: German version: A study on cancer pain. *Pain, 29,* 195–207.

Kolanowski, A. M. (1990). Restlessness in the elderly: The effect of artificial lighting. *Nursing Research, 39,* 181–183.

Kolcaba, K. Y. (1991). A taxonomic structure for the comfort concept. *Image: Journal of Nursing Scholarship, 23,* 237–240.

Krupp, L. B., Alvarez, L. A., LaRocca, N. G., & Scheinberg, L. C. (1988). Fatigue in multiple sclerosis. *Archives of Neurology, 45,* 435–437.

Laframboise, J. M. (1989). The effect of relaxation training on surgical patients' anxiety and pain. In S. G. Funk, E. Tornquist, M. T. Champagne, L. A. Copp, & R. A. Wiese (Eds.), *Key aspects of comfort* (pp. 155–159). New York: Springer Publishing Co.

Lang, N. M., & Marek, K. D. (1991). The policy and politics of patient outcomes. *Journal of Nursing Quality Assurance, 5*(2), 7–12.

Lanier, D. C., & Stockton, P. (1988). Clinical predictors of outcomes of acute episodes of low back pain. *Journal of Family Practice, 27,* 483–489.

Lazersfeld, P. (1955). Foreword. In H. Hyman (Ed.), *Survey design and analysis*. New York: Free Press.

Leidy, N. K. (1990). A structural model of stress, psychosocial resources, and symptomatic experience in chronic physical illness. *Nursing Research, 39,* 230–235.

Levin, R. F., Malloy, G. B., & Hyman, R. B. (1987). Nursing management of postoperative pain: Use of relaxation techniques in female cholecystectomy patients. *Journal of Advanced Nursing, 12,* 463–472.

Lohr, K. N. (1988). Outcome measurement: Concepts and questions. *Inquiry, 25,* 37–50.

Maiani, G., & Sanavio, E. (1985). Semantics of pain in Italy: The Italian version of the McGill Pain Questionnaire. *Pain, 22,* 399–405.

Malone, M. D., & Strube, M. J. (1988). Meta-analysis of non-medical treatments for chronic pain. *Pain, 34,* 231–244.

Marek, K. D. (1989). Outcome measurement in nursing. *Journal of Nursing Quality Assurance, 4*(1), 1–9.

McCorkle, R., Benoliel, J. Q., Donaldson, G., Georgiadou, F., Moinpour, C., & Goodell, B. (1989). A randomized clinical trial of home nursing care for lung cancer patients. *Cancer, 64,* 1375–1382,.

McCorkle, R., Benoliel, J. Q., & Georgiadou, F. (1989). The effects of home care on patients' symptoms, hospitalizations, and complications. In S. G. Funk, E. Tornquist, M. T. Champagne, L. A. Copp, & R. A. Wiese (Eds.), *Key aspects of comfort* (pp. 303–312). New York: Springer Publishing Co.

McMillan, S. C. (1989). The relationship between age and intensity of cancer-related symptoms. *Oncology Nursing Forum, 16,* 237–241.

McMillan, S. C., & Williams, F. A. (1989). Validity and reliability of the constipation assessment scale. *Cancer Nursing, 12,* 183–188.

McQuay, H. J., Carroll, D., & Moore, R. A. (1988). Postoperative orthopaedic pain: The effect of opiate premedication and local anaesthetic blocks. *Pain, 33,* 291–295.

Melzack, R. (1975). The McGill Pain Questionnaire: Major properties and scoring methods. Pain, *1,* 277–299.

Moran, K. J. (1989). The effects of self-guided imagery and other-guided imagery on chronic low back pain. In S. G. Funk, E. Tornquist, M. T. Champagne, L. A. Copp, & R. Wiese (Eds.), *Key aspects of comfort* (pp. 160–165). New York: Springer Publishing Co.

Murphy, S. A. (1989). Multiple triangulations: Applications in a program of nursing research, *Nursing Research, 38,* 294–297.

Nadzam, D. M. (1991). The agenda for change: Update on indicator development and possible implications for the nursing profession. *Journal of Nursing Quality Assurance, 5*(2), 18–22.

Nelson, T. S., & Planchock, N. Y. (1989). The effects of transcutaneous electrical nerve stimulation (TENS) on postoperative patients' pain and narcotic use, In. S. G. Funk, E. Tornquist, M. T. Champagne, L. A. Copp, & R. A. Wiese (Eds.), *Key aspects of comfort* (pp. 140–144). New York: Springer Publishing Co.

Norman, G. R. (1989). Issues in the use of change scores in randomized trials. *Journal of Clinical Epidemiology, 42,* 1097–1105.

Piper, B. F. (1989). Fatigue: Current bases for practice. In S. G. Funk, E. Tornquist, M. T. Champagne, L. A. Copp, & R. A. Wiese (Eds.), *Key aspects of comfort* (pp. 187–198). New York: Springer Publishing Co.

Piper, B. F., Lindsey, A. M., & Dodd, M. J. (1987). Fatigue mechanisms in cancer patients: Developing nursing theory. *Oncology Nursing Forum, 14*(6), 17–23.

Piper, B. F., Lindsey, A. M., Ferketich, S., Paul, S. M., & Weller, S. (1989). The development of an instrument to measure the subjective dimension of fatigue. In S. G. Funk, E. Tornquist, M. T. Champagne, L. A. Copp, & R. A. Wiese (Eds.), *Key aspects of comfort* (pp. 199–207). New York: Springer Publishing Co.

Polit, D. F., & Hungler, B. P. (1983). *Nursing research: Principles and methods.* Philadelphia: Lippincott.

Radvila, A., Adler, R. H., Galeazzi, R. L., & Vorkauf, H. (1987). The development of a German language (Berne) pain questionnaire and its application in a situation causing acute pain. *Pain, 28,* 185–195.

Rauen, K. K., & Holman, J. B. (1989). Pain control in children following tonsillectomies: A retrospective study. *Journal of Nursing Quality Assurance, 3*(3), 45–53.

Renfroe, K. L. (1988). Effect of progressive relaxation on dyspnea and state anxiety in patients with chronic obstructive pulmonary disease. *Heart and Lung, 17,* 408–413.

Rettig, R. (1991). History, development and importance to nursing of outcomes research. *Journal of Nursing Quality Assurance, 5*(2), 13–17.

Roper, W. L., Winkenwerder, W., Hackbarth, G. M., & Krakauer, H. (1988). Effectiveness in health care: An initiative to evaluate and improve medical practice. *New England Journal of Medicine, 319,* 1197–1201.

Ross, D. (1990). Constipation among hospitalized elders. *Orthopedic Nursing, 9*(3), 73–77.

Schaefer, K. M. (1990). A description of fatigue associated with congestive heart failure: Use of Levine's conservation model (NLN Publication No. 15-2350). In M. E. Parker (Ed.), *Nursing theories in practice* (pp. 217–237). New York: National League for Nursing.

Schnelle, J. F., Traughber, B., Sowell, V. A., Newman, D. R., Petrilli, C. O., & Ory, M. (1989). Prompted voiding treatment of urinary incontinence in nursing home patients: A behavior management approach for nursing home staff. *Journal of the American Geriatrics Society, 37,* 1051–1057.

Schwartz, R., Moody, L., Yaraneti, H., & Anderson, G. C. (1987). A meta-analysis of critical outcome variables in non-nutritive sucking in pre-term infants. *Nursing Research, 36,* 292–297.

Stewart, A. L., Greenfield, S., Hays, R. D., Wells, K., Rogers, W. H., & Berry, S. (1989). Functional status and well-being of patients with chronic conditions. *Journal of the American Medical Association, 262,* 907–913.

Tarlov, A. R., Ware, J. E., Greenfield, S., Nelson, E. C., Perrin, E., & Zubkoff, M. (1989). The medical outcomes study. An application of methods for monitoring the results of medical care. *Journal of the American Medical Association, 262,* 925–930.

Tilden, V. P., Nelson, C. A., & May, B. A. (1990). Use of qualitative methods to enhance content validity. *Nursing Research, 39,* 172–175.

Tollison, C. D., Kriegel, M. L., & Satterthwaite, J. R. (1989). Comprehensive treatment of acute and chronic low back pain: A clinical outcome comparison. *Orthopaedic Review, 18,* 59–64.

Vanderiet, K., Adriaensen, H., & Carton, H. (1987). The McGill Pain Questionnaire constructed for the Dutch language (MPQ-DV): Preliminary data concerning reliability and validity. *Pain, 30,* 395–408.

Verbrugge, L. M., & Ascione, F. J. (1987). Exploring the iceberg: Common symptoms and how people care for them. *Medical Care, 25,* 539–561.

Voith, A. M., Frank, A. M., & Pegg, J. S. (1989). Validation of fatigue as a nursing diagnosis. In R. M. Carroll-Johnson (Eds.), *Classification of nursing diagnoses: Proceedings of the eighth conference* (pp. 453–458). Philadelphia: Lippincott.

Wall, P. D. (1988). The prevention of postoperative pain. *Pain, 33,* 289–290.

Waltz, C. F., Strickland, O. L., & Lenz, E. R. (1991). *Measurement in nursing research* (2nd ed.). Philadelphia: Davis.

Webster-Stratton, C., & Fjone, A. (1989). Interactions of mothers and fathers with conduct problem children: Comparison with a nonclinic group. *Public Health Nursing, 6,* 218–223.

Welch, C. E., & Grover, P. L. (1991). An overview of quality assurance. *Medical Care, 29,* AS8–28.

Wells, K. B., Stewart, A., Hays, R. D., Burman, A., Rogers, W., Daniels, M., Berry, S., Greenfield, S., & Ware, J. (1989). The functioning and well-being of depressed patients: Results from the medical outcomes study. *Journal of the American Medical Association, 262,* 914–919.

Werley, H. H., & Lang, N. (1988). *Identification of the nursing minimum data set.* New York: Springer Publishing Co.

Wilkie, D. J. (1990). Cancer pain management: State of the art nursing care. *Nursing Clinics of North America, 25,* 331–343.

Wilkie, D. J., Savedra, M. C., Holzemer, W. L., Tesler, M. D., & Paul, S. M. (1990). Use of the McGill Pain Questionnaire to measure pain: A meta-analysis. *Nursing Research, 39,* 36–41.

Williams, R. C. (1988). Toward a set of reliable and valid measures for chronic pain assessment and outcome research. *Pain, 35,* 239–251.

Woods, N. F. (1987). Premenstrual symptoms: Another look. *Public Health Reports* (102 Supplement), 106–112.

Chapter 7

The Role of Nurse Researchers Employed in Clinical Settings

KARIN T. KIRCHHOFF
COLLEGE OF NURSING AND UNIVERSITY HOSPITAL UNIVERSITY OF UTAH

CONTENTS

The focus of this review is the research published on the role of nurse researchers employed in clinical settings. One major study was done; several smaller subsequent studies followed, primarily of a regional nature.

The role of nurse researcher employed in the clinical setting is a relatively new one. Federal facilities such as the Walter Reed Army Institute for Research, associated with the Walter Reed General Hospital (Werley, 1962), and the Veteran's Administration Hospitals in 1963 (Cross, 1977) were among the first to implement the role.

These positions were few until the late 1970s and early 1980s. Dr. Susan Boehm organized a group of clinical nurse researchers that began to meet biennially in 1979 during the American Nurses Association Council of Nurse Researchers conference. At these meetings members discussed their positions, shared job descriptions, and mentored those considering such a position. At more recent meetings the topics have included research utilization strategies, appropriateness of various funding mechanisms for clinical nurse researchers (CNRs), and reports of research on CNRs.

The 1979 listing contained 28 names; a few did not hold titles within a clinical setting. By 1983 there were approximately 50 names on the list with research titles and clinical affiliations. Dr. Karin Kirchhoff assumed leadership of the group at that time.

Although there were many strong statements in the literature about the need for research by investigators in academic settings, support for research by those in clinical settings was not as frequent. However, in 1980 the American Society for Nursing Service Administrators (ASNSA), later known as the American Organization of Nurse Executives, published a position statement, "The Role of the Nursing Service Administrator in Nursing Research," supporting the position of a research coordinator who would be part of the nursing administrative staff (ASNSA, 1980). Both the conduct and use of research in hospitals was strongly supported in this statement.

The American Hospital Association (AHA) (AHA, 1985), in the *Nurse Executive Management Strategies,* published a section entitled "Integration of Nursing Research into the Practice Setting." The economic constraints in health care were seen as an incentive for integrating nursing research into the practice setting. Ways of structuring the research program within the nursing department were described; the functional model and the line and staff model were compared as structural designs to accept a research position. The use of a department or division was the third program design described. Support for the research functions despite type of design was strong. Expectations were set for three program functions: setting of program objectives to reflect departmental commitment to practice-based research, arrangements for research project implementation, and development of protocols to meet needs of the nursing department as well as the health care institution.

METHODS OF REVIEW

A search through *Index Medicus* and the *Cumulative Index to Nursing and Allied Health Literature* augmented personal bibliographies on research in hospitals, the roles of the nurse researcher employed in clinical settings, and nursing administration and research. A computer search was performed for the time period January 1983 through February 1992. The period of 1980 to 1983 was searched manually. Key terms were *nursing research, clinical nursing research,* and *research personnel.* Additionally nursing textbooks were examined for relevant research. Contacts in the special-interest group, Nurse Researchers Employed in Clinical Settings, within the American

Nurses Association Council of Nurse Researchers, were used to augment the completed search for "in press," unpublished, or missed research articles.

Although there is considerable literature on the topic of research in hospitals that will not be reviewed in this chapter, most of it is of an advocacy nature—advice about how to do research (Davis, 1981) or reports of how it has been done at a single institution (Kirchhoff, 1985; Stetler, 1984). Surveys have shown an increase in the conduct (Pettengill, Knafl, Bevis, & Kirchhoff, 1988) and use (Pettengill et al., 1988; Wake, 1990) of research in U.S. hospitals and also in Canadian hospitals (Thurston, Tenove, & Church, 1990). An instrument to assess a department of nursing's readiness to participate in research has been developed (Egan, McElmurry, & Jameson, 1981) and questions have been suggested for an assessment of an agency's philosophy of nursing and a nurse's fit within it (Rempusheski, 1991). Suggestions about how to involve staff nurses in research abound (Davis, 1981; Hoare & Earenfight, 1986; Stetler, 1983).

The literature related to the role of the nurse researcher employed in a clinical setting or about research programs in hospitals is similar to many case reports. Some of that literature is included if it is of a theoretic nature or is written by an incumbent of such a position about their experiences or recommendations from their experiences.

ROLE OF NURSE RESEARCHER EMPLOYED IN CLINICAL SETTING

A chapter from the perspective of role theory was published by Mayer (1983) on this role because it was not only new for the profession but also for the employing organizations and other researchers. Strategies, activities, and a job description were included to assist with role taking and role making.

In 1983 the Division of Nursing, United States Public Health Service (Grant no. 5 R01 NU0087) funded Knafl, Bevis, and Kirchhoff to study the nurse researcher role in a clinical setting. All of the data-based publications on a national scale have come from this study. Because that study was an in-depth qualitative study on topics related to the development of the role, separate articles were written on each of the topics.

One of the key issues in the definition of these role incumbents is that they receive at least a portion of their salary from the clinical setting in contrast to those who receive all of their salary from an academic setting but conduct research in the clinical setting. For ease of use CNR will be used for those who receive salary from the clinical setting for research as has been done in earlier publications (Hagle, Kirchhoff, Knafl, & Bevis, 1986).

The early literature describing the qualifications and responsibilities of the CNR had been anecdotal and prescriptive; it reflected the opinions of those CNRs in the position or nurse administrators who had hired them (Knafl, Bevis, & Kirchhoff, 1987a). Because the role was relatively new and most incumbents were the first of their kind, a study was developed to document the themes by which the role was enacted and negotiated by the incumbent and the chief nurse executive (CNE). This study was grounded conceptually and methodologically in a framework of symbolic interactionism.

Data were collected from 34 CNRs and their 31 respective CNEs. Three CNEs had two CNRs each. Inclusion of a CNR in the study required at least 50% employment as a CNR and at least 6 months in the position. The 1983 list of CNRs was screened to find those meeting the inclusion criteria; those included were asked if they were aware of others who might meet the criteria to have the largest possible sample. Thirty-seven CNRs met the criteria; 34 agreed to participate, and one was not interviewed because she was an investigator in the study.

CNRs and CNEs were interviewed by telephone using a semistructured interview between July and December 1983. Transcriptions of all interviews were coded using the following broad categories: organizational context, role activities, role relationships, role development, role performance, and advice to others.

The following information was gathered within the organizational context category. Sixteen (52%) of the institutions had instituted the position in the last 5 years. Most CNRs (71%) had a direct reporting relationshp with the CNE but did not have a budget (62%). Most CNRs (76.5%) had a secretary but did not have professional personnel reporting to them (59%). CNEs (74%) described the strategies they used to both assure viability of the role and integrate the CNR into the organization (Knafl et al., 1987a).

Role activities and relationships was another category. The typical CNR spent half of the work time in research and the other half in administration and staff development (research inservice and consultation). In addition to research activities the CNRs engaged in quality assurance activities, program evaluation, and research utilization. One half of the studies in which the CNRs were engaged were categorized as related to clinical practice (Knafl et al., 1987a).

Enactment of a New Role

Role development was another category of information that was sought in the study. Both CNEs and CNRs believed that they had contributed to the role of the CNR. The CNR shaped the role by convincing others of the importance of nursing research; the CNE provided the structure and support for the activities of the CNR (Knafl et al., 1987a).

Role performance was examined because the incumbents had been in their position for at least 6 months. Both groups evaluated the performance in the CNR role in highly positive terms, although the criteria used in assessment differed. Some focused internally on the organizational contribution, some focused externally on the contribution to science, and some focused on both. CNEs tended to be internally focused, whereas CNRs tended to be both. Roles, organizational contexts, and activities differed across the 31 settings, but the overall impression was that of success. There seemed to be no right way to define and develop the role, but the individual CNR's style and the organizational context need to be considered (Knafl et al., 1987a). Seventy percent of the CNR-CNE pairs had different perceptions of the CNR role, but the differences did not lead to conflict about role enactment (Knafl, Hagle, Bevis, Faux, & Kirchhoff, 1989).

Strategies for Success

Through coding of interview data the following four major goals for successful enactment of the CNR role were identified:

1. Promote interest of the nursing staff in nursing research
2. Increase CNR's autonomy and control over position and activity
3. Demonstrate contribution of nursing research to the organization
4. Convey acceptability as an individual

The CNRs conveyed a need to become part of the organization in this goal. Related strategies were used to accomplish this. For the first goal the strategies included increasing CNR visibility and increasing the staff interest and involvement in research. Strategies used by the CNR to meet the second goal of increasing autonomy were influencing the structure of the position, the budget, and setting limits on involvement. The CNR was involved in communicating outcomes of nursing research and selecting a visible first project to accomplish the third goal of demonstrating nursing research's contribution. The fourth goal, mentioned by 38% of the CNRs, had strategies relating to good interpersonal skills as corroborated by Dennis and Strickland (1987), and being seen on work shifts other than day.

The CNEs had goals of assuring the viability of the position in the hospital, integrating the CNR, and fostering a research climate (Knafl, Hagle, Bevis, & Kirchhoff, 1987). The goals identified by both groups were consistent; this reflected a valuing of nursing research. Because their goals were developmental and focused on the role as well as the activities, they were modified by Schutzenhofer (1991) to focus more on staff nurse activities. These findings for successful research programs are corroborated by Smeltzer and Hinshaw (1988).

Research Activities

The 34 CNRS in this study reported more than 200 projects in which they were involved at the time of the interview. Most of these studies (51%) were initiated by nurses in the institution. Most CNRs (76%) spent their time primarily involved in research. The type of involvement was categorized in one of three models of role enactment: the traditional scientist model in which the CNR takes responsibility for both identifying needed research and conducting it, the associate model in which the CNR takes the lead in either but not both, and the facilitator model in which the CNR works to prepare other nurses to carry out the research. Use of the facilitator model was associated with a large quantity of more ongoing studies (Knafl, Bevis, & Kirchhoff, 1987b).

The findings from this study were reported in a series of publications. They are valid because the sample included almost all known incumbents at the time. The findings were well received by the CNRs at the biennial meeting in 1985, following completion of the study. The number of persons in the role has increased dramatically; some categorizations and separate analyses will be possible should another study be done. For example, those with joint appointments could be compared with those who have only hospital responsibilities. Additional topics could be addressed such as strategies for involving staff nurses in research, focus of the research activities (conduct and utilization), and amount of funding.

The results of this study were contrasted with the various recommendations for the position as published in the literature. Although a doctorate has been agreed on, the benefits of a research and statistical background were compared with those from an extensive clinical background. The personal qualities of the CNR listed in the literature and by the respondents were the most similar of these contrasts; interpersonal relationships were critical in this position. The CNE's sense of organizational commitment was evidenced in the study by the financial support of the position, provision of secretarial support, and direct reporting relationship to the CNE. This support also was evidenced in the literature as summarized by Hagle and colleagues (1986).

Issues in which there was less agreement in the literature and among the

CNRs included whether the position should be line or staff (Mayer, 1983), the way to structure the position, and organizational placement (Kirchhoff, 1981). Various combinations were evident; the research responsibilities were at times associated with responsibilities for quality assurance (Larson, 1983), education, infection control, or other types of evaluative functions. How the researcher was selected (Cronenwett, 1986) and used (Baker, 1978; Cronenwett, 1985; Lawson, 1988) determines the type of potential outcomes for the nursing department.

Wallace and Ventura (1991) listed topics to be considered in the job interview of a CNR: organizational issues, role issues, goals of the program, employment practices, and facilities and resources. When all of these have been satisfactorily discussed, both the CNE and the CNR will have a good foundation for a future positive relationship. All of the required resources and financial requirements should be considered before hiring the CNR. These have been well outlined by Lawson (1988).

The preparation of such an individual is now receiving attention (Dennis, 1991; Lawson, 1989). Dennis (1991) suggested ways to tailor the usual doctoral program to meet the unique educational and experiential needs of those preparing to become CNRs.

The only other study of the CNR role was conducted on a sample at six agencies in the eastern United States and consisted of 10 researchers (Dennis & Strickland, 1987). The advantages of combinations of responsibilities within the clinical setting as well as various ways to augment part-time employment as a CNR were outlined. The different potential foci of the role, administrative or clinical, will pose issues for preparation and selection of the CNR.

PRODUCTIVITY

Although Knafl and associates (1987b) measured aspects of CNR productivity, little additional information has been obtained. Although CNRs have been studied for productivity, they have usually been included as part of other groups, and their data are not presented separately. Part-time CNRs can be lost by being included in studies of faculty productivity without being identified as a subgroup (Megel, Langston, & Creswell, 1988) or in studies of nursing research units (International Council of Nurses, 1984) without the units in hospitals receiving a separate categorization. At other times the number of CNRs may be too small a subsample, that is, 5 of 49 research facilitators (McArt, 1987) to make meaningful comments about the group.

In a telephone survey of Los Angeles Directors of Nursing, 33% ($n = 6$) of the facilities had a nurse researcher; those facilities indicated that moderate to extensive levels of research were being conducted. In contrast the remainder without nurse researchers reported little or no nursing research activity (Betz, Poster, Randell, & Omery, 1990). Other questions were asked about the current research status at each clinical site. In answer to a question about the ideal nursing research program, the most frequent response was "having a nurse researcher."

PROGRAM REPORTS

Descriptions of single programs in hospitals (Campbell & Chulay, 1990; Hegedus & Marino, 1989; Hinshaw & Smeltzer, 1987; Hunt & Waudby, 1990; Keefe & Biester, 1988; Kirchhoff, 1985; Lindeman, 1973; Marchette, 1985; Rempusheski & Chamberlain, 1989; Schutzenhofer, 1991; Stark, 1989) were found and models for how these programs could be structured have been proposed (Engstrom, 1984; Smeltzer & Hinshaw, 1988). Recommendations have been published about how to develop such programs by those who were responsible for them (Chance & Hinshaw, 1980; Lawson, 1987; Mackay, Grantham, & Ross, 1984; Marchette, 1985; Padilla, 1979). Rosswurm (1992) described the development of her program, which is conceptualized as integrating quality improvement with the conduct and use of research.

The use of collaboration as a model across clinical settings was promoted by Stanford and eight other agencies (Zalar, Welches, & Walker, 1985). Courses and consultation were offered as well as a sharing of resources and facilities. Networking among three Boston hospitals to promote a nursing research program was supported by the local Sigma Theta Tau chapter (Hunt et al., 1983). The process of networking was described as idea initiation, role clarification, negotiation, integration, and creativity. Keefe, Pepper, and Stoner (1988) described how the three hospitals linked their research program with a College of Nursing Center for Nursing Research.

Several issues about the optimal structure of the research program within the nursing service department of clinical agencies are unresolved. Should the CNR be "line" or "staff"? With line authority, there is legitimate power; with a staff position there could be expert power. Should the researcher be a director of nursing research with equal status with the other directors of nursing or a research coordinator? Is there one model that will work in all settings, or is it site specific? Should the position be coupled with other administrative responsibilities? If yes, then the researcher will be less productive in facilitating studies. If no, then the researcher may be the first position to be cut when there are budget problems. Should there be a separate budget for research that gives a greater sense of control and more Hays points (if that is the system used) for setting salary ranges? Time is saved, however, by not having a separate budget and the vulnerability to budget cuts might be lessened.

Whether the position should be structured with an academic appointment is another major issue. With an academic appointment, the researcher has colleagues with whom to dialogue and the potential to access needed resources. The appointment usually brings with it some level of time commitment, which could detract from research productivity. However the position is structured, the researcher needs to have a career as well as a job. The career includes time for one's own research and other professional activities. The job will already have long hours that will reduce the energy and time remaining for the career. The usual mechanisms for peer review in career progression are limited unless there also is a faculty appointment; however, faculty may not fully understand the implications of the CNR role.

ORGANIZATIONAL ATTRIBUTES

A Delphi study of the important institutional attributes for success of a nursing research program yielded 53 attributes. The compatibility of research with the agency's mission statement, the CNE support for research and "hard" money support, resources for the program, and the researcher as a dynamic facilitator were the top ranked (Snyder-Halpern, 1991). The top-outcome indicators of successful nursing research programs were the publications, departmentally funded projects that are completed and published, the reward system, the support of the members of the Department of Nursing, and the integration of the research program into the department.

A second Delphi survey by the same investigator was undertaken to validate the 53 attributes from the first study. The top five attributes for success of research programs were (a) the CNE demonstrates enthusiasm and personal support for research, (b) the CNE demonstrates respect for nursing research, (c) the CNR's position is funded by the organization, (d) the CNE values nursing research, and (e) the department's philosophy reflects a value of nursing research (R. Snyder-Halpern, personal communication, March 2, 1992). Also these were categorized in round 3 according to an organizational model of analysis as inputs, transformation process, or outputs. How the panelists interpreted the attributes may influence how they categorized them.

If the CNE's enthusiasm is seen as a response to success rather than a prerequisite, it will be categorized as an output rather than an input. What is yet unanswered is: What are the minimal resources or organizational attributes required for success in the initiation of a research program? Are there institutions that should not initiate such a position until changes are made?

DIRECTIONS FOR FUTURE RESEARCH

Another national survey is needed. Now that the population of CNRs is larger, cross-classifications by type of research program or type of appointment is possible. The factors affecting greater satisfaction for the incumbents and the CNEs could be identified. The institutional characteristics could be assessed and their influence on research productivity outlined.

How these individuals and their institutions evaluate the CNR's productivity needs to be explicated. Is it in terms of numbers of studies or publications or grants, or is it in less quantifiable terms such as morale of the staff, pride in its resources and accomplishments, or the effectiveness of administrative and clinical decisions that have been supported by research? What is the impact of this position on quality of care, especially when the CNR is administratively responsible for that function? What are the effects of such a position on turnover and retention? Conversely, how many of the affected nursing staff have decided to return to school for further education?

When CNRs have left positions, what have been the consequences to the institution? How often has a replacement been made? Is the sample size of this group large enough to draw conclusions about reasons for departure?

An initial database exists for the CNR group. A longitudinal study would be appropriate because participants in the first study were relatively new in their positions.

REFERENCES

American Hospital Association (1985). Strategies: Integration of nursing research into the practice setting. *Nurse executive management strategies* (pp. 1–12). Chicago: Author.

American Society for Nursing Service Administrators (1980). *The role of the nursing service administrator in nursing research*. Chicago: Author.

Baker, V. E. (1978). Nursing administration and research. *Nursing Leadership, 1,* 5–9.

Betz, C. L., Poster, E., Randell, B., & Omery, A. (1990). Nursing research productivity in clinical settings. *Nursing Outlook, 38,* 180–183.

Campbell, G. M., & Chulay, M. (1990). Establishing a clinical nursing research program. In J. G. Spicer & M. Robinson (Eds.), *Managing the environment in critical care nursing* (pp. 52–60). Baltimore, MD: Williams & Wilkins.

Chance, H. C., & Hinshaw, A. S. (1980). Strategies for initiating a research program. *Journal of Nursing Administration, 10*(3), 32–39.

Cronenwett, L. R. (1985). Hiring a nurse researcher. *Journal of Nursing Administration, 15*(10), 5–7.

Cronenwett, L. R. (1986). Selecting a nurse researcher. *Journal of Nursing Administration, 16*(1), 7–8.

Cross, E. D. (1977). Nursing research in the Veteran's Administration. *Nursing Research, 26,* 250–252.

Davis, M. Z. (1981). Promoting nursing research in the clinical setting. *Journal of Nursing Administration, 11*(2), 22–27.

Dennis, K. E. (1991). Components of the doctoral curriculum that build success in the clinical nurse researcher role. *Journal of Professional Nursing, 7,* 160–165.

Dennis, K. E., & Strickland, O. L. (1987). The clinical nurse researcher: Institutionalizing the role. *International Journal of Nursing Studies, 24*(1), 25–33.

Egan, E. C., McElmurry, B. J., & Jameson, H. M. (1981). Practice-based research: Assessing your department's readiness. *Journal of Nursing Administration, 11*(10), 26–32.

Engstrom, J. L. (1984). University, agency, and collaborative models for nursing research: An overview. *Image: Journal of Nursing Scholarship, 16,* 76–80.

Hagle, M. E., Kirchhoff, K. T., Knafl, K. A., & Bevis, B. E. (1986). The clinical nurse researcher: New perspectives. *Journal of Professional Nursing, 2,* 282–288.

Hegedus, K. S., & Marino, B. L. (1989). The nursing research program at Children's Hospital, Boston. *Journal of Nursing Administration, 19*(6), 9–10.

Hinshaw, A. S., & Smeltzer, C. H. (1987). Research challenges and programs for practice settings. *Journal of Nursing Administration, 17*(7–8), 20–26.

Hoare, K., & Earenfight, J. (1986). Unit-based research in a service setting. *Journal of Nursing Administration, 16*(4), 35–40.

Hunt, V., Stark, J. L., Fisher, F., Hegedus, K., Joy, L., & Woldum, K. (1983). Networking: A managerial strategy for research development in a service setting. *Journal of Nursing Administration, 13* (7–8), 27–32.

Hunt, V., & Waudby, E. (1990). The nursing research model at St. Elizabeth's Hospital, Boston. *Journal of Nursing Administration, 20*(10), 4–5.

International Council of Nurses (1984). Survey of nursing research units: ICN report. *International Nursing Review, 31*(4), 116–121.

Keefe, M. R., & Biester, D. J. (1988). Developing a research program in a clinical setting. *Journal of Pediatric Nursing, 3,* 269–272.

Keefe, M. R., Pepper, G., & Stoner, M. (1988). Toward research-based nursing practice: The Denver collaborative research network. *Applied Nursing Research, 1,* 109–115.

Kirchhoff, K. T. (1981). Information exchange: Request for assistance. *Western Journal of Nursing Research, 3,* 421–423.

Kirchhoff, K. T. (1985). Employed for research in the clinical setting. In K. E.

Barnard & G. R. Smith (Eds.), *Faculty practice in action* (pp. 201–211). Kansas City, MO: American Academy of Nursing.

Knafl, K. A., Bevis, M. E., & Kirchhoff, K. T. (1987a). Development and enactment of a new role. [Newsletter]. *Council of Nurse Researchers, 14,* 1–4.

Knafl, K. A., Bevis, M. E., & Kirchhoff, K. T. (1987b). Research activities of clinical nurse researchers. *Nursing Research, 36,* 249–252.

Knafl, K. A., Hagle, M. E., Bevis, M. E., Faux, S. A., & Kirchhoff, K. T. (1989). How researchers and administrators view the role of the clinical nurse researcher. *Western Journal of Nursing Research, 11,* 583–592.

Knafl, K. A., Hagle, M. E., Bevis, M. E., & Kirchhoff, K. T. (1987). Clinical nurse researchers: Strategies for success. *Journal of Nursing Administration, 17*(10), 27–31.

Larson, E. (1983). Combining nursing quality assurance and research programs. *The Journal of Nursing Administration, 13*(11), 32–35.

Lawson, L. L. (1987). Developing a research structure within the nursing department. *Journal of Nursing Administration, 17*(11), 6–7.

Lawson, L. L. (1988). Functions of the nurse researcher. *Journal of Nursing Administration, 18,* 8–9, 23.

Lawson, L. L. (1989). Developing investigators who will generate clinically relevant science. *Journal of Nursing Administration, 19*(1), 6–7.

Lindeman, C. A. (1973). Nursing research: A visible, viable component of nursing practice. *Journal of Nursing Administration, 3*(2), 18–21.

MacKay, R. C., Grantham, M. A., & Ross, S. E. M. (1984). Building a hospital nursing research department. *Journal of Nursing Administration, 14*(7–8), 23–27.

Marchette, L. (1985). Developing a productive nursing research program in a clinical institution. *Journal of Nursing Administration, 15*(3), 25–30.

Mayer, G. G. (1983). The clinical nurse-researcher: Role-taking and role-making. In N. L. Chaska (Ed.), *The nursing profession: A time to speak* (pp. 216–223). New York: McGraw-Hill.

McArt, E. W. (1987). Research facilitation in academic and practice settings. *Journal of Professional Nursing, 3,* 84–91.

Megel, M. E., Langston, N. F., & Creswell, J. W. (1988). Scholarly productivity: A survey of nursing faculty researchers. *Journal of Professional Nursing, 4,* 45–54.

Padilla, G. V. (1979). Incorporating research in a service setting. *Journal of Nursing Administration, 9*(1), 44–49.

Pettengill, M. M., Knafl, K. A., Bevis, M. E., & Kirchhoff, K. T. (1988). Nursing research in midwestern hospitals. *Western Journal of Nursing Research, 10,* 705–717.

Rempusheski, V. F. (1991). Incorporating research role and practice role. *Applied Nursing Research, 4,* 46–48.

Rempusheski, V. F., & Chamberlain, S. L. (1989). Nursing research image at Beth Israel Hospital, Boston. *Journal of Nursing Administration, 19*(10), 6–7.

Rosswurm, M. A. (1992). A research-based practice model in a hospital setting. *Journal of Nursing Administration, 22*(3), 57–60.

Schutzenhofer, K. K. (1991). Scholarly pursuits in the clinical setting: An obligation of professional nursing. *Journal of Professional Nursing, 17,* 10–15.

Smeltzer, C. H., & Hinshaw, A. S. (1988). Research: Clinical integration for excellent patient care. *Nursing Management, 19*(1), 38–40, 44.

Snyder-Halpern, R. (1991). Attributes of service-based nursing research programs useful for decision-making. *Nursing Administration Quarterly, 15*(4), 82–84.

Stark, J. L. (1989). A multiple-strategy based research program for staff nurse involvement. *Journal of Nursing Administration, 19*(9), 7–8.

Stetler, C. B. (1983). Nurses and research: Responsibility and involvement. *National Intravenous Therapy Association 6,* 207–212.

Stetler, C. B. (1984). *Nursing research in a service setting.* Reston, VA: Reston.

Thurston, N. E., Tenove, S. C., & Church, J. M. (1990). Hospital nursing research is alive and flourishing! *Nursing Management, 25*(5), 50–54.

Wake, M. M. (1990). Nursing care delivery systems: Status and vision. *Journal of Nursing Administration, 20*(5), 47–51.

Wallace, K. G., & Ventura, M. R. (1991). Planning the interview for a clinical nurse researcher. *Journal of Nursing Administration, 21*(12), 54–59.

Werley, H. (1962, March). Promoting the research dimension in the practice of nursing through the establishment and development of a department of nursing in an institute of research. *Military Medicine,* 219–231.

Zalar, M. K., Welches, L. J., & Walker, D. D. (1985). Nursing consortium approach to increase research in service settings. *The Journal of Nursing Administration, 15*(7–8), 36–41.

PART III

Research on Nursing Education

Chapter 8

Nurse-Midwifery Education

CLAIRE M. ANDREWS
FRANCES PAYNE BOLTON SCHOOL OF NURSING
CASE WESTERN RESERVE UNIVERSITY

CAROL E. DAVIS
COLLEGE OF NURSING UNIVERSITY OF SOUTH CAROLINA

CONTENTS

Nurse-midwifery education in the United States has now entered a 7th decade. Built on early apprenticeship models for ensuring safety and excellence of practice, nurse-midwifery schools in the second 50 years continue in experiental traditions established by early leaders such as Mary Breckinridge (Lubic, 1982). Content delivery, however, has evolved from tutorial, on-site

The authors acknowledge the contribution to this chapter by Gail Mitchell, Ph.D.

instruction to include modular, off-campus, and community-based self-paced learning. Published research findings to support evolution of nurse-midwifery education, to serve as a foundation for programmatic methods and curricular design, and to guide delivery of instruction are almost nonexistent. A call by Baxter in 1980, "Nurse-midwifery research is needed . . . in nurse-midwifery education" (p. 1) was followed by several reports in the literature. The focus of this chapter is to examine critically those studies that have been done and to report newer nurse-midwifery educational models that have been described in the literature. A historical overview of nurse-midwifery education and research is provided. Finally, reported findings are used as a stimulus for identifying emerging trends and the impact of sociologic and political issues on nurse-midwifery education.

SELECTION OF STUDIES FOR REVIEW

Cooper (1982) described the integrative research review as the synthesis of separate empiric findings into a coherent whole. The intent of the authors was to conduct such a review on the topic of nurse-midwifery education research.

To retrieve information on the topic of nurse-midwifery education research, the reviewers conducted the following computer and visual searches of nursing and allied health English literature using the following key words: nursing, midwifery, education, and research.

Computer searches were done of *Cumulative Index of Nursing and Allied Health Literature* for the dates 1983 to 1991; Doctoral Dissertation Abstracts for the period from 1900 to 1991; and Psychological Abstracts from 1974 to 1991. Visual searches were done of the *Cumulative Index of Nursing and Allied Health Literature* from 1956 to 1983 and of the *International Nursing Index* from 1966 to 1983.

Additionally, the ancestry approach was used to track former studies cited in reference lists (Cooper, 1982). These various methods of retrieving literature on nurse-midwifery education research produced a total of only seven published research reports. Of the more than 300 articles reviewed on nurse-midwifery education, most were focused on explication of multiple problems and concerns, teaching strategies and curriculum models, anecdotal descriptions of clinical experiences, philosophic issues, testing and certification, faculty shortages, problems in academia, and funding issues.

REPORTED RESEARCH ON NURSE-MIDWIFERY EDUCATION

Reported research in nurse-midwifery education was grouped into the following categories: (a) investigations of characteristics of applicants seeking admission to nurse-midwifery programs or personality characteristics associated with success in nurse-midwifery programs ($n = 2$); (b) investigations of needs of knowledge with attitudes of student nurse-midwives ($n = 2$); (c) testing or certification research ($n = 2$); and (d) one feasibility study on an intercampus model for graduate education in nurse practitioner–midwifery ($n = 1$). Additionally, three anecdotal reports of different program evaluations are included to analyze existing opinion about innovative educational approaches in nurse-midwifery.

Characteristics of Applicants and Successful Students

Two studies were found that explored characteristics of applicants to and successful students in nurse-midwifery programs. Warpinski and Adams (1979) conducted a survey to "obtain information on applicants to nurse-midwifery educational programs . . . so that recommendations could be made concerning future planning for nurse-midwifery education in the United States" (p. 5). The researchers sought empiric data to support claims that applicants to nurse-midwifery educational programs exceeded available positions. A researcher-developed questionnaire was completed on 649 submitted applications from 16 nurse-midwifery programs in the United States. A matching process eliminated 130 duplicate applications, leaving a total sample of 519 questionnaires representing different applicants.

Findings indicated 83.4% of applicants applied to only one program. Descriptive statistics were presented on variables of gender, race, marital status, number of children, geographic location, citizenship, grade-point average, graduate record examination, and nursing background. Chi-square and *t*-test analyses were conducted to determine differences on dependent variables between applicants to certificate programs and applicants to master's programs. There were 238 applicants for 74 places in graduate programs and 310 applicants for 66 places in certificate programs. Based on these findings, the researchers recommended development of nurse-midwifery educational programs especially in states where no programs existed. Warpinski and Adams (1979) concluded with the following recommendations: (a) integrating certificate programs into formal educational systems; (b) providing credit for prior experience and learning; (c) instituting part-time study; and (d) establishing registered nurse (RN) to master's of science in nursing (MSN) programs in universities.

This descriptive survey provided valuable information about multiple characteristics of applicants to nurse-midwifery educational programs. Major limitations of the report are related to the researcher-developed questionnaire. First, the questionnaire was never fully described. Second, the researchers stated the questionnaire was pretested by two persons who filled out questionnaires to identify problems with interpretation and response. Discussion of reliability of the tool was limited to this pretest with subsequent revisions. Investigators did not identify persons who filled out the questionnaires at the 16 program sites nor did they mention if these persons received any uniform instruction in completing the questionnaires.

The surplus of applicants for available placements in nurse-midwifery programs changed dramatically from 1980 to 1990 for traditional nurse-midwifery education programs. Rooks, Carr, and Sandvold (1991) reported that "although the number of students entering nurse-midwifery education programs increased to 231 in 1989, 9% of the places in our educational programs were not filled last year" (p. 125). This decrease in applicants contributed to the current shortage of nurse-midwives and focused attention on recruitment issues.

Bry and Marsico (1980) launched a study to determine whether success in nurse-midwifery education and practice was related to specific personality characteristics. The fact that some nurses successfully completed a nurse-midwifery program without going into practice after graduating, at a time when such practitioners were desperately needed, prompted this investigation.

Researchers used the California Psychological Inventory (CPI) (Gough, 1956) to measure characteristics of 36 RN students enrolled in two nurse-midwifery programs, one certificate and one master's degree. The CPI was administered somewhere between decision to apply and completion of first year of the program. "Success" in nurse-midwifery was defined by four criteria: (a) completion of the program, (b) completion within a specified time, (c) completion without the faculty becoming concerned, and (d) entry into practice within 6 months of graduation. Of the 36 students, 19 were classified as successful based on established criteria. Stepwise discriminate analysis was computed using the 18 CPI scale scores and age as independent variables. Success was the dependent variable. Findings indicated 94% of subjects were correctly classified based on the Socialization, Dominance, Tolerance, and Self-Control subscales of the CPI. Based on subscale characteristics, Bry and Marsico (1980) described the potential nurse-midwifery student and successful practitioner as an individual who conforms to social mores, takes initiative once understanding is reached, is accepting and nonjudgmental of people and places, and is not impulsive in actions. The investigators concluded with a call for studies to validate predictive value of the CPI for identifying nurse applicants who would not only complete their nurse-midwifery education but who would then enter practice.

The major weakness of this study was the extremely small sample size coupled with 19 independent variables for statistical analysis. Nunnally (1978) recommended 30 subjects per independent variable for statistical regression and cautioned that 10 subjects per variable in factor analysis presents serious problems. The sample in this study consisted of 36 subjects. Bry and Marsico (1980) did acknowledge the very preliminary nature of the study. Another limitation of this research was that differences between subjects based on type of program were not addressed.

Identification of Needs and Attitudes Toward the Learning Experience

Walsh and Jaspan (1990) conducted a study to identify perceived learning needs of lay midwives entering nurse-midwifery education programs and to explore attitudes that may influence the learning experiences of these students. The impetus to do this study was the reported decline of applications to nurse-midwifery education programs. A survey questionnaire was used for this descriptive research. The instrument was developed by the investigators who identified variables that may influence (a) student-educator relationships, (b) attitudes toward midwifery practice, and (c) attitudes toward educational approaches in nurse-midwifery education. The instrument is not fully described with the exception of the attitudinal survey. There is some evidence of validity, but reliability of the instrument is not addressed.

Two types of respondants were sought: nurse midwifery educators (in American College of Nurse-Midwives [ACNM] accredited programs) and nurse-midwives who were lay midwives when they entered nurse-midwifery education programs. The report did not state if the second group were recent graduates or not. Time since graduation may well have influenced responses. The sample did not include lay midwives who were currently enrolled in a nurse-midwifery education program. This is a weakness when considering the stated purpose of the study.

The investigators wrote to nurse-midwifery program directors of the 24 ACNM-accredited programs. Twenty-one program directors agreed, and the survey was sent to the respective nurse-midwifery faculty. Of the 116 surveys sent, 63 (54%) were returned for analysis. Certified nurse-midwives who were lay midwives when they entered a nurse-midwifery program were identified from an advertisement that was placed in two midwifery journals, word of mouth, and personal referrals. Twenty-one surveys were sent, and 13 (62%) were returned. The small sample size is a limitation.

Nurse-midwife educators stated that, compared with traditional nurse-midwifery students, the lay midwife nurse-midwifery students relied on experience and intuition for decision making rather than scientific method/systematic data collection; were reluctant to use technology-based interventions when appropriate; and were not socialized into the medical-nursing world. The lay midwife nurse-midwifery students perceived themselves as differing from traditional students. They believed they were stronger in midwifery skills; were weaker in areas not usually addressed in lay midwifery preparation (i.e., pharmacology, high-risk pregnancies); needed to learn the language of medicine; and had greater needs regarding complex management.

Nurse-midwifery educators tended to have positive attitudes toward lay-midwife nurse-midwifery students. Between 25% and 50% conveyed some negative remarks regarding their worth and abilities as students.

Knowledge and Attitudes About Sex

Using a descriptive, exploratory survey design, Greener and Reagan (1986) investigated student nurse-midwives' knowledge and attitudes about human sexuality. These researchers postulated that nurse-midwives have a sound knowledge base, and an open, accepting attitude, which must adequately manage problems and concerns of families. Two parts (attitudes and knowledge) of the Sex Knowledge and Attitudes Test (Preliminary Technical Manual, 1979) and a demographic and background questionnaire were distributed to 320 nurse-midwife students enrolled in nurse-midwifery programs throughout the United States.

The response rate was 55% (179) with 34% returned by students in certificate programs and 66% returned by students in master's programs. Measures of central tendency were reported on sociodemographic and educational data. Each subject received five raw scores on the Sex Knowledge and Attitudes Test, which were analyzed using Pearson product moment correlation. The researchers also computed *t*-tests on selected variables to determine significant differences between groups.

Significant positive relationships were reported between knowledge and some but not all attitudes. More knowledgeable students were more liberal in attitude toward autoerotic activities but not toward premarital and extramarital heterosexual relations or abortion. Sexual myths were rejected more frequently by students with more education. Prior education in human sexuality was shown to increase knowledge but not necessarily to influence attitude; however, less knowledgeable students were less tolerant and vice versa. When groups were compared on the basis of age, marital status, length of time in nursing, or level in nurse-midwifery program, no significant differences were found. Significant differences were accounted for, however, when groups were compared on religion, educational level, degree of urbanization, type of midwifery program, and prior education in human sexuality.

Greener and Reagan (1986) concluded that, in general, nurse-midwife students were knowledgeable about human sexuality but views about abortion were generally conservative. The researchers addressed limitations of the study related to lack of information about nonrespondents. Content limitations of the instrument to only four areas of human sexuality led researchers to recommend further pre–postexperimental studies for evaluating the value of human sexuality education as relates to unique needs of nurse-midwifery students. The investigators suggested further research to establish a knowledge base about the role of knowledge and attitude toward human sexuality for nurse-midwives who counsel families.

Testing and Certification

Fullerton and Thompson (1985) reported findings from a study "designed to test the feasibility of using entry-level certification examination as a tool for reevaluation of competence (recertification)" (p. 72). The researchers specifically looked at differences on scores between first-time and midcareer candidates, differences between nurse-midwives according to career focus (practice, administration, education), and differences according to demographic indices.

An initial intent to conduct stratified random sampling was not possible so researchers settled for 82 first-time candidates and 62 volunteers in the recertification category. The desired stratification of one faculty, two administrators, and five practitioners also was not achieved in the volunteer sample. All subjects completed the American College of Nurse-Midwives National Certification Examination (Form 980). This essay format test assesses cognitive knowledge and judgment in six areas of nurse-midwifery practice: antepartum, intrapartum, postpartum, newborn, family planning and well-women gynecology, and professional issues.

Data were analyzed using a one-way analysis of variance between the four research groups (i.e., three categories of recertification candidates and first-time candidates). Mean score performance on the six subscales of the examination was identified as the criterion variable. Significant differences were found among the four groups in performance on all subscales except postpartum.

Fullerton and Thompson (1985) reported that mean scores for the recertification group were significantly less than first-time candidate means. Failure rate for the recertification candidates was reported to be higher than the 12% of first-time candidates. The faculty subgroup of recertification subjects scored consistently higher in all six subareas than the administration group with the practitioner scoring in between.

Findings, although limited by nonrandom nature of the sample, indicated that for nurse-midwives involved in practice and education, competency was maintained according to written criteria. Investigators endorsed recertification as a valid measure for assessing cognitive competency over time. Recommendations for future research were centered on the need to develop creative ways for determining the practical skills component of competency. Also addressed was the need for criterion-referenced scoring, concurrent validity of examination process, and peer review and self-assessment strategies needed for assuring continued competency.

Fullerton, Howell, and Kim (1986) tested the feasibility of using single-response multiple choice as an alternative format to the essay response traditional format for the ACNM certification examination. The multiple-choice format was constructed by members of the ACNM Division of Examiners and was originally piloted with eight certified nurse-midwives who were on the committee but who had not been involved in test construction. Further revisions produced the final 92-item multiple-choice format that was administered to 138 volunteer candidates who were ready to sit for the ACNM certification examination.

Item analysis procedures for determining difficulty, discriminatory power, and effectiveness of distractors were computed. Four of the 92 test items exceeded acceptable levels of difficulty, and 13 of the 92 items were shown to be poor discriminators. The reliability index using the Kuder Richardson formula, was .73, which was judged sufficient to use the examination. To determine if subject performance was independent of examination format, each candidate's scores from the two examinations were plotted against each other. Analysis of variables indicated no significant differences among subjects on either format as a result of sociodemographic variables.

The correlation between multiple-choice scores and essay scores was $r = 0.30$, which was interpreted as a modest relationship. Fullerton and associates (1986) concluded that a reliable multiple-choice test was constructed, but equivalence with the traditional pen-and-paper formation was not established. The researchers suggested that knowing the multiple choice did not really count may have influenced student performance attitudes. A recommendation for further exploration of possible alternative formats was proposed.

Intercampus Feasibility Study

A feasibility study was conducted by Weiss, McLain, and Fullerton (1988) to determine the possibility of developing a collaborative intercampus network for graduate studies in nursing. A critical need for practitioners in primary care and nurse-midwifery in the San Diego area, coupled with inadequate educational opportunities, activated educators in the Primary Care Nurse

Practitioner Program at the San Diego School of Medicine to expand educational opportunities by negotiating a collaborative MSN venture with the University of California at San Francisco School of Nursing.

The goal of educators to develop a viable model for the intercampus MSN was accomplished through efforts of an advisory committee with representatives from both campuses. Data were collected through interview with select individuals (faculty, administrators, students); review of documents (curriculum materials, policies, relevant literature); and consultation with a National League for Nursing accreditation expert.

An intercampus model was accepted and administrative, curricular, fiscal, and faculty criteria established. Additionally, an evaluation plan was established. The intercampus model was found to have both strengths and limitations. Strengths were identified as increased enrollments, increased number and variety of clinical sites, increased graduate practitioners to serve the community, and increased collegial relationships among faculty, The San Diego campus was particularly valued for providing rich practice experiences for nurse-midwives. Limitations related to the difficulties with travel for some students, the time and effort required for ensuring congruent philosophies and curricula between programs, unequal resources, complex lines of communication and collegiality for intercampus students, and the challenge of developing efficient policies and procedures for processing information. Overall, the intercampus model was described as an extremely viable option for increasing educational opportunities for graduate nursing students.

NONRESEARCH PROGRAM EVALUATIONS

Two accounts of off-campus pilot projects were described in the literature (Farr & Funches, 1982; Lonsdale, Murdaugh, & Stiles, 1982). These reports, although not research based, provide valuable accounts of possible collaborative opportunities that can result from efforts of committed individuals. Farr and Funches (1982) described a joint program between the nurse-midwifery program at the School of Allied Health Professions at the College of Medicine and Dentistry in Newark, New Jersey, with the McTammany Nurse-Midwifery Center, Inc., located in Reading, Pennsylvania. The nurse-midwives were providers of full-service private practice with deliveries equally distributed among home, hospital, and birthing center. This nurse-midwifery certificate program was 1 year in length and used a modular-based curriculum. Practicing nurse-midwives initiated the collaborative off campus effort out of desire to participate in quality nurse-midwifery education. They knew they could provide students with a rich experience of midwifery practice managed by nurses. The program in New Jersey was limited by dependence on medical center placements for student experiences. Farr and Funches (1982) presented details of the pilot off-campus experience and the success of two students. Evaluations from both agencies and students were positive.

Similarly, Lonsdale and colleagues (1982) described the collaborative efforts between Su Clinica Familiar, a nurse-midwifery clinic in Texas, with the Georgetown University Midwifery Education Program in Washington, D.C. A successful certificate program was implemented for a 1-year period to expand clinical sites for students and increase midwifery practice to the community served by Su Clinica. The program ended after 1 year because of a change in focus at the university, but the authors provide valuable suggestions for others embarking on collaborative efforts to enhance nurse-midwifery education. Yates (1983) described an accredited refresher program at Booth Maternity Center in Philadelphia. The unique philosophy and modular program provided a rich individualized learning experience for nurse-midwives. Unique needs of the refresher student in nurse-midwifery were highlighted. Yates defined success of the program in terms of successful certification of graduates, and the high percentage (79%) of refreshers who were employed in practice.

CRITICAL ANALYSIS OF RESEARCH IN NURSE-MIDWIFERY EDUCATION

The state of research-generated knowledge in nurse-midwifery education is extremely limited but not without value. The fledgling status of nurse-midwifery education research, as indicated by this review, has substantiated important areas of concern.

Researchers have been concerned about maximizing the benefit from limited student placement in nurse-midwifery programs by identifying possible characteristics linked to success to recruit students most likely to excel. They have been concerned about methods to make certification testing as efficient and reliable as possible, and ensure competency for existing practitioners. And, perhaps most evident, is their concern to establish and evaluate alternative educational models including community-based sites for nurse-midwife students. Students require experience in nonmedical practice settings that focus on labor and birth as an uncomplicated experience for healthy women and their families. Research identifying and evaluating the different practice patterns characteristic of graduates with experience in the different practice sites will be invaluable. These concerns parallel the concerns of nurse-midwifery educators not conducting research and the changing nature of nurse-midwifery as it unfolds in the United States.

HISTORICAL PERSPECTIVE OF NURSE-MIDWIFERY EDUCATION AND RESEARCH

The trajectory of education and research in nurse-midwifery is displayed in Table 8.1. The first program to prepare graduate nurses in nurse-midwifery was started in 1932 at The Maternity Center Association School of Nurse-Midwifery in New York (Hsia, 1982). Growth was slow in ensuing decades. By 1960, there were only seven programs for nurse-midwives (Dempkowski, 1982). The 1970s, however, witnessed a rapid expansion of federally funded nurse-midwifery programs (Hsia, 1982). By 1981, there were 21 training programs (Dempkowski, 1982), and by 1985 there were 25 programs: 16 graduate and 9 certificate programs (Raisler, 1987). In 1991, there were 34 programs: 22 graduate, 10 certificate, and 2 precertification programs (Roberts, 1991).

The first mention of a specific research project related to nurse-midwifery education appeared in the literature in 1975 from the Northeast Regional Council on Education for Nurse-Midwives. One of the priority projects identified by this council was research to determine personality characteristics of successful nurse-midwifery students. Beebe (1977) emphasized the need to search for admission criteria that best predicted motivation and success for professional midwifery practice. Warpinski and Adams published their study on the characteristics of applicants to nurse-midwifery programs in 1979. This was followed by the Bry and Marsico (1980) research proposing specific personality characteristics of successful nurse-midwifery students.

In 1977, Marsico addressed the need to move clinical experiences of nurse-midwives from traditional medical center practice to alternative birthing centers. She called for research investigating professional outcomes of professional responsibility and confidence for students between groups of nurses who completed clinical experience in medical centers versus midwifery practice centers.

By the early 1980s, the calls for research became more frequent. Baxter (1980) claimed nurse-midwifery was suffering from lack of research in three main areas: maternal-fetal outcomes, specific clinical practices, and nurse-

Table 8.1 Historical Overview of Nurse-Midwifery Events, Education, and Research

Year	*Event*	*Curriculum/ intervention*	*Research*
1932	Maternity Center Association School of Nursing—first program to prepare graduate nurses to become nurse-midwives	Tutorial method of instruction and apprenticeship	
1939	Frontier Nursing Service opened school of nurse-midwifery		
1947	First master's of nursing with certificate in nurse-midwifery at Catholic University of America (closed 1968)		
1960	Nurse-midwifery practice severely restricted in United States; only three jurisdictions provide for nurse-midwifery practice		
1965	Nine active schools in United States		
1970	Success of the Frontier Nursing Service and Maternity Center Association led to rapid expansion of programs with federal funding; acute shortage of faculty	Modular curriculum initiated; learning outcomes in form of measurable objectives; student viewed as active learner	
1975			Northeast Regional Council on Education for nurse-midwifery; development of clinical challenge exams for terminal behaviors
1977	Call to search for admission criteria that measure motivation and maturity for success in professional practice; call to move clinical experiences out of traditional medical centers		

1979	Core competencies in nurse-midwifery developed by Educational Committee of the American College of Nurse-Midwifery		Survey research on characteristics of applicants in nurse-midwifery educational programs
1980	Educational programs for nurse-midwifery now at 21; currently 2,000 nurse-midwives		Research on personality characteristics associated with success in learning and practicing nurse-midwifery
1982	Call for research to evaluate effect of current educational systems and possible educational alternatives		
1982	Twenty-three educational programs; financial cutbacks and shortage of faculty; call to develop innovative educational programs and off-campus and part-time experiences for learning and challenge examinations		Two reports of successful off-campus nurse-midwifery educational programs; one report on refresher program
1984	Community Based Nurse-Midwifery Education Program established by Maternity Center Association, Frances Payne Bolton School of Nursing, National Association of Childbearing Centers, and Frontier Nursing Service	Marketing model of education; principles of adult learning; student viewed as consumer; modular, self-directed learning; challenge examinations	
	Repeated concerns to move clinical experiences out of medical centers		
1985	Twenty-six basic educational programs in nurse-midwifery	Provision of educational opportunities that do not require students to leave families and communities	Research testing recertification in nurse-midwifery
			Research exploring knowledge and attitudes of student nurse-midwives on human sexuality

Table 8.1 *(continued)*

Year	*Event*	*Curriculum/ intervention*	*Research*
			Research assessing alternative to essay format of certification examination
1988	First 16 students admitted to Community-Based Nurse-Midwifery Education Program		Feasibility study for collaborative intercampus model for graduate studies in nurse-midwifery
1989	Four thousand nurse-midwives in United States		
1991	Number of new graduates increases after decade of decline; more placements than applicants; need for intense recruitment; call to support certificate programs and non-MSN programs; call for research to compare outcomes of various nurse-midwifery educational programs		
1992	Thirty-four nurse-midwifery programs; largest nurse-midwifery class to date admitted to Community Based Nurse-Midwifery Education Program (CNEP), 140 students		

midwifery education. Corbett and Marsico (1981) posited that faculty were not rewarded in traditional academic settings and that nurse-midwifery education was suffering in medical centers dominated by the biomedical, high-technology approach to labor and delivery. The need to explore alternatives in education was particularly emphasized in the first half of the 1980s (Corbett & Marsico, 1981; Elder, 1984; Hsia, 1982; Hurzeler, 1981; Kaplan, 1981). The following year, articles describing off-campus student-faculty experiences emerged in the literature (Farr & Funches, 1982; Lonsdale et al.,

1982). These case-study–type reports indicated collaboration between academic and practice settings was possible and that outcomes were most promising.

In 1984, additional cutbacks in funding for nurse-midwifery education forced closure of several nurse-midwifery schools (University of Mississippi Medical Center, St. Louis University Graduate Program, and University of Arizona Nurse-Midwifery Program) (Varney, 1987). Educational literature in this era focused on needs to expand options for learning through part-time study and challenge examinations (Elder, 1984). Again, inadequacy of medical center clinical experiences was cited as a major concern. The Frontier School of Nurse-Midwifery and Family Nursing rose to the challenge and initiated a major collaborative effort to combine university resources with clinical resources in nurse-midwifery community birthing centers. A community-based nurse-midwifery educational program (CNEP) was established through the joint efforts of the Maternity Center Association in New York, the Frances Payne Bolton School of Nursing at Case Western Reserve University, the National Association of Childbearing Centers, and the Frontier Nursing Service (Ernst, 1989). In 1988, the first 16 students were admitted into CNEP and interest in the program was reported as exceedingly high (Ernst, 1989). This is evidenced by the admission of 92 students in 1991 and 140 students in 1992.

Between 1985 and 1988, four of the five studies presented earlier emerged in the literature. While it appeared that a trend for more research was emerging, the expected increase in research activities has not been sustained. Paine and Greener (1989), reporting on the 1987–1988 ACNM Needs Assessment Survey, indicated that only 21 (2.8%) of the 748 nurse-midwives listed research in nurse-midwifery education as most important. Fifty percent of the responses indicated issues of safety, quality, and outcomes of practice were most valuable. The concern for safe, quality practice is understandable, but the 2.8% of persons who listed research in education as most important is alarmingly small given the plethora of documented concerns about nurse-midwifery education. Another explanation for the dearth of research in nurse-midwifery education could be that program and evaluative research is now occurring and has not yet reached the literature. A more likely explanation is the paucity of doctoral-prepared nurse-midwives interested in nurse-midwifery education research.

NEED FOR DOCTORAL-EDUCATED NURSE-MIDWIVES

Several authors have addressed consequences of the lack of doctoral-prepared nurse-midwives (Corbett & Marsico, 1981; Raisler, 1987). Raisler suggested

"Our profession has been notably reluctant to accept the doctorate as the necessary qualification for faculty and clinical practice leadership" (1987, p. 1). If nurse-midwifery is a specialty in its own right, with a unique knowledge base, it must have doctoral-prepared scholars to establish and extend a scientific and theoretically sound knowledge base.

IMPACT OF MEDICAL CENTER PRACTICE ON NURSE-MIDWIFERY EDUCATOR

The diverging philosophic approaches of medicine and nurse-midwifery are also taking a toll on nurse-midwifery education. Hsia (1982) stated that when medicine encouraged women to deliver their babies in hospitals in the 1950s, nurse-midwives lost their hold on professional autonomy. For two decades nurse-midwifery practice was restricted to hospital practice in New York State (Hsia, 1982). Even the advent of hospital-based birthing rooms did not significantly alter the medicalization of labor and birth.

Corbett and Marsico (1981) and Elder (1984), to name just two sources, have drawn attention to the problems of medical center clinical sites for educating nurse-midwives. The off-campus projects described earlier indicate viable alternatives, but competition for resources and shortage of academically prepared faculty severely impact further development of such projects. The intercampus model between the San Diego School of Medicine and the University of California at San Francisco School of Nursing clearly led the way to a new era in nurse-midwifery education.

DIRECTIONS FOR FUTURE RESEARCH

Undoubtedly, research in nurse-midwifery is mandated on this eve of the 21st century. Educators must build programs and develop curricula based on evaluative outcomes. While research guides practice, research findings must also form the foundation for further programs. The authors offer the following 10 foci of critical areas deserving of investigation: research-based program evaluation; replication-extension predictors for successful graduates who practice; research comparing outcomes from different programs; research exploring barriers to higher education; research evaluating quality of life-health for families cared for by nurse-midwives educated in alternative birthing centers;

philosophic research (for theory generation and values clarification in nurse-midwifery); qualitative research that explores professional satisfaction in practice and academia; qualitative research that explores why certified nurse-midwives leave practice or choose not to go into nurse-midwifery practice following graduation; research on recruitment and retention issues; and research exploring specific learning needs of nurse-midwife students.

REFERENCES

Baxter, L. (1980). Thoughts on nurse-midwifery and research. *Journal of Nurse-Midwifery, 25*(3), 1–2.

Beebe, J. E. (1977). The future of nurse-midwifery education: Survival of the profession. *Journal of Nurse-Midwifery, 12*(3), 16–19.

Bry, B. H., & Marsico, C. N. (1980). Personality characteristics associated with success in learning and practicing nursing-midwifery. *Journal of Nurse-Midwifery, 25*(3), 11–15.

Cooper, H. M. (1982). Scientific guidelines for conducting integrative research reviews. *Review of Educational Research, 52,* 291–302.

Corbett, M. A., & Marsico, T. (1981). Faculty burn-out in nurse-midwifery education. *Journal of Nurse-Midwifery, 26*(5), 32–36.

Dempkowski, A. (1982). Future prospects of nurse-midwifery in the United States. *Journal of Nurse-Midwifery, 27*(2), 9–15.

Elder, N. (1984). Nurse-midwifery education—Present and future perspectives at FNS. *Frontier Nursing School, Quarterly Bulletin,* 60(2), 19–24.

Ernst, K. (1989). CNEP—A pilot community-based nurse-midwifery education program. *Frontier Nursing Service Quarterly Bulletin, 65*(1), 1–4.

Farr, M. M., & Funches, J. M. (1982). A successful pilot off-campus nurse-midwifery program. *Journal of Nurse-Midwifery, 27*(3), 31–36.

Fullerton, J. T., Howell, B. B., & Kim, P. T. (1986). Assessment of one alternative to an essay format certification examination. *Journal of Nurse-Midwifery, 31*(2), 105–108.

Fullerton, J. T., & Thompson, J. E. (1985). Recertification in nurse-midwifery: A critical analysis of use of a written examination. *Journal of Nurse-Midwifery, 30*(2), 71–78.

Gough, H. G. (1956). *California Psychological Inventory*. Palo Alto, CA: Consulting Psychologists Press.

Greener, D., & Reagan, P. (1986). Sexuality: Knowledge and attitudes of student nurse-midwives. *Journal of Nurse-Midwifery, 31*(1), 30–37.

Hsia, L. (1982). Fifty years of nurse-midwifery education: Reflections and perspectives. *Journal of Nurse-Midwifery, 27*(4), 1.

Hurzeler, C. (1981). Use of the certified nurse-midwife in the education of the lay-midwife. *Journal of Nurse-Midwifery, 26*(3), 57–59.

Kaplan, K. B. (1981). A faculty fellowship at maternity center association: An innovative approach in nurse-midwifery continuing education. *Journal of Nurse-Midwifery, 26*(2), 27–29.

Lonsdale, L., Murdaugh, A., & Stiles, D. (1982). Su Clinica Familiar—Georgetown University pilot project. *Journal of Nurse-Midwifery, 27*(5), 25–33.

Lubic, R. W. (1982). Nurse-midwifery education—the second 50 years. *Journal of Nurse-Midwifery, 25*(5), 5–9.

Marsico, T. (1977). The role of administrator. *Journal of Nurse-Midwifery, 22*(3), 19–22.

Nunnally, J. C. (1978). *Psychometric theory* (2nd ed.). New York: McGraw-Hill.

Paine, L. L., & Greener, D. L. (1989) Nurse-midwives speak out on research: Results of the 1987–88 Needs Assessment survey: II. *Journal of Nurse-Midwifery, 34*(2), 66–70.

Preliminary Technical Manual, Sex Knowledge and Attitudes Test, 2nd ed. (1979). Unpublished report available from the Center for the Study of Sex Education in Medicine, 4025 Chestnut Street, Philadelphia, PA 19104.

Raisler, J. (1987). Nurse-midwifery education, issues for survival and growth. *Journal of Nurse-Midwifery, 32*(1), 1–3.

Roberts, J. (1991). An overview of nurse-midwifery education and accreditation. *Journal of Nurse-Midwifery, 36*(6), 1–4.

Rooks, J. P., Carr, K. C., & Sandvold, I. (1991). The importance of nonmaster's degree options in nurse-midwifery education. *Journal of Nurse-Midwifery, 36*(2), 124–130.

Varney, H. (1987). *Nurse-midwifery* (2nd ed.). Boston: Blackwell Scientific.

Walsh, L. U., & Jaspan, A. L. (1990). Lay-midwife to nurse-midwife: Perceived learning needs and attitudes toward the learning experience. *Journal of Nurse-Midwifery, 35*(4), 204–213.

Warpinski, D. H., & Adams, C. J. (1979). Characteristics of applicants to nurse-midwifery educational programs. *Journal of Nurse-Midwifery, 24*(3), 5–9.

Weiss, S., McLain, B., & Fullerton, J. (1988). A collaborative intercampus model for graduate studies in primary care nursing. *International Journal of Nursing Studies, 25*, 261–270.

Yates, S. A. (1983). A refresher program for nurse-midwives: The Booth experience. *Journal of Nurse-Midwifery, 28*(3), 11–17.

PART IV

Research on the Profession of Nursing

Chapter 9

AIDS-Related Knowledge, Attitudes, and Risk for HIV Infection Among Nurses

Joan G. Turner
University of Alabama School of Nursing
University of Alabama at Birmingham

CONTENTS

The first reports of what would later be identified as AIDS appeared in the literature in 1981. With identification of a causative agent, human immunodeficiency virus (HIV), and subsequent development of HIV antibody tests, the spread of HIV infection could be monitored. In the first decade of the epidemic, there was exponential growth in the number of reported cases of AIDS as the epidemic spread into different population groups and geographic areas. The cumulative number of cases in the United States for the 10-year period exceeded 179,000, of which 63% were reported to have died (Centers for Disease Control [CDC], 1991c). The number of AIDS cases reflects only the severest clinical manifestations of HIV infection, however. Estimates made in 1991 placed the number of HIV-infected individuals in the United States at 800,000 to 1.2 million, with an estimated 8 to 10 million infected adults worldwide (CDC, 1990, 1991b).

From the outset, nurses have given care to persons with AIDS (PWAs) in many settings. As the epidemic expanded, the need for HIV-related knowledge and fears about occupational risks to caregivers has affected the profession of nursing. Various health care professionals have described or attempted to change the cognitive and affective responses to care of HIV-infected persons. Several disciplines and governmental bodies have tried to establish the numeric risks associated with accidental occupational exposure to blood and body fluids which contain HIV. The purpose of this report is to present a critical review of the research literature related to nurses' knowledge, attitudes, and workplace risk relative to AIDS and HIV infection.

For this review, the authors operationalized terms as follows: (a) *AIDS* subsumes the natural history of HIV infection beginning with the high-risk individual and environment plus the geographic prevalence of HIV, and ending with the disability and death of the infected individual; (b) *knowledge* refers to cognitive processes including recall and use of information and concepts, (c) *attitudes* refer to affective responses based on beliefs or perceived feelings that may or may not influence behavior; (d) *risk* refers to increased susceptibility to HIV infection, and (e) *nurse* refers to registered nurse (RN).

METHODS OF REVIEW

An initial computer search using MEDLINE was conducted using the index words "acquired immunodeficiency syndrome," "nurses," and "nursing" for the period October 1988 through March 1991. Additionally, a manual search was done of the *CINAHL* for the same period under the heading "acquired immunodeficiency syndrome." The period from 1985 to October 1988 had previously been searched for an earlier review article (Turner, 1990). The bibliographies of five other related review articles provided a partial cross-check on the completeness of the library-based search (All, 1989; Cohen, 1988; Larson, 1988; Larson & Ropka, 1991; Swanson, Chenitz, Zalar, & Stoll, 1990). Only articles in English-language nationally circulated publications were included in the review.

When appropriate titles were located, the article was retrieved and examined to determine whether it met the selection criteria for this review. First, the article had to qualify as a research report, and second, only studies involving RNs as subjects were used.

To qualify as a research report, the manuscript had to reflect the five major research elements recommended by Cooper (1982), which are evidence of problem formation, data collection, evaluation, analysis, and interpretation. The scientific merit of each study was reviewed according to criteria elaborated by Duffy (1985).

A total of 26 manuscripts were used in which researchers examined AIDS-related knowledge and attitudes among RNs. Additionally, 10 studies were included wherein the subjects were students studying to become RNs. Nurse subjects included in these studies came from nearly all clinical specialities and from diverse geographic settings in the United States, Canada, Great Britain, and Australia. All but six of these articles were atheoretic descriptive designs. Fourteen other nursing studies were reviewed on universal precautions (UP) and risk for HIV infection associated with occupational exposure.

Nurses' AIDS-related Knowledge and Attitudes

An implied assumption of the research on knowledge and attitudes is that nurses with adequate AIDS-related knowledge will be more capable of rendering quality care to HIV-infected individuals and will provide supportive and counseling services to those at risk. However, this review challenges the validity of this assumption because there is an ever increasing quantity of new information to be learned and the caregivers' affective responses are very complex.

Studies in this section are grouped according to method of sample selection and study design. The first section includes reports in which samples were selected by convenience. The major foci were fear of contagion, homophobia, and specific AIDS-related knowledge deficits. In the second section, studies in which researchers began with random selection are presented, and in the third section intervention studies are reviewed.

Surveys With Convenience Samples. An early survey of nurses' AIDS-related attitudes and knowledge was conducted in a New York City hospital (Blumenfield, Smith, Milazzo, Seropian, & Wormser, 1987). No reliability or validity data were given for the 10-item instrument. The response rate was 33% (n = 107) in July 1983 before education sessions and 56% (n = 191) in January 1984 after completion of education, but it was not clear if all nurse subjects were RNs. Investigators reported that fear of caring for homosexual and male prisoners owing to the fear of AIDS decreased significantly after the inservice training. However, on the posttest about 50% of subjects believed AIDS could be transmitted to caregivers despite precautions, and 39% said they would request a transfer if they had to care for PWAs routinely (Blumenfield et al., 1987).

In another early study, Wallack (1989) collected data in 1985 on nurses and physician house-staff regarding AIDS-related anxieties using a 79-item, investigator-designed tool. Sixty-seven physician house-staff and 172 nurses comprised the convenience sample. It was unclear whether all nurse subjects were RNs. Sixty-five percent (n = 43) of house-staff and 63% (n = 108) of nurses believed they were at risk for AIDS even with infection precautions, and 53% said they sometimes avoided performing procedures on PWAs because of fear of contagion.

Almost 50% of subjects felt anger toward homosexuals and blamed that group's promiscuity for causing the epidemic. One-third (n = 57) of nurses thought gay men with AIDS had only themselves to blame for being ill. Wallack (1989) concluded that the AIDS crisis has led health care workers to "confront their own attitudes toward homosexuality" (p. 509).

Just before 1985, a survey was conducted at a large urban teaching hospital that examined homophobia among that institution's physicians and nurses. The purpose of the study was to "investigate whether the AIDS epidemic may have activated underlying anxieties and fueled negative attitudes" among health care professionals (Douglas, Kalman, & Kalman, 1985, p. 1311). A total of 261 RNs working on medical units or in the emergency room and 91 physician house officers were invited to participate. The response rates were 35% (n = 91) and 41% (n = 37), respectively. Subjects completed a questionnaire designed to measure attitudes about homosexuality. The questionnaire used was a preexisting tool entitled the Index of Homophobia Scale (IHP) for which reliability and validity previously were established (Douglas et al., 1985).

Investigators reported that mean scores for both nurses and physicians fell in the low-grade homophobic range with no statistically significant differences between the two groups. However, women respondents were significantly more homophobic than men. Subjects who had a friend or relative who was homosexual were less homophobic than those who did not. One of 37 physicians (3%), and 11 of 90 nurses (12%) agreed that "homosexuals who contract AIDS are getting what they deserve" (p. 1310). Although the Douglas et al. (1985) study had numerous investigator-identified limitations, such as a responder versus nonresponder bias and lack of a control group, it has been referenced in most subsequent research relative to homophobia among nurses and other health care professionals.

In a 1986 survey of health care workers in which 183 out of 208 respondants (89%) were RNs, Barrick (1988) used a variety of standardized and investigator-developed instruments to examine attitudes toward homosexuals and PWAs. Positive attitudes toward homosexuals and comfort in caring for PWAs were found to be significantly associated. Barrick (1988) noted the lack of a comparison group and that subjects' responses may have been affected by factors such as social desirability. Recommendations for further research included the need for replication and for intervention designs focusing on attitude change.

A group of researchers in Australia also examined health professionals' attitudes toward homosexuality and AIDS (Hunt, Waddell, & Robathan, 1990). All health professionals at a pediatric teaching hospital were invited to complete a questionnaire designed to measure homophobia and AIDS phobia. The final sample of 446 (response rate 55%) included 238 nurses. The investigators found that, as a group, nurses scored lower on the AIDS phobia and homophobia scales compared with physicians or other health professionals.

Using Lazarus's theory of coping and adaptation, four nurse researchers surveyed 134 perinatal nurses' AIDS-related knowledge and attitudes (Prince, Beard, Ivey, & Lester, 1989). Subjects were recruited from five midwestern hospitals. Forty percent (n = 53) said they did not know that HIV had been found in human breast milk, and only one half (n = 67, 50%) knew that most children with HIV infection were infected through perinatal transmission. More than one third (36%) thought they were being exposed to HIV in daily work activities, and only 24% (n = 32) would have volunteered to care for an HIV-infected infant. Subjects' most frequently reported fear related to AIDS was exposure to the HIV virus in an emergency patient care situation.

In a survey on a convenience sample of 120 RNs employed at a large teaching hospital in Tennessee, Morgan and Treadway (1989) used a previously developed tool for which no reliability or validity information was given. They reported that misinformation on modes of HIV transmission was prevalent, although more highly educated nurses generally had higher levels of AIDS-related knowledge.

The purpose of a study conducted in Baltimore was to compare critical care nurses in a teaching hospital (TH) with their cohorts in a community hospital (CH) on AIDS-related knowledge, attitudes, and concerns. Forty-two subjects in the TH (84%) and 48 (96%) in the CH participated (Damrosch, Abbey, Warner, & Guy, 1990). TH nurses had more favorable attitudes, but a sizable percentage in the TH (n = 19, 45%) and the CH (n = 31, 65%) indicated that they would refuse to care for PWAs if given a choice. Because 90% of all subjects (n = 81) made a perfect score on the knowledge test, investigators expressed concern that the items had been "too easy" and urged revision of the test. The authors cautioned against generalization of findings, but suggested that nurses' attitudes may be related to differing characteristics of the work settings (Damrosch et al., 1990). Caution is also warranted owing to the small sample size in only one hospital.

Baird and Beardslee (1990) distributed 1,000 questionnaires to nurses from three northeastern Colorado hospitals. Information regarding the reliability and validity of the investigator-designed instrument was included in the report. Their purpose was to use the survey results to design continuing-eduation programs.

Fifty-two percent (n = 515) of the 1,000 questionnaires were returned.

Nurses were more knowledgeable about transmission modalities and infection control precautions than about human sexuality, drug abuse, and appropriate risk-reduction counseling. More knowledge about HIV was significantly related to positive attitudes toward PWAs, and negative beliefs about homosexuality and drug abuse related to more negative attitudes about AIDS care. Investigators concluded that RNs need to be sensitized and educated relative to the issues of sexuality and homosexuality, history taking, and counseling, and that the affective learning domain must be included in AIDS-related education (Baird & Beardslee, 1990).

Fear of contagion and homophobia were two recurring themes in this group of studies. The inference was that such feelings influenced nurses' responses to PWAs. The generalizability of these findings is limited by the convenience method of sample selection, respondent-nonrespondent bias, the cross-sectional versus longitudinal study designs, and concerns about the instrumentation. It would be difficult to make definitive comparisons between study findings because the instrumentation was different in each survey. Only five of nine authors mentioned the reliability and/or validity of their instrument.

The second major finding of the studies in this section was specific knowledge deficits regarding HIV infection. That focus can also be noted for many of the studies presented in the next section.

Studies With Random Selection. As part of a nationwide survey of nurses in the United States, 68% (n = 194) of randomly invited community health nurses (CHNs) volunteered to participate in a survey of AIDS-related knowledge and information deficits (Flaskerud, 1988). Subjects responded to a pretested 80-item instrument. After analysis of those data collected in 1986 and 1987, the investigator reported that subjects who anticipated seeing a PWA and those with less educational preparation needed more information and knowledge. At least 75% of respondents asked for more information on a wide variety of AIDS-related topics such as transmission in the workplace, infection control precautions, safer sexual practices, psychosocial care of clients, and ethical issues in client care.

Flaskerud (1988) suggested that attitudes toward PWAs are improved by knowledge, and that nurses should provide clear guidelines for infection control, tangible support services, and clear legal and ethical guidelines. Limitations included: sampling was from the membership list of only one national organization, the respondents were more educated than the national norm, and they were overrepresented from states with a high incidence of AIDS cases.

As part of the same national survey, 233 psychiatric nurses were randomly selected from the membership list of the American Nurses' Association Council of Psychiatric–Mental Health Nurses and invited to participate. A total of 180 (77.2%) completed questionnaires. Seventy-five percent needed more information on (a) transmission risk in the workplace and appropriate precautions, (b) neuropsychiatric syndromes, and (c) psychosocial issues. Flaskerud (1989) concluded that new AIDS-related developments occur constantly so educational efforts must be ongoing.

A survey conducted to help develop AIDS-specific continuing education was given to American oncology nurses in 1986–87. A questionnaire containing 109 items on AIDS-related knowledge and experience was mailed to 1,006 randomly selected members of the Oncology Nursing Society (Jacob, Ostchega, Grady, Gallaway, & Kish, 1990). A total of 692 oncology nurses (70%) responded and reported that they had experience in some aspects of care, such as the terminally ill and their families, but needed more preparation to respond adequately to the general needs of PWAs. They wanted more clinical and nursing care knowledge of specific manifestations of HIV infection (Jacob et al., 1990).

Haughey, Scherer, and Wu (1989) invited a randomly selected sample of 1,100 nurses in upstate New York to participate in a survey to assess AIDS-related knowledge including the epidemiology, pathophysiology, transmission, and treatment of AIDS. A total of 581 (51%) completed the investigator-designed knowledge test. The total mean score was slightly less than 70% correct. Fifty-four percent of nurse respondents were unaware that infection control guidelines had been issued for health care workers, and one half (51%) were unaware that used needles should not be recapped.

In a separate report, Scherer, Haughey, and Wu (1989) examined quantitative and qualitative data from this random sample of New York nurses on attitudes toward PWAs. Consistent with Douglas and associates (1985), they found that care of PWAs was complicated by negative attitudes toward homosexuality. Instrument reliability and validity were addressed, but no study limitations were identified, even though responder versus nonresponder bias was likely (Scherer et al., 1989).

In a survey in England in the fall of 1986, Stanford (1988) measured district nurses' AIDS-related knowledge and attitudes. Eighty-five nurses from each of two districts were randomly selected; the response rates were 79% (n = 67) and 72% (n = 62) yielding a total sample of 129. Subjects' attitudes were generally positive but specific knowledge deficits included modes of transmission and appropriate precautions. The investigator concluded that subjects' knowledge level was unsatisfactory.

In an effort to identify English community health nurses' experience and beliefs related to AIDS, investigators invited a stratified random sample of 5,243 to participate in a mail survey (Bond, Rhodes, Phillips, Setters, Foy & Bond, 1990) that yielded a 74% response rate (n = 3797). Most respondents lacked confidence about providing health education, counseling, and terminal care. Only 3 of 10 knowledge questions were answered correctly by 75% of subjects. Those with inservice education achieved significantly higher scores than those who had no such education. Only 10% (n = 388) knowingly had cared for a PWA or HIV-infected client, but 28% had experience with individuals at high risk for infection (Bond et al., 1990).

Kerr and Horrocks (1990) mailed questionnaires on AIDS-related knowledge and attitudes to a sample of 400 nurses in Nova Scotia. Subjects were randomly selected from 5,400 nurses working in obstetrics, pediatrics, and medical-surgical areas in the province. The response rate was 45% (n = 179). Subjects responded to a seven-part instrument in which four of the seven parts were researcher developed. Three sections were developed and piloted by other investigators, but reliability and validity of the various components were not discussed.

Subjects had trouble selecting groups at highest risk for HIV infection and 45% (n = 80) believed the cause of AIDS was unknown. More knowledgeable respondents were less homophobic, and the more homophobic and AIDS phobic had children and lacked experience with PWAs (Kerr & Horrocks, 1990). Further, nearly 70% said the "existence of AIDS made nursing a high risk occupation" (p. 127). Most believed in the right of PWAs to have quality care, but 12% (n = 22) said they would definitely refuse to care for PWAs. Another 40% (n = 72) would use excessively conservative isolation techniques on PWAs. The investigators suggested development and testing of educational programs that effect attitude change along with knowledge gain (Kerr & Horrocks, 1990).

Using change theory as a theoretic framework, van Servellen, Lewis, and Leake (1988) surveyed nurses who had cared for PWAs to assess AIDS-related attitudes, fears, and knowledge as a preparatory step to designing educational offerings. Out of 3,000 randomly invited California nurses, 1,203 (42%) participated. More than one half (n = 645, 53.6%) said that nurses should be permitted to refuse to care for PWAs. Even though these nurses lived in California, which has a high number of PWAs and HIV seropositivity, only 122 (11.9%) correctly identified all AIDS-related symptoms. Also, 91.3% (n = 1,098) did not routinely take sexual histories, and only 17.5% (n = 210) explained methods to decrease risk of exposure to HIV. The investigators concluded that nurses need education on the etiology, symptoms, and treatment of AIDS and they recommended that future studies address and alter negative attitudes and beliefs toward PWAs (van Servellen et al., 1988).

A survey of physicians during the same period and using similar instrumentation (van Servellen, Lewis, & Leake, 1990) differed in that telephone interviews were conducted with the primary care physicians. No explanation for the different data collection techniques was offered nor was it addressed as a limitation in interpreting the results or comparing the physician and nurse data.

Physicians and nurses were similar; both groups could identify those at high risk for HIV infection. All subjects had trouble identifying *low-risk* individuals and neither group exercised adequate counseling practices with patients who were at risk for HIV infection. Compared with physicians, nurses were more likely to work with PWAs, were more uncomfortable caring for gay male patients, attended fewer educational programs on AIDS, and had less knowledge about the epidemiology and clinical findings associated with AIDS. The investigators stipulated the need for research that reports *actual* knowledge deficits and attitudinal barriers before designing educational programs (van Servellen et al., 1990).

In an interdisciplinary study, psychologists and nurses used three standardized instruments and clinical vignettes to determine if PWAs were stigmatized in a negative manner (Kelly, St. Lawrence, Hood, Smith, & Cook, 1988). Although this study focused on attitudes, the purpose was to define areas that would be amenable to educational strategies and ultimately to improve the psychologic comfort of nurses and PWAs. Out of 500 randomly invited nurses in Mississippi and surrounding areas, of which 91% were RNs, 166 (32.3%) volunteered to participate. Subjects' responded to one of four vignettes. The investigators subsequently reported that homosexual patients, regardless of illness, were evaluated as more deserving of what happened to them. In fact, homosexual patients were stigmatized with negative attitudes and attributions similar to those shown toward PWAs. Investigators suggested that nurses with such negative attitudes and perceptions would be unlikely to establish open and nonjudgmental caring relationships with PWAs and homosexual patients with any diagnosis (Kelly et al., 1988).

Using 600 volunteer nurse subjects from a relatively wide geographic region with a high incidence of AIDS, Forrester (1990) examined the relationship among AIDS-related risk factors such as whether the patient was homosexual or an intravenous drug user (IVDU), medical diagnosis (AIDS vs. non-AIDS) and do-not-resuscitate orders. Subjects were randomly assigned to one of six experimental groups with each group responding to a different vignette. Unlike Kelly and associates (1988), Forrester (1990) reported that whether or not the patient was described as gay or as an IVDU did not influence nurse subjects' attitudes about how aggressive the patient's treatment should be.

The purpose of most studies was to identify AIDS-related knowledge needs of nurses to be used in designing educational programs. Both general and specialty-specific information needs for nurses in various clinical settings were identified, as was fear of contagion and homophobia. Generalizibility of the results is once again limited by the cross-sectional design of the studies. In addition, attempts at random selection fell short with only 32% to 79% response rates. Also, less than half (n = 5) addressed instrument reliability or validity.

Intervention Studies. Although many investigators identified educational needs and attitude deficits, few educational intervention studies were found. Young (1988) reported an educational intervention in which all 22 RN subjects significantly improved on the cognitive section, but 50% ($n = 11$) demonstrated no change in attitudes. The other half demonstrated more positive attitudes toward homosexuality on the posttest. Young (1988) noted that helping nurses understand their negative feelings toward homosexuality might help them understand "the possible risks that such prejudices carry for their clients" (p. 10). Young emphasized the need for control groups to improve study design and for long-term follow-up to see if changes seemingly effected through educational intervention would last over time.

In a quasi-experimental design with an attitudinal framework developed by Fishbein and Ajzen, RNs in a three-county area in northern Alabama participated in a seminar on general AIDS-related knowledge and attitude resolution towards PWAs. The control group ($n = 49$) was pretested, did not attend the seminar, and was posttested in 30 days. The experimental group ($n = 149$) was pretested at the onset of the seminar, posttested immediately after participation, and then again in 30 days (Turner, Gauthier, Ellison, & Greiner, 1988). There were no significant differences between the two groups on pretest scores. For the experimental group, the general AIDS knowledge score increased significantly on the posttest and then rose slightly on the 30-day retest, and their attitudes were significantly more positive on posttest. For controls, knowledge also increased on posttest and attitudes were more positive. The authors suggested that simply taking the pretest may have raised consciousness and motivated individual learning in control subjects. The more knowledgeable subjects were, the more positive were their attitudes on pre- and posttest (Turner et al., 1988).

In another educational intervention study conducted in the spring and summer of 1988, a convenience sample of 125 California nurses participated in an AIDS-related workshop. There was no control group. Subjects were pretested and posttested using a structured questionnaire that measured AIDS-related knowledge and attitudes. Subjects were retested again 2 to 3 months after the educational offering. Flaskerud, Lewis, and Shin (1989) reported that those who had not cared for a PWA made greater gains in pretest/posttest knowledge and retained these gains on retest. Overall, there were significant gains in knowledge and positive attitudes, and subjects retained knowledge and positive attitudes in the retest period.

Young, Koch, and Preston (1989) reported from then-extant literature that the fear of homosexuality, unlike the fear of AIDS itself, was based on moral judgments. On that premise, they designed an educational intervention to improve knowledge and change attitudes toward AIDS and homosexuality and constructed an instrument that was used as a pretest, posttest, and

3-month retest. Their supporting conceptual framework was Fishbein and Ajzen and their assumption was if attitudes are learned, a process of affective education can produce attitude change in motivated subjects.

Participating in the original workshop, which included a variety of teaching methods, were 170 RNs and 30 other allied health workers; however, only 56 subjects completed all three phases of the project. Knowledge scores improved and attitudes were less negative toward HIV-infected individuals on posttest. Nurses demonstrated more willingness to care for PWAs and those who were least fearful and most willing showed more positive attitudes post intervention than those who were most fearful and least willing to change. The investigators noted limitations such as no control group and inability to generalize to other nurses (Young et al., 1989).

Armstrong-Esther and Hewitt (1990) reported that direct education increased knowledge and liberalized self-reported attitudes toward AIDS and care of PWAs in a group of 60 Canadian RNs enrolled in a baccalaureate nursing program. In the one-group design, nurses were pretested and then posttested 4 months later. The instruction regarding AIDS was part of an epidemiology course. A previous epidemiology class served as a reference group. The investigators noted that they could provide evidence about *actual* versus stated behavior, but this observation is true of all methods that use self-report.

Synthesis of these findings indicates that educational interventions can produce positive changes in subjects' self-reported knowledge and attitudes but leaves unanswered whether changes in knowledge and attitudes result in changes in actual behavior. All of the samples were convenience, and only two of five studies had control or reference groups.

Studies of Nursing Students. There were a few studies on AIDS-related attitudes and knowledge among nursing students. Nursing students had significant knowledge deficits related to AIDS, concerns about providing care to PWAs, and unfavorable attitudes toward PWAs (Armstrong-Esther & Hewitt, 1989; Bowd & Loos, 1987; Lester & Beard, 1988). As much as 50% of some convenience samples of nursing students thought that practicing nurses should be able to refuse to care for PWAs (Wiley, Heath, & Acklin, 1988). Some investigators concluded that educational interventions produced a positive impact on knowledge and attitudes among nursing students (Brown et al., 1990; Goldenberg & Laschinger, 1991; Klisch, 1990; Lawrence & Lawrence, 1989), but others said students questioned the adequacy of their preparation to provide care to PWAs (Cassells & Redman, 1989; Haughey, Scherer, & Wu, 1990).

Other Studies of Health Care Workers. Finally, a number of studies focused on AIDS-related knowledge and attitudes among a variety of health care workers. These studies included a subsample of RNs but are not reviewed in detail here because findings were only reported for the total group and not for members of the various participating disciplines (Gordin, Willoughby, Levine, Gure & Neill, 1987; Henry, Campbell, & Willenbring, 1990; O'Donnell & O'Donnell, 1987; Royce & Birge, 1987; Searle, 1987; Valenti & Anarella, 1986; Wertz, Sorenson, Leibling, Kessler, & Heeren, 1987.

OCCUPATIONAL EXPOSURE RISK AND UNIVERSAL PRECAUTIONS

In an effort to protect all health care workers (HCWs) against occupational exposure to blood-borne diseases such as HIV, the CDC published guidelines for practice in 1987, 1988, and 1989, that have become known as Universal Precautions (UPs). They are "universal" in the sense that under these guidelines, all care recipients are considered potentially infected and infectious regardless of diagnosis or presentation (CDC, 1991a). Also in public recognition of the occupational risk that blood-borne diseases pose for all HCWs, the Occupational Safety and Health Administration (OSHA) has mandated that all employers (including health care facilities) take specific steps to protect their employees against accidental exposure. These steps include education in the use of UPs and ready access to necessary equipment. These guidelines became regulatory in December, 1991 (OSHA, 1991).

Numerous authors have reported that compliance to the CDC OSHA guidelines is poor (Becker, Janz, Band, Bartley, Snyder, & Gaynes, 1990; Geberding et al., 1987; Gruber et al., 1989; Hartnett, 1987; Kelen, DiGiovanna, Bisson, Kalainov, Silvertson, & Quinn, 1989; Loewen, Dhillon, Willy, Wesley, & Henderson, 1989; Makulowich, 1988; O'Kane, 1988; Wertz et al., 1987). Thousands of exposures to blood and body fluids that may contain pathogens such as HIV have been documented in the United States. As of early 1991, CDC was aware of 25 HCWs in the United States who seroconverted to HIV following an occupational exposure to HIV. In addition, 16 other workers with suspected occupationally acquired HIV infection were reported. However, seroconversion after a specific exposure incident could not be documented in this group (CDC, 1991a).

In 1988 the CDC estimated that the risk of infection from an HIV-positive needlestick was less than 1%; and that the risk from exposure to nonintact skin was far less than 1% (CDC, 1988). When prospective study results became available, CDC reported (199a) that the risk of HIV transmission due to a single occupational percutaenous exposure to HIV-infected blood was, on the average, 0.3%; (upper limit of the 95% confidence interval 0.6%). Transmission of HIV after a mucous membrane or skin exposure to HIV-infected blood has been reported and, although the exact risk is unknown, based on studies to date, the upper limit of the 95% confidence interval after mucous membrane or skin contact was estimated to be between 0.03% and 0.09% (CDC, 1991a).

Knowledge, Attitudes, and Practices Related to UPs

A nationwide survey of certified nurse midwives (CNM) was conducted to determine (a) the type and frequency of blood and body fluid exposures they experienced, and (b) the degree to which they used UPs (Loewen et al., 1989). The response rate was 60.2% for a total sample of 1784. First, 65.1% (n = 1161) reported having been soaked through to the skin with amniotic fluid or blood at least once in the past 6 months, and 25% (392) reported five or more such exposures. Facial splashes were reported by 50% and almost 17% had an eye splash at least once in the past 6 months. Sixty-two percent (n = 1107) reported torn gloves during procedures, and 158 reported two to five needlesticks in this time period. However, because it was not clearly operationalized on the survey tool, these needlesticks could have involved either clean or used needles.

Second, only 55.1% (n = 983) said they used UPs in their practice, but investigators reported that some of these subjects answered factual questions about UPs incorrectly. Over one third (n = 685, 38.4%) felt that UPs were unnecessary and others said UPs decreased dexterity and interfered with the midwife–client relationship. Many of these CNMs practice predominantly in urban settings where HIV infections are likely to be high (Loewen et al., 1989).

Gruber and associates (1989) reported that the 231 RNs in their convenience sample had a mean 64% correct response rate regarding appropriate practice of UPs and found no relationship between knowledge about UPs and practice of UPs. These investigators concluded that although basic information was essential, compliance would have to address psychosocial and motivational aspects.

Wiley and associates (1990) found that 18% of their 323 nurse subjects did not follow UPs routinely and 17% of subjects believed infection control guidelines were not completely protective. Those who had sustained an accidental occupational exposure (n = 64) were more likely to endorse universal testing for all inpatients and were also more likely to consider changing specialities and/or professions because of HIV-related risks (Wiley, Heath, Acklin, Earl, & Barnard, 1990).

Although compliance to UPs in the United States is variable, medical and political communities in other countries have not espoused UP guidelines. For example, the Australian Medical Association has been publicly opposed to UP because they find the concept of considering all patients potentially HIV-infected to be wasteful due to the cost of barrier equipment such as gloves, gowns, masks, and goggles (Hunt et al., 1990). A potential justification for such barriers was illustrated in a survey of nurses at a community hospital in Australia. Nielson (1988) reported that 62% of 66 subjects (n = 41) said they frequently had unprotected skin contact with blood or secretions containing blood and 53% (n = 35) said that they stuck themselves with used needles or sharps at least once a year.

As a part of UP guidelines, CDC officials recommended that needles not be recapped after use. A study of recapping practices among 110 physicians and 91 nurses (n = 201) at four large hospitals in Michigan concluded that the practice of recapping was related to inadequate knowledge (Becker et al., 1990). They concluded that inservice education must address preexisting behaviors and tailor education programs to the different needs of learners (Becker et al., 1990).

The relationship between education and compliance to UP remains unclear. Fahey, Koziol, Banks, and Henderson (1991) reported that the incidence of accidental cutaneous exposures significantly decreased after subjects participated in training specific to UPs, and Hixon, Thomason, and Nodhturft (1990) reported that UP practices by hospital personnel increased after a 4-hour educational program. However, in a longitudinal study of the relationship between reports of needlestick injuries and regular inservice education, Linneman, Cannon, DeRonde, and Lanphear (1991) found that inservice infection control programs from 1986 to 1989 failed to reduce reported needlestick injuries. Talan & Baraff (1990) found that educational programs to improve both knowledge and practice of UPs by nursing personnel ultimately produced no statistically significant improvements in UP practices. Further, the educational program had no effect on long-term general knowledge. They concluded by noting that the practice of UPs was far from universal in their setting (Talan & Baraff, 1990).

At this point, it is unclear how to effect any consistent changes in use of UPs. In fact, researchers at the national level have taken two divergent approaches to the problem. For example, some say the behavior of professionals cannot be changed, and as a result, are looking at ways to make the health care environment safer. Others believe health care worker attitudes and behaviors can be changed by use of appropriate theoretic frameworks and experimental designs.

SUMMARY AND RECOMMENDATIONS FOR FUTURE RESEARCH

A review of the literature on nurses' AIDS-related knowledge, attitudes, and risk for HIV infection contains several pervasive themes. First, nurse-subjects in the studies had severe gaps in AIDS-related knowledge. Care of PWAs is rapidly becoming a nursing specialty; therefore, the more relevant question may, in fact, be: "Do nurses whose primary client population is PWAs have adequate specialized knowledge?" There were no studies on AIDS-nurse specialists.

Initial preparation in nursing is as a generalist, so the pressing question for nursing as a discipline is to determine whether nurse-generalists have the basic knowledge needed to (a) protect against transmission of blood-borne diseases, (b) care for the occasional PWA in collaboration with the specialist, and (c) effectively engage in nursing skills that might involve risk reduction counseling or advocacy for the worried well, HIV-infected clients and their families, and/or significant others. The literature reviewed on nurse-generalists indicates that they do not have the requisite knowledge or skills required to provide quality care to HIV-infected persons.

A second fact emerging from this review is that many of the reports were needs assessments rather than research studies. Even when the project was designed to be research there were deficits in operationalization of terms, review of the literature, use of conceptual or theoretical models, subject selection, data collection methods, and establishing reliability and validity of instruments. The study designs were predominantly descriptive and almost uniformly cross-sectional. In most of the studies reviewed, the review of past research was cursory. Not a single study that addressed nurses' implementation of UPs looked back at the literature on nurse and health care worker compliance to isolation guidelines in the past. If such a review had been attempted, it would have become clear that numerous earlier studies have documented that compliance with infection control guidelines historically has been poor (Kelen, 1990; Kelen et al., 1991).

Only six studies of all those reviewed mentioned a conceptual framework, and more often than not, findings and discussion were not related back to the conceptual components. Further, in only 12 of 25 studies on nurses' knowledge and attitudes were subjects invited by randomization. In addition, the response rates ranged from 32.2% to 79%, so selection was not actually random. Only two of five intervention studies used a control group.

In all studies on knowledge, attitudes, and practice of UPs, nurse subjects self-reported data, but the possibility of their responses being affected by social desirability bias was rarely stated as a limitation. Reliability and/or validity of instruments were discussed in less than one-third of the studies.

In an earlier review, Larson (1988) found no research articles on HIV infection with nurses as first authors during the period January 1983 to April 1987. For this review, a group of articles focused on nurses was found. Clearly the quantity of research by nurses on HIV infection has increased. However, the methodological issues discussed above limit the generalizability of the results of the studies reviewed and make comparisons of studies difficult. Similar methodological limitations have been noted by other reviewers (Larson & Ropka, 1991; Swanson et al., 1990).

In the past 10 years, HIV infection has emerged as a global health problem. The World Health Organization has estimated that by the year 2000, 40 million people may be affected by the pandemic if current trends continue (CDC, 1991b). As the AIDS/HIV epidemic continues to expand in scope and complexity, the impact on nurses and the nursing profession also will increase and become more diverse. With new treatment modalities extending life expectancy and with HIV infection becoming more geographically and socially diverse, nurses in all areas of specialization will be confronted with clients in various stages of HIV infection. The research presented here has identified knowledge deficits, attitudes, and beliefs that may adversely affect the quality of care provided to PWAs and may increase nurses' occupational risk of exposure. Future research in this area must focus on the design and evaluation of effective intervention strategies to meet nurses' needs for knowledge, skills, and values-clarification as caregivers of persons with HIV infection.

REFERENCES

All, A. (1989). Health care workers' anxieties and fears concerning AIDS: A literature review. *The Journal of Continuing Education in Nursing, 20,* 162–165.

Armstrong-Esther, C., & Hewitt, W. (1989). Knowledge and perception of AIDS among Canadian nurses. *Journal of Advanced Nursing, 14,* 923–938.

Armstrong-Esther, C., & Hewitt, W. (1990). The effect of education on nurses' perception of AIDS. *Journal of Advanced Nursing, 15,* 638–651.

Baird, S. C., & Beardslee, N. Q. (1990). Developing an inservice program on acquired immunodeficiency syndrome (AIDS). *Journal of Nursing Staff Development, 6,* 269–274.

Barrick, B. (1988). The willingness of nursing personnel to care for patients with acquired immune deficiency syndrome: A survey study and recommendations. *Journal of Professional Nursing, 4,* 366–372.

Becker, M. H., Janz, N. K., Band, J., Bartley, J., Snyder, M. B., & Gaynes, R. P. (1990). Noncompliance with Universal Precautions Policy: Why do physicians and nurses recap needles? *American Journal of Infection Control, 18,* 232–239.

Blumenfield, M., Smith, P. J., Milazzo, J., Seropian, S., & Wormser, G. P. (1987). Survey of attitudes of nurses working with AIDS patients. *General Hospital Psychiatry, 9,* 58–63.

Bond, S., Rhodes, T., Phillips, P., Setters, J., Foy, C., & Bond, J. (1990). HIV infection and AIDS in England: The experience, knowledge and intentions of community nursing staff. *Journal of Advanced Nursing, 15,* 249–255.

Bowd, A. D., & Loos, C. H. (1987). Nursing students' knowledge and opinions concerning AIDS. *Nursing Papers/Perspectives in Nursing, 19*(4), 11–20.

Brown, Y., Calder, B., & Rae, D. (1990). The effect of knowledge on nursing students' attitudes toward individuals with AIDS. *Journal of Nursing Education, 29,* 367–372.

Cassells, J., & Redman, B. (1989). New baccalaureate graduates in care of AIDS patients: Perceptions of preparedness and information accessibility. *Journal of Continuing Education in Nursing, 20,* 156–161.

Centers for Disease Control. (1987). Recommendations for prevention of HIV transmission in health-care settings. *Morbidity and Mortality Weekly Report, 36,* 35–185.

Centers for Disease Control. (1988). AIDS and HIV update: Acquired immunodeficiency syndrome and human immunodeficiency virus infection among health-care workers. *Morbidity and Mortality Weekly Report, 37,* 229–234, 239.

Centers for Disease Control. (1989). Guideline for prophylaxis against *pneumocystis carinii* pneumonia for persons infected with human immunodeficiency virus, *Morbidity and Mortality Weekly Report, 38,* 1–37.

Centers for Disease Control. (1990). HIV prevalence estimates and AIDS case projections for the United States: Report based upon a workshop. *Morbidity and Mortality Weekly Report, 39*(RR-16).

Centers for Disease Control. (1991a). Estimates of the risk of endemic transmission of hepatitis B virus and human immunodeficiency virus to patients by the percutaneous route during invasive surgical and dental procedures. Atlanta, GA: U. S. Department of Health and Human Services (Draft distributed to participants at the CDC hearing, January 30, 1991).

Centers for Disease Control. (1991b). The HIV/AIDS epidemic: The first 10 years. *Morbidity and Mortality Weekly Report, 40,* 357.

Centers for Disease Control. (1991c). Update: Acquired immunodeficiency syndrome-United States, 1981–1990. *Morbidity and Mortality Weekly Report, 40,* 358–363, 369.

Cohen, F. L. (1988). Acquired immunodeficiency syndrome research in critical care: A critical review and future directions. *Focus on Critical Care, 15*(4), 30–35.

Cooper, H. M. (1982). Scientific guidelines for conducting integrative research reviews. *Review of Educational Research, 52,* 291–302.

Damrosch, S., Abbey, S., Warner, A., & Guy, S. (1990). Critical care nurses' attitudes toward, concerns about, and knowledge of the acquired immunodeficiency syndrome. *Heart & Lung, 19,* 395–400.

Douglas, C. J., Kalman, C. M., & Kalman, T. P. (1985). Homophobia among physicians and nurses: An empirical study. *Hospital and Community Psychiatry, 36,* 1309–1311.

Duffy, M. E. (1985). A research appraisal checklist for evaluating nursing research reports. *Nursing and Health Care, 6,* 539–547.

Fahey, B. J., Koziol, D. E., Banks, S. M., & Henderson, D. (1991). Frequency of nonparenteral occupational exposures to blood and body fluids before and after universal precautions training. *The American Journal of Medicine, 90*(9), 145–147.

Flaskerud, J. (1988). Community health nurses' AIDS information needs. *Journal of Community Health Nursing, 5,* 149–157.

Flaskerud, J. (1989). Psychiatric nurses' needs for AIDS information. *Perspectives in Psychiatric Care, 25*(3), 3–9.

Flaskerud, J., Lewis, M., & Shin, D. (1989). Changing nurses' AIDS-related knowledge and attitudes through continuing education. *The Journal of Continuing Education in Nursing, 20,* 148–154.

Forrester, D. A. (1990). AIDS-related risk factors, medical diagnosis, do-not-resuscitate orders and aggressiveness of nursing care. *Nursing Research, 39,* 350–354.

Gerberding, J., Bryant-LeBlanc, C., Nelson, K., Moss, A., Osmond, D., Chambers, H., Carlson, J., Drew, W., Levy, J., & Sande, M. (1987). Risk of transmitting the human immunodeficiency virus, cytomegalovirus and hepatitis B virus to health care workers exposed to patients with AIDS and AIDS-related conditions. *Journal of Infectious Diseases, 156*(1), 1–8.

Goldenberg, D., & Laschinger, H. (1991). Attitudes and normative beliefs of nursing students as predictors of intended care behaviors with AIDS patients: A test of the Ajzen-Fishbein theory of reasoned action. *Journal of Nursing Education, 30,* 119–126.

Gordin, F. M., Willoughby, A., Levine, L., Gure, L., & Neill, K. (1987). Knowledge of AIDS among hospital workers: Behavioral correlates and consequences. *AIDS, 1*(3), 183–188.

Gruber, M., Beavers, F., Johnson, B., Brackett, M., Lopez, T., Feldman, M., & Ventura, M. (1989). The relationship between knowledge about acquired immunodeficiency syndrome and the implementation of universal precautions by registered nurses. *Clinical Nurse Specialist, 3,* 182–185.

Hartnett, S. M. (1987). A hospital-wide AIDS education program. *Journal of Continuing Education in Nursing, 18,* 64–67.

Haughey, B., Scherer, Y., & Wu, Y. (1989). Nurses' knowledge about AIDS in Erie County, New York: A research brief. *The Journal of Continuing Education in Nursing, 20,* 166–168.

Haughey, B., Scherer, Y., & Wu, Y. (1990). AIDS education and patient care experiences of senior nursing students in Buffalo, NY: A research brief. *Journal of Nursing Education, 29,* 234–235.

Henry, K., Campbell, S., & Willenbring, K. (1990). A cross-sectional analysis of variables impacting on AIDS-related knowledge, attitudes, and behaviors among employees of a Minnesota teaching hospital. *AIDS Education and Prevention, 2*(1), 36–47.

Hixon, A. K., Thomason, S. S., & Nodhturft, V. L. (1990). Evaluating quality and ongoing improvement of clinical practice following HIV/AIDS education. *Journal of Nursing Quality Assurance, 5*(1), 61–72.

Hunt, L., Waddell, C., & Robathan, G. (1990). AIDS: Attitudes and education. *The Australian Journal of Advanced Nursing, 7*(3), 28–33.

Jacob, J. G., Ostchega, Y., Grady, C., Gallaway, L. J., & Kish, J. P. (1990). Self-assessed learning needs of oncology nurses caring for individuals with HIV-related disorders: A national survey. *Cancer Nursing, 13,* 246–255.

Kelen G. (1990). Human immunodeficiency virus and the Emergency Department: Risks and risk protection for health care workers. *Annals of Emergency Medicine, 19,* 242–248.

Kelen, G., Bennecoff, T., Kline, R., Green, G., & Quinn, T. (1991). Evaluation of two rapid screening assays for the detection of human immunodeficiency virus—Infection in Emergency Department Patients. *American Journal of Emergency Medicine, 9,* 416–420.

Kelen, G. D., DiGiovanna, T., Bisson, L., Kalainov, D., Sivertson, K. T., & Quinn, T. C. (1989). Human immunodeficiency virus infection in emergency department patients. *Journal of the American Medical Association, 262,* 516–522.

Kelly, J. A. St. Lawrence, J. S., Hood, H., Smith, S., & Cook, D. (1988). Nurses' attitudes toward AIDS. *The Journal of Continuing Education in Nursing, 19,* 78–83.

Kerr, C. I., & Horrocks, M. J. (1990). Knowledge, values, attitudes and behavioural intent of Nova Scotia nurses toward AIDS and patients with AIDS. *Canadian Journal of Public Health, 81,* 125–128.

Klisch, M. L. (1990). Caring for persons with AIDS: Student reactions. *Nurse Educator, 15*(4), 16–20.

Larson, E. (1988). Nursing research and AIDS. *Nursing Research, 37,* 60–62.

Larson, E., & Ropka, M. E. (1991). An update on nursing research and HIV infection. *Image: Journal of Nursing Scholarship, 23,* 4–12.

Lawrence, S., & Lawrence, R. (1989). Knowledge and attitudes about acquired immunodeficiency syndrome in nursing and non-nursing groups. *Journal of Professional Nursing, 5,* 92–101.

Lester, L. B., & Beard, B. J. (1988). Nursing students' attitudes toward AIDS. *Journal of Nursing Education, 27,* 399–404.

Linnemann, C. C., Cannon, C., DeRonde, M., & Lanphear, B. (1991). Effect of educational programs, rigid sharps containers, and universal precautions on reported needlestick injuries in healthcare workers. *Infection Control and Hospital Epidemiology, 12,* 214–219.

Loewen, N. L., Dhillon, G., Willy, M. E., Wesley, R., & Henderson, D. K. (1989). Use of precautions by nurse-midwives to prevent occupational infections with HIV and other blood-borne diseases. *Journal of Nurse-Midwifery, 34,* 309–317.

Makulowich, G. S. (1988). Implementing CDC guidelines for infection control. *AIDS Patient Care, 2*(1), 14–17.

Morgan, K. J., & Treadway, J. (1989). Surveying nursing staff's attitudes about AIDS. *AIDS Patient Care, 3*(5), 34–38.

Nielsen, C. (1988). AIDS: Attitudes and risks in the occupational setting. *The Australian Journal of Advanced Nursing, 5*(2), 46–52.

Occupational Safety and Health Administration. (1991, December 6). Occupational exposure to bloodborne pathogens. 29 CFR Part 1910.1030 [Docket No. H-370]. *Federal Register, 56,* 64004–64179.

O'Donnell, L., & O'Donnell, C. R. (1987). Hospital workers and AIDS: Effect of in-service education on knowledge and perceived risks and stresses. *New York State Journal of Medicine, 87,* 278–280.

O'Kane, P. M. (1988). Developing an AIDS program—Why some hospitals resist. *AIDS Patient Care, 1*(3), 28–30.

Prince, N. A., Beard, B. J., Ivey, S., & Lester, L. (1989). Perinatal nurses' knowledge and attitudes about AIDS. *Journal of Obstetric, Gynecologic, and Neonatal Nursing, 18,* 363–369.

Royce, D., & Birge, B. (1987). Homophobia and attitudes towards AIDS patients among medical, nursing and paramedical students. *Psychological Reports, 61,* 867–870.

Scherer, Y. K., Haughey, B. P., & Wu, Y. W. (1989). AIDS: What are nurses' concerns? *Clinical Nurse Specialist, 3,* 48–54.

Searle, E. S. (1987). Knowledge, attitudes, and behaviour of health professionals in relation to AIDS. *Lancet, 1,* 26–28.

Stanford, J. (1988). Knowledge and attitudes to AIDS. *Nursing Times, 84*(24), 47–50.

Swanson, J. M., Chenitz, C., Zalar, M., & Stoll, P. (1990). A critical review of human immunodeficiency virus infection—and acquired immunodeficiency syndrome related research: The knowledge, attitudes, and practice of nurses. *Journal of Professional Nursing, 6,* 341–355.

Talan, D., & Baraff, L. (1990). Effect of education on the use of universal precautions in a university hospital emergency department. *Annals of Emergency Medicine, 19,* 1322–1326.

Turner, J. G. (1990). Acquired immunodeficiency syndrome. In J. J. Fitzpatrick, R. L. Taunton, & J. Q. Benoliel (Eds.), *Annual Review of Nursing Research* (Vol. 8, pp. 195–210). New York: Springer Publishing Co.

Turner, J. G., Gauthier, D. K., Ellison, K. J., & Greiner, D. (1988). Nursing and AIDS: Knowledge and attitudes. *American Association of Occupational Health Nurses Journal, 36,* 274–277.

Valenti, W., & Anarella, J. (1986). Survey of hospital personnel on the understanding of the acquired immunodeficiency syndrome. *American Journal of Infection Control, 14,* 60–63.

Van Servellen, G. M., Lewis, C. E., & Leake, B. (1988). Nurses' responses to the AIDS crisis: Implications for continuing education programs. *The Journal of Continuing Education in Nursing, 19,* 4–8.

Van Servellen, G., Lewis, C. E., & Leake, B. (1990). The limitations of generic AIDS educational programs for the health professions. *The Journal of Continuing Education in the Health Professions, 10,* 223–236.

Wallack, J. J. (1989). AIDS anxiety among health care professionals. *Hospital and Community Psychiatry, 40,* 507–510.

Wertz, D. C., Sorenson, J. R., Liebling, L., Kessler, L., & Heeren, T. C. (1987). Knowledge and attitudes of AIDS health care providers before and after educational programs. *Public Health Reports, 102,* 248–254.

Wiley, K., Heath, L., & Acklin, M. (1988). Care of AIDS patients: Student attitudes. *Nursing Outlook, 36,* 244–245.

Wiley, K., Heath, L., Acklin, M., Earl, A., & Barnard, B. (1990). Care of HIV-infected patients: Nurses' concerns, opinions, and precautions. *Applied Nursing Research, 3,* 27–33.

Young, E. W. (1988). Nurses' attitudes toward homosexuality: Analysis of change in AIDS workshops. *The Journal of Continuing Education in Nursing, 19,* 9–12.

Young, E. W., Koch, P., & Preston, D. (1989). AIDS and homosexuality: A longitudinal study of knowledge and attitude change among rural nurses. *Public Health Nursing, 6,* 189–196.

PART V

Other Research

Chapter 10

Family Unit-Focused Research: 1984–1991

Ann L. Whall
Carol J. Loveland-Cherry
School of Nursing,
University of Michigan

CONTENTS

As a field of knowledge expands, cataloging, classification, description, and analysis of the content of that field of knowledge begin. The substantive knowledge known as family research in nursing or family nursing research is currently being classified and evaluated. In Feetham's (1984) examination of family research within nursing from the earliest efforts through 1983, several important aspects of this literature were identified. Feetham specified two major categories of research: family research that focused on the family unit and family-related research that focused on individual members within the family. In a further explication of the types of research, Feetham (1991) argued that family unit research is focused on the family as a whole and is transactional in nature in contrast to a focus on linear relationships between family members using data obtained from individuals. For the current review, research that focused on the family unit (i.e., measured family system variables) was included. Research that focused primarily on a family member or aspects of a specific illness, with the family unit as context or secondary/discussant variable, was considered as family-related research and not included in the review.

Since Feetham's (1984) review, there has been an exponential growth in family research in nursing. Specific subcategories, for example, family adaptation to chronic illnesses in children (Austin, 1991) and family caregiving (Given & Given, 1991), have been reviewed in other volumes of the *Annual Review of Nursing Research (ARNR)*. Based on an extensive examination of the literature within nursing, many citations that could be classified as family-related research were located. It was further concluded that there was sufficient growth in family unit research for examination of the latter category alone. In all likelihood other categories will be identified and examined in the future as subtopic areas within family-related and family unit research. It was determined, in this effort, to focus as Feetham had on research that could be described as family unit research.

There have been several attempts in the past within nursing to classify family research. Some of the schema used are those identified by Feetham (1984), Meister (1984), Murphy (1986), Whall (1981), and Whall and Fawcett (1991). Whall (1981) used the following categories: family unit research, research on dyadic family interactions, research on family negotiating within the environment, and research on individuals within families. Five categories were delineated by Meister (1984): theoretic perspectives on the family, natural family transitions, family and health, family and illness, and family and public policy.

Murphy (1986) identified the following categories as those that nursing shares with other disciplines: health maintenance and coping in healthy families; family response to illness; family transitions and evolving family structures; family interface with other social systems; family and public policy; and cross-cultural family research. Whall and Fawcett (1991) drew on these classification attempts and used these categories to address the state of the science and art in family research in nursing: family nursing theory issues, changes in family structure, healthy families, and the impact of illness on the family. For this chapter, the data were used to generate the categories for the review, and the resulting categories resemble those of Murphy. The categories used for this review are family transitions and evolving structure (with five subcategories); cross-cultural family research; family "needs" studies (with four subcategories), and methodologic studies.

The process that was used to identify published family research in nursing was stepwise in nature. The *Cumulative Index of Nursing Studies* was reviewed for the target period, 1984 to 1991, for journal articles; books and dissertation research were excluded. A computerized MEDLINE search as well as a hand search of several major family journals external to nursing (*Family Relations, Family Process, Journal of Marriage and the Family,* and *Family Review*) also were used. Only journals published in the United States and only articles written in English were selected. After redundancies were eliminated, articles that were not research were eliminated. The resulting list was compared with an unpublished review of family research in nursing for the years 1985 to 1989 (personal communication, Nancy Trigar-Artinian). This initial process resulted in a list of 199 articles that were concerned with families and were reports of research.

The next goal was to exclude articles that did not have the family unit as the major focus. Thus articles were excluded in which the family as a whole was not discussed, data on more than two family members (such as husband and wife), were not collected or in which family-focused instruments were not used. Because other ARNR chapters have reviewed family caregiving, family adaptation to chronic illness in children, childhood bereavement, and family violence, a decision was made to exclude all articles that could be identified as falling within these areas. Therefore, research focused primarily on spousal and other dyadic relationships, such as caregiver/patient, as well as that focused on family bereavement and violence (such as elder abuse), were excluded. Moreover a nurse author needed to be identified as a member of the group authoring the article. From the 199 articles, 51 were identified as having a family unit focus as defined for this review.

Each of the articles selected for its family unit focus was analyzed in terms of design, theoretic/conceptual framework, conceptualization/definition of family unit; in addition sample size/type, major variables, and instruments used were noted to describe the studies. These questions also were addressed: Is the term "family" defined? Is the study design appropriate? Is there conceptual congruence between the instruments and analysis? Are the findings appropriate given the study intent and methods? Not all these findings could be presented in this chapter; selected findings were, therefore, used to describe trends and patterns within categories.

FAMILY TRANSITIONS AND EVOLVING FAMILY STRUCTURES

The health-related consequences of family structure were a major focus within this overall category. Studies in this category are discussed in the following subcategories.

Postdivorce Adjustment in Families

Five studies (Bryan, Coleman, Ganong, & Bryan, 1986; Ganong & Coleman, 1991; Pett & Vaughan-Cole, 1986; Siebert, Ganong, Hagemann, & Coleman, 1986; Webster-Stratton, 1989) examined aspects of postdivorce adjustment for parents and children. These studies reflect the concern, evident in the larger literature on divorced families, regarding the potential for negative consequences for both parents and children. The results in general are consistent with other literature and contribute to nursing's knowledge of the fastest growing family form in the United States, the single-parent family.

Several studies of single-parent families have focused on the impact of divorce on parents and children. Pett and Vaughan-Cole (1986), for example, examined the impact of economic pressures on social and emotional functioning of divorced custodial parents. The changes in social status were more extreme for female custodial parents; they experienced lower incomes and more fluctuation in income, with those in the lowest income group initially having the greatest changes. The results supported the negative impact of a precarious economic situation for many female-headed, single-parent families and the need for assistance to improve their financial status.

Webster-Stratton (1989) studied the effects of divorce on support, conflict, mothers' and fathers' perceptions of children's adjustment, parenting behaviors, and child conduct problems. The sample was recruited from a parenting clinic and included those maritally supported, maritally distressed, and single parents. Mothers' low marital satisfaction was significantly correlated with behavior problems of children and high parenting stress. For fathers, low marital satisfaction was related to higher parenting stress. Single mothers reported more child behavior problems and higher parenting stress. Observations of mother–child interactions demonstrated that single mothers used more commands, criticisms, and questions, and that these children were less compliant and more deviant. All mothers reported perceiving male children as having more problems than female children. However, single mothers perceived more problems with daughters than did other mothers. The findings are important for they support the stresses experienced by single-parent families and the consequences for children in these families.

A variety of examinations of the consequences of divorce and remarriage are evident in the program of research of Ganong and Coleman (Bryan et al., 1986; Ganong & Coleman, 1986, 1991; Siebert et al., 1986). One component of this program of research has examined the negative stigma associated with stepfamilies, and the effects of family structure on perceptions of stepparents and stepchildren (Bryan et al., 1986; Siebert et al., 1986). The researchers found that stepparents were viewed more negatively than were married and widowed parents and that children in stepfamilies and single-parent families were viewed more negatively than those in other family types. The authors concluded support for the notion that family structure acts as a cue for stereotyping. The implications for nurses working with these families relate to the potential negative bias.

Health in Single-Parent Families

Three studies specifically examined health and health behaviors in single-parent families. Duffy (1986) described primary prevention behaviors of female-headed, single-parent families and identified barriers to practice of health behaviors. Data were collected using interviews, a health diary, and a card sort. All families described doing at least one primary prevention behavior regularly, primarily behaviors related to use of the health care system and behaviors to maintain one's health. Women identified several barriers to primary prevention including time, money, needing support, not feeling good about the behavior, never thinking about the behavior, and needing more information.

Hanson (1986) studied characteristics of health in single-parent families. A significant negative correlation between social-economic status and children's health was demonstrated. In addition, children living with fathers had lower physical health scores than those living with mothers. Social support was positively related to parents' mental health and children's overall health; communication was positively related to parents' mental health and to children's physical and mental health. Religiousness was related to children's overall and physical health.

Loveland-Cherry (1986) used Pratt's (1976) Energized Family Model to examine the differences in health behaviors in single-parent and two-parent families. The sample was recruited from community groups. There were no significant differences in nutrition, sleep, or exercise behaviors for individuals in the two types of families. However, different family factors were related to health behaviors in the two types of families. In single-parent families, there were positive correlations between mothers' use of positive socialization practices, and mothers' and total family's health practices. Children's involvements in activities outside the home were positively related to their own and total family health practices. In two-parent families, mothers' use of aversive control with children was positively correlated with total family health practices. Children's participation in activities outside the home was positively correlated with their own and total family personal health practices. Family socioeconomic status and health training efforts by parents were not significantly related to health practices.

These studies reflect a growing but limited concern within nursing regarding the potential impact of the single-parent family on health. Clearly, the complex pressures on female-headed families that may negatively affect health promotion and maintenance activities are of concern. The findings do not as yet present a clear picture of whether a single-parent family structure compromises the health and health behaviors of members. Comparative studies between single- and two-parent families provide beginning explanations of how families promote health in their members.

Employment and Family Stress

Considerable debate regarding the effects of dual-wage-earner family structure on family and individual outcomes is evident in the literature. Two-income families were the targeted group when Sund and Ostwald (1985) examined relationships between family stress and personal and life-style-related variables. Relationships between stress levels and life-style variables were evident. Older parents and older children had lower family stress scores, and the higher the income satisfaction, satisfaction with child care, and flexibility in leisure activities, the lower the stress score.

Another study (Youngblut, Loveland-Cherry, & Horan, 1991) investigated the effects of maternal employment, mothers' degree of choice, and satisfaction with employment status on family functioning and the development of preterm infants. No significant differences in family function or child development by maternal employment status were found. However, better motor development scores were evident in infants of mothers who reported having more choice in employment decisions than in infants of mothers reporting less choice. Results of these two studies (Sund & Ostwald, 1985; Youngblut et al., 1991) suggest that the employment status of the mother may not be as critical as other factors, such as choice in employment decisions and resources.

The stress of unemployment has potential negative consequences for family members. Friedemann (1987) examined the effects of fathers' unemployment on family members. Relationships were examined between economic indicators and child factors, parent factors, and parent-child factors. Economic setbacks in families were negatively correlated with peer acceptance of a child, and economic variables were found to be related to fathers' depression scores. Troubled marital relationships were related to mothers' and fathers' depression scores.

Krach (1990) investigated the financial strain in farm families as well as perceptions of filial responsibility and affection for aged parents. Although most of the subjects had inadequate incomes, feelings of filial responsibility remained strong as financial resources decreased and frequent satisfying contact between family and aged relatives continued. Continued use of the Double ABCX Model of Family Stress in three of these studies (Friedemann, 1987; McCubbin & Patterson, 1983; Sund & Ostwald, 1985) suggests that it is a useful framework for understanding the impact of economic stressors on family health.

Intergenerational Families

Increasing numbers of three-generation families are existent in the United States; two qualitative studies examined the patterns of interaction in these families. The roles of grandmothers in assisting their grandchildren to cope with problems were the subject of a study reported in two articles (Flaherty, 1988; Flaherty, Facteau, & Garver, 1987). This study, one of the few with a sample of other than white subjects, explored the functions of grandmothers in caring for the children of their adolescent daughters in black families. The family was defined as consisting of a grandmother, her biologic daughter, and the daughter's infant. Qualitative analysis yielded seven grandmother functions: managing, caretaking, coaching, assessing, nurturing, assigning, and patrolling, in descending order of occurrence.

Lund, Feinhauer, and Miller (1984) examined problems identified by families when an elderly grandparent resided in the family home. Content analysis of the elderly family members' responses to open-ended items dealing with specific difficulties indicated few major problems but also ambivalent feelings. Some dissatisfaction—with such things as a feeling of loneliness, lack of friends, and absence of enough meaningful roles—was evident. The investigators stressed the lack of uncertainty expressed by the elders regarding how other family members viewed them. Overall, the adult caregiver children responded positively about their elderly parent and their living situation. The most common problem identified by the families was lack of communication within the family. The grandchildren identified problems with being able to stay away from home overnight, lack of space, communication, and difficulty with personal behaviors of the grandparent. The families were more able to identify problems than solutions.

Family Stress During Transition to Parenthood

Transition to parenthood has continued to be viewed as a stressful period for families. Several nurse researchers (Brown, 1986; Mercer & Ferketich, 1990; Mercer, Ferketich, DeJoseph, May, & Sollid, 1988; Pridham & Zavoral, 1988) have examined this transitional period from a stress-coping perspective. In a cross-sectional study, Brown (1986) compared social support, stress, and health in expectant couples. Models for predicting health were different for mothers and fathers. While partner support and stress were critical factors for both mothers and fathers, chronic illness and support from others also were important predictors of mothers' health.

The Mercer and Ferketich program of research focuses on family stress during transition to parenthood (Mercer & Ferketich 1990; Mercer et al., 1988; Mercer, May, Ferketich, & DeJoseph, 1986). This team of researchers developed a model that predicted family functioning in groups of expectant parents. A sample of high-risk mothers and their partners, and low-risk mothers and their partners were interviewed during the 24th to 34th week of the pregnancy. It was hypothesized that high-risk women and partners experiencing antenatal hospitalization would report less optimal family functioning than the low-risk group and that expectant partners would report similar levels of family functioning. The findings supported that high-risk women reported significantly less optimal family functioning than low-risk women, but only high-risk women's partners reported perceptions of similar levels of family functioning. Low-risk men reported significantly less discrepant family functioning.

A second study (Mercer & Ferketich, 1990) was a follow-up of the same sample at 8 months postpartum using the same theoretic model. The proposed model had relatively low predictive power among groups. Respecified, empiric models had moderate to strong explanatory power for family functioning. Overall, results indicated that different explanatory models may be active for mothers and fathers and for high-risk women versus other groups. Further, perceived support was more predictive of family functioning than was received support. Of special note was the use of causal modeling to expand the understanding of the complexity of variables related to family functioning during this transition period.

Pridham and Zavoral (1988) addressed family support available for mothers of new infants. The researchers posed questions to mothers on availability of help with household tasks and infant care from fathers, grandparents, and others. Perceived support versus received support was a major focus. Biweekly interviews of mothers and log keeping were used. The framework guiding the study was that of family stress/coping. This study was unusual in that it focused on household tasks and a log-keeping interview format across time.

Commonalities are evident in this first category of studies related to family transitions and evolving family structures. Studies modified and extended existing theories and existing conceptual frameworks, often that of stress/coping. The focus also was often on the consequences of a transition or structural change in relation to family health. Fairly large sample sizes are found in this category along with a survey design emphasis. Development of middle-range family theory that is focused on maintaining health during these transitional events is one clear outcome of the studies in this category. Several needs for further research are evident after the review of this group of studies: replication of studies, the interrelating of studies, cross-analyses of instruments used to address family stress and coping, the fostering of continuing programs of research and second-generation programs of research, as well as the need to make clear the definitions of family that are used in each study so that clearer comparisons of results (such as meta-analysis) may be made.

CROSS-CULTURAL FAMILY RESEARCH

Little attention to culturally, ethnically, or racially diverse families was evident in the nursing literature for the selected period. Only two family unit–focused studies that explicated the ethnocultural aspects of specific groups of families were found for this period. Using a general system theory orientation, Dechesnay (1986) addressed Jamaican families; a participant observation technique was used to collect data. Dominant forms of family structure were identified: nuclear, patriarchal-patrifocal, matrifocal, and quasi-matrifocal. The first type was characterized by traditional sex-role expectations; the second type evidenced some matriarchal sex-role expectations; the third structure included those single mothers and children who lived in the mother's or maternal grandmother's home but had fathers who visited. The investigator concluded that matrifocal and quasi-matrifocal types of families should be considered as lying within the range of healthy families, contrary to the view of the Eurocentric model. This study demonstrates the need for health professionals to consider variables related to cultural preference and to be concerned about ethnocentric conclusions that may be drawn from a dominant cultural perspective.

The second study was published in two parts (Erkel, 1985a, 1985b) and focused on community health nurses' views of service to low-income black, Mexican-American, and white families. The study was conceptualized within a cultural conflict framework and used both a participant observation and survey method. Community health nurses and a maternal-child health consultant were recruited from visiting nurse districts with predominantly black, Mexican-American, or white populations. Respondents identified more major problems in delivering care to Mexican-American families than to white or black families, but the difference was not statistically significant.

More family unit studies that are focused on cultural variability are needed to understand adequately cultural preference in health and illness; it seems evident that the relevance and effectiveness of nursing practice depends on such knowledge. The knowledge needed to prepare nurses to work effectively and appropriately with culturally diverse families is an area that needs to be further developed. Qualitative family studies would seem to provide an important avenue for this research.

FAMILY NEEDS STUDIES

Many family needs studies examined perceptions and feelings of families with a member with a critical illness, often cardiovascular disease or cancer. The variables of interest often were descriptions of family emotional needs during the illness (Artinian, 1989; Boykoff, 1986; Daley, 1984; Gillis, 1984; Hinds, 1985; Leske, 1986; Lewandowski & Jones, 1988; Lynn-McHale & Bellinger, 1988; Norris & Grove, 1986). Some of these studies continued earlier work on family needs, for example, Molter's (1979) work. Dracup and Brau (1978), and Hampe (1975) used the Critical Care Family Needs Inventory (CCFNI) developed by Molter and Leske; the Norris and Grove (1986) questionnaire of perceived needs of families of critically ill patients also was used in several studies. Only one qualitative study (Titler, Cohen, & Craft, 1991) was found that explored family needs.

Across studies there are similarities in family perceived needs during severe illnesses. Some of these needs are relief of anxiety, information, need to be with the patient, need to be helpful to the patient, need for support and ventilation, and assurance that the patient is receiving competent, compassionate care (Boykoff, 1986; Daley, 1984; Leske, 1986; Price, Forrester, Murphy, & Monaghan, 1991). For families of individuals with cancer, who lived at home, needs were more specific: providing physical care, financial need, affective/psychologic needs, and respite needs (Hinds, 1985).

Several studies compared nurses' perceptions of family needs to those of the family members (Forrester, Murphy, Price, & Monaghan, 1990; Jacono, Hicks, Antonioni, O'Brien, & Rasi, 1990; Lynn-McHale & Bellinger, 1988; Norris & Grove, 1986). Findings across studies consistently indicated that nurses were only moderately accurate in identifying the family's perception of their needs; families and nurses identified different needs and different levels of needs. Nurses were more accurate, however, when it came to evaluating family satisfaction levels.

In this family needs/perceptions of needs category, there is evidence of replication and building of a knowledge base regarding needs of families. In fact, a consensus regarding common family needs supports the readiness to move to intervention studies. As in other categories, cultural differences were not usually noted.

Family Needs During Illness

One study (Mishel & Murdaugh, 1987) addressed the needs that family members of heart transplant recipients experience. Data were collected using an open-ended question format during support groups. The themes that emerged were immersion, passage, and negotiation, which as a group were entitled "redesigning the dream." The themes corresponded with the three states of cardiac condition, the waiting, hospitalization, and recovery.

Dyck and Wright (1985) examined the expectations of relatives of hospitalized cancer patients regarding nursing care. The patients were in one of three stages: diagnostic, recurrent, or terminal cancer. Many family members in the total sample did not expect the nurse to do much for them, whereas more than a third of the sample indicated that honest information from the nurse was important, and about a fourth of the sample indicated they thought such information was beyond the scope of the nurse's role. Most family members expressed satisfaction with the nursing care they received. Families identified desirable traits for nurses as competence, compassion, friendliness, cheerfulness, and genuineness.

Lewandowski and Jones (1988) had families of patients with cancer rank a series of nursing interventions as least and most helpful at different times during the illness. The most helpful interventions focused on providing information regarding the patient's care, letting members talk about feelings, and crying with families.

In two studies (Halm, 1990; Sigsbee & Geden, 1990), interventions were directed at decreasing anxiety in family members. Halm (1990) found that support groups were effective in reducing anxiety of adult family members during a relative's critical illness. In the second study, cardiopulmonary resuscitation was taught to family members of hospitalized cardiac patients and family members of nonhospitalized cardiac patients (Sigsbee & Geden, 1990). Family members demonstrated a significant decline in anxiety over three time periods.

Dracup (1984) addressed the psychologic risks and benefits of teaching cardiopulmonary resuscitation to family members of patients at high risk for sudden death. Control theory provided the theoretic structure for the study. There were significant differences in patient outcome measures across time.

Flodquist and Singer (1984) addressed nurses working with families in an intensive care unit (ICU). Nurses from one ICU attended educational sessions and nurses from a comparison unit did not. Results indicated that, for the nurses in the educational sessions, there were significant opinion changes. The nurses from the intervention unit evidenced a positive change in the total number of activities related to family members.

Chaves and Faber (1987) examined the effect of an education-orientation program on family members' psychologic stress and physiologic responses. There were significant differences in mean heart rate for the experimental group: the heart rates were lower after the education-orientation program.

Reduction of Stress in Families of Critically Ill Individuals

This group of studies focuses on the family's perception of and reaction to the illness event. The illnešs events covered a broad range of physical and psychologic illness: botulism (Hardin & Cohen, 1988), coronary bypass surgery (Gilliss, 1984; Gilliss, Sparacino, Gortner, & Kenneth, 1985), vascular disease (Leavitt, 1990), severe head injury (Mirr, 1991), ventilator-dependent adults (Smith, Mayer, Parkhurst, Pertkins, & Pingleton, 1991), and four studies focused on various aspects of individuals with psychiatric problems and their families (Hughes, Joyce, & Staley, 1987; Johnson, 1986; Rose, Finestone, & Bass, 1985; Wilk, 1988).

Other than the use of crisis theory (Dyck & Wright, 1985; Hardin & Cohen, 1988), stress theory (Gilliss, 1984; Gilliss et al., 1985), and Roy's Model (Smith et al., 1991), no consistent use of theoretic frameworks was evident in this group of studies. Both qualitative (Artinian, 1989) and quantitative studies identified sources of stress for families: fear of losing the family member patient; numbness/panic; insensitivity and impersonalization; family relations; financial strain; family member distress; lack of intrafamily support; and lack of control/feeling of not knowing outcomes.

The program of research with families of individuals who have undergone coronary aretery bypass surgery by Gilliss and colleagues (Gilliss, 1984; Gilliss et al., 1985) is noteworthy in that it is one of a few that have moved to an intervention stage. Family stress theory provides the framework for the program of research. Results indicated higher levels of stress in spouses than patients, although stress levels of patients and spouses were positively correlated. Sources of stress included waiting for the surgery and lack of control of hospital events. Three categories of factors were identified as contributing to the medical or surgical treatment choice: severity of illness; events leading to the decision for treatment; and features of the treatment. Most surgical respondents identified family and friends as being supportive of the decision and were more likely to identify joint husband-wife decision making. Surgical patients and their families experienced more restrictions in their activities and more disruption in family patterns and routines. They also reported more frequent contact with nurses who were often the primary source of information. Based on the results of this study, a clinical trial is in progress (Gilliss, Neuhaus, & Hauck, 1990).

Families and Infectious Diseases

Only one study examined family reactions to an infectious disease. Results of the longitudinal study of the psychosocial responses of family members of victims of a botulism outbreak identified anxiety and depression as the major psychologic reactions (Hardin & Cohen, 1988). Two types of anxiety identified were death anxiety and anxiety as a response to loss of control. Families also reported anxiety characterized by a sense of helplessness, fear of the unknown, and fear of being responsible for the physical care of the patients. The most frequently identified support were spouses, prayer, talking with a friend, and a sense of humor. Professional staff was identified as a support but not as frequently as anticipated.

Families and Mental Illness

Historically, interest in the mental health of families was centered on identifying eitiologies of schizophrenia (Bateson & Jackson, 1968). This focus has changed both within and external to nursing to a broader perspective.

Stuart, Laraia, Ballenge, and Lydiard (1990) addressed childhood family experiences of women with bulimia and depression. The findings supported significant differences in the perception of family "growing-up" experiences by women with these conditions and the control group.

Recently interventions with the family environment as a therapeutic milieu have been considered. Although the number of these studies is limited, they highlight the needs of families and also offer support for the viability of developing family-focused mental health interventions.

Measures of critical dimensions of the family environment, except for cohesion, were not significantly different for families in which the young chronically mentally ill adult lived in the home compared with those where the adult lived outside the home (Wilk, 1988). The role of the family in terms of improved outcomes for psychiatric patients is not clear. For example, there were no significant differences in readmission occurrences for psychiatric patients by extent of involvement of the family (Hughes et al., 1987). Results emphasized family interest in the control of the patient's behaviors, the need to talk to others experiencing a similar event, and feelings of isolation (Rose et al., 1985), and the sometimes minimal expectations that families have for patients (Johnson, 1986).

Williams, Elder, and Griggs (1987) studied the effects of family training on child behavior and parent satisfaction. Forty-seven family members who stayed at a short-term facility for behavioral/developmental problems self-reported data on the child behavior and parent satisfaction. Of the parents responding, all reported moderate to high satisfaction with treatment. Children's fears and inhibitions improved as did aggressive antisocial behavior, the former showing more improvement than the latter. For the children for whom preadmission and follow-up data were available, most showed a decrease in total behavior problems. The results suggested short-term effects of the training program. The authors recommended further evaluation using a prospective research design.

It can be said that common theoretic approaches evident in studies of families and illness include crisis theory (Dyck & Wright, 1985; Hardin & Cohen, 1988; Leske, 1986; Lynn-McHale & Bellinger, 1988); stress and coping (Artinian, 1989; Gilliss 1984; Gilliss et al., 1985; Hinds, 1985; Rose et al., 1985); adaptation (Lewandowski & Jones, 1988); and Minuchin's Structural Family Theory (Boykoff, 1986). Although both qualitative and quantitative approaches were evident, the latter was predominant. The studies were largely descriptive, correlational, and cross-sectional in nature. Samples were primarily those of convenience and were recruited from clinical populations. Studies of families in this overall needs category often used small samples, used multiple frameworks, and were concerned primarily with family perceptions and reactions. The conditions/illnesses that form the backdrop for this group of studies are disparate in nature. Replication of studies focused on a specific illness event would assist with generalization across studies. A more consistent identification of the theoretic framework and specific attention to the definition of family would also assist in cross-evaluation and meta-analysis of results.

METHODOLOGIC STUDIES

Several studies were reviewed that reported on the development of instruments to measure family variables. Two of the instruments are for use with families with critically ill members, the area of family nursing research that has the greatest number of publications. The Gortner Values in the Choice of Treatment Inventory (Gortner, Hudes, & Zyzanski, 1984; Gortner & Zyzanski, 1988) measures values related to the choice of treatment (i.e., the choice of surgical or medical treatment for coronary artery disease). The original instrument was developed by Gortner and used with a convenience sample of 15 surgical bypass patients (Gortner, Shortridge, Baldwin, & Sparacino, 1980). Following initial testing, a 20-item, two-factor (autonomy and beneficence) instrument resulted. The revised instrument was piloted with convenience samples of surgical bypass patients and patients treated medically for coronary artery disease and their family members. A revision of the inventory resulted in a 16-item scale and another revision in a 12-item scale. Factor analysis confirmed the two-factor structure, with similar solutions for patients and families. The agreement between patient and families appears to be greater for beneficence than for autonomy.

The second instrument, the CCFNI, developed by Molter (1979) and Leske (1986, 1991), is widely used to assess family needs. The results of three studies (Coutu-Wakulczyk & Chartier, 1990: Leske, 1991; Macey & Bouman, 1991) are consistent in supporting the reliability: coefficient alpha of .91 for a French version and .92 for the English version. Evaluation of the instrument using the Gunning Fog Index indicated that persons with a 9th-grade reading level could read and understand the CCFNI. Some redundancies among need statements have been found and a suggestion has been made to eliminate or combine some of the items.

The Family Research Interest Group of the Midwest Nursing Research Society developed the Family Dynamic Measure over a 5-year period (Lasky et al., 1985). Based on a review of 14 existing instruments, a total of 112 items were developed to frame questions on six dimensions of family life. Content validity was established using a panel of experts and pilot testing. After revisions, a 55-item Likert-type format was piloted with three groups to address reliability and validity. Two subscales, Individuation-Enmeshment and Flexibility-Rigidity consistently had alpha levels less than .70; reliabilities for all other subscales were greater than .70.

Hymovich (1984) developed the Chronicity Impact and Coping Instrument: Parent Questionnaire (CICI:PQ) to address the impact of a child's chronic illness on parents. The conceptual framework of the instrument was a modification of a framework developed earlier by Hymovich (1979). There are four components to the framework: developmental tasks of individuals and families; variables that influence the effect of a child's chronic illness on the family; coping strategies used by family members; and the intervention needed by families. The CICI:PQ addresses the second and third components of this framework. Based on the early work, a 500-item questionnaire was developed. The instrument was piloted with three different samples, with revisions after each pilot. The result was a 167-item questionnaire with three subscales measuring stressors, coping strategies, and values/attitudes/beliefs.

The final methodologic study examined the reliability and validity of the Family Environment Scale (Moos, 1979; Moos, Insel, & Humphrey, 1979; Moos & Moos, 1986), a widely used family instrument (Loveland-Cherry, Youngblut, & Leidy, 1989). Confirmatory factor analysis did not establish the three dimensions proposed for the instrument. Exploratory factor analysis resulted in a two-factor solution similar to those reported in the literature. Recommendations based on the findings included (a) using a Likert-type response format rather than the dichotomous format given for the instrument; (b) caution regarding three subscales because of reliabilities less than .70; and (c) possibly redefining the subscales based on analysis of the items.

Other articles that deserve mention are two that discuss issues related to scoring and analyzing family data (Jacobsen, Tulman, & Lowery, 1991; Uphold & Strickland, 1989). Both address approaches to analyzing data from more than one respondent. Uphold and Stickland clearly and concisely review the pros and cons of the various approaches to combining data from members of families. The article by Jacobsen, Tulman, and Lowery does not specifically deal with family data, but gives an excellent discussion of issues related to analysis of paired data; a situation common to family research when more than one family member are respondents.

Finally, an important body of work is the theory and instrument development efforts of McCubbin and Thompson (1987). Their continuing refinement of the ABCX Model of Family Stress (Hill, 1958) has resulted in the T-Double ABCX Model of Family Stress (McCubbin, 1988; McCubbin & McCubbin, 1987). As the model has evolved, a series of instruments to measure concepts in the model also have been developed. The work with this model and the accompanying instrumentation is a significant contribution to family research in nursing; both the model and the instruments are now widely used.

Although there are few studies in the methodology category for the chosen period, these are important efforts. The instruments and their underlying theory are consistent with the perspective of nursing and are essential for this developing area. Commonalities among these methodologic efforts are as yet minimal. However, there is promise that these methodologic efforts are the first of many, and commonalities across instruments will emerge.

DIRECTIONS FOR FUTURE RESEARCH

The number of family-unit studies in nursing has increased dramatically since the time of Feetham's review in 1984 to the present family unit–focused review of 1984 to 1991. Although still disparate in subject matter, commonalities are beginning to emerge. Persistent questions pertain to assisting families coping with illness events. Not focused primarily on the illness, a health perspective is emerging. Middle-range family theory is a product of these studies. However, there remains one persistent theoretic issue, that is, the unit of analysis, the family, is very often not explicitly defined.

The studies for the most part are not replication efforts, and thus the results are still in need of further examination. Programs of research are evident (e.g., Gillis et al., 1985, 1990; McCubbin et al., 1989: Mercer et al., 1988). The methods are not diverse, and primarily quantitative approaches are used; most studies are descriptive or exploratory in nature. Intervention studies are found primarily in the area of assisting families in the hospital setting to cope with illness in family members. In addition, more attention needs to be given to understanding how family health is promoted and maintained.

As with Feetham's review, the recommendation again is made to define explicitly the theoretic framework for each study so that analysis and evaluation of the theory underlying these studies and outcomes of these studies is facilitated. Such explication would facilitate the use of meta-analysis.

REFERENCES

Artinian, N. T. (1989). Family member perceptions of a cardiac surgery event. *Focus on Critical Care, 16*, 301–308.

Austin, J. K. (1991). Family adaptation to a child's chronic illness. In J. J. Fitzpatrick, R. L. Taunton, & A. K. Jacox (Eds.), *Annual Review of Nursing Research* (pp. 103–120). New York: Springer Publishing Co.

Bateson, B., & Jackson, D. (1968). Some varieties of pathogenic organization. In D. Jackson (Ed.), *Communication, family and marriage* (pp. 200–215). Palo Alto: Science and Behavior Books.

Boykoff, S. L. (1986). Visitation needs reported by patients with cardiac disease and their families. *Heart and Lung, 15*, 573–584.

Brown, M. A. (1986). Social support, stress, and health: A comparison of expectant mothers and fathers. *Nursing Research, 35*, 72–76.

Bryan, L. R., Coleman, M., Ganong, L. H., & Bryan, S. H. (1986). Person perception: Family structure as a cue for stereotyping. *Journal of Marriage and the Family, 48*(1), 169–174.

Chavez, C. W., & Faber, L. (1987). Effect of an education-orientation program on family members who visit their significant other in the intensive care unit. *Heart and Lung, 16*, 92–99.

Coutu-Wakulczyk, G., & Chartier, L. (1990). French validation of the critical care family needs inventory. *Heart and Lung, 19*, 186–192.

Daley, L. (1984). The perceived immediate needs of families with relatives in the intensive care setting. *Heart and Lung, 13,* 231–237.

Dechesnay, M. (1986). Jamaican family structure: The paradox of normalcy. *Family Process, 25,* 293–300.

Dracup, K. (1984). Consequences of cardiopulmonary resuscitation training for family members of high-risk cardiac patients. *Heart and Lung, 13,* 296.

Dracup, K., & Breu, C. (1978).Using nursing research findings to meet the needs of grieving spouses. *Nursing Research, 27,* 212–216.

Duffy, M. E. (1986). Primary prevention behaviors: The female-headed one-parent family. *Research in Nursing and Health, 9,* 115–122.

Dyck, S., & Wright, K. (1985). Family perceptions: The role of the nurse throughout an adult's cancer experience. *Oncology Nursing Forum, 12*(5), 53–56.

Erkel, E. A. (1985a). Conceptions of community health nurses regarding low-income Black, Mexican American and white families: I. *Journal of Community Health Nursing, 2*(2), 99–107.

Erkel, E. A. (1985b). Conceptions of community health nurses regarding low-income Black, Mexican American and white families: II. *Journal of Community Health Nursing, 2*(2), 109–118.

Feetham, S. L. (1984). Family research: Issues and directions for nursing. In H. H. Werley & J. J. Fitzpatrick (Eds.), *Annual Review of Nursing Research,* pp. 3–26. New York: Springer Publishing Co.

Feetham, S. (1991). Conceptual and methodological issues in research of families. In A. L. Whall & J. Fawcett (Eds.), *Family theory development in nursing: State of the art and science* (pp. 55–68). Philadelphia: Davis.

Flaherty, M. J. (1988). Seven caring functions of black grandmothers in adolescent mothering. *Maternal-Child Nursing Journal, 17,* 191–207.

Flaherty, M. J., Facteau, L., & Garver, P. (1987). Grandmother functions in muitigenerational families: An exploratory study of black adolescent mothers and their infants. *Maternal-Child Nursing Journal, 16,* 61–73.

Flodquist, G., & Singer, S. (1984). Increasing staff sensitivity to family needs. *Heart and Lung, 13,* 196–297.

Forrester, D. A., Murphy, P. A., Price, D. M., & Monaghan, J. F. (1990). Critical care family needs: Nurse-family member confederate pairs. *Heart and Lung, 19,* 655–661.

Friedemann, M. (1987). Families of unemployed workers: Need for nursing intervention and prevention. *Archives of Psychiatric Nursing, 1,* 81–89.

Ganong, L., & Coleman, M. (1986). A comparison of clinical and empirical literature on children in stepfamilies. *Journal of Marriage and Family, 48,* 309–318.

Ganong, L. H., & Coleman, M. (1991). Remarriage and health. *Research in Nursing and Health, 14,* 205–211.

Gilliss, C. L. (1984). Reducing stress during and after coronary artery bypass surgery. *Nursing Clinics of North America, 19,* 103–112.

Gilliss, C. L. (1991). Family nursing research, theory and practice. *Image: Journal of Nursing Scholarship, 23,* 19–22.

Gilliss, C. L., Neuhaus, J., & Hauck, W. (1990). Improving family functioning after cardiac surgery: A randomized trial. *Heart and Lung, 19,* 648–654.

Gilliss, C. L., Sparacino, P. S., Gortner, S. R., & Kenneth, H. Y. (1985). Events leading to the treatment of coronary artery disease: Implications for nursing care. *Heart and Lung, 14,* 350–356.

Given, B. A., & Given, C. W. (1991). Family caregiving for the elderly. In J. J. Fitzpatrick, R. L. Taunton, & A. K. Jacox (Eds.), *Annual Review of Nursing Research* (pp. 77–101). New York: Springer Publishing Co.

Gortner, S. R., Hudes, M., & Zyzanski, S. J. (1984). Appraisal of values in the choice of treatment. *Nursing Research, 33,* 319–324.

Gortner, S. R., Shortridge, L., Baldwin, A., & Sparacino, P. A. (1980). Ethical influences on family decisions regarding election of treatment. In *Ethical dimensions of nursing research,* Scholarly Nursing Leadership Series (pp. 114–133). Baltimore: University of Maryland School of Nursing.

Gortner, S. R., & Zyzanski, S. J. (1988). Values in the choice of treatment: Replication and refinement. *Nursing Research, 37,* 240–244.

Halm, M. (1990). Effects of support groups on anxiety of family members during critical illness. *Heart and Lung, 19,* 62–71.

Hampe, S. (1975). Needs of the grieving spouse in a hospital setting. *Nursing Research, 24,* 113–120.

Hanson, S. M. (1986). Healthy single parent families. *Family Relations, 35,* 125–132.

Hardin, S. B., & Cohen, F. L. (1988). Psychosocial effects of a catastrophic botulism outbreak. *Archives of Psychiatric Nursing, 2,* 173–184.

Hill, R. (1958). Generic features of families under stress. *Social Casework, 39*(2–3), 32–52.

Hinds, C. (1985). The needs of families who care for patients with cancer at home: Are we meeting them? *Journal of Advanced Nursing, 19,* 575–581.

Hughes, L., Joyce, B., & Staley, D. (1987). Does the family make a difference? *Journal of Psychosocial Nursing, 25*(8), 9–13.

Hymovich, D. P. (1979). Assessment of the chronically ill child and family. In D. P. Hymovich & M. U. Barnard (Eds.), *Family health care* (Vol. 1, 2nd ed.) (pp. 280–293). New York: McGraw-Hill.

Hymovich, D. P. (1984). Development of the Chronicity Impact and Coping Instrument: Parent questionnaire (CICI:PQ). *Nursing Research, 33,* 218–222.

Jacobsen, B. S., Tularan, L., & Lowery, B. J. (1991). Three sides of the same coin: The analysis of paired data from dyads. *Nursing Research, 40,* 359–363.

Jacono, J., Hicks, G., Antonioni, C., O'Brien, K., & Rasi, M. (1990). Comparison of perceived needs of family members between registered nurses and family members of critically ill patients in intensive care and neonatal intensive care units. *Heart and Lung, 19,* 72–78.

Johnson, S. W. (1986). Mutual expectations: How family members view the social role of the mental health center client. *Journal of Psychosocial Nursing, 24*(10), 35–36.

Krach, P. (1990). Filial responsibility and financial strain: The impact on farm families. *Journal of Gerontological Nursing, 16,* 38–41.

Lasky, P., Buckwalter, K. C., Whall, A., Lederman, R., Speer, J., McLane, A., King, J. M., & White, M. A. (1985). Developing an instrument for the assessment of family dynamics. *Western Journal of Nursing Research, 7,* 40–57.

Leavitt, M. B. (1990). Family recovery after vascular surgery. *Heart and Lung, 19,* 486–490.

Leske, J. S. (1986). Needs of relatives of critically ill patients: A follow-up. *Heart and Lung, 15,* 189–193.

Leske, J. S. (1991). Internal psychometric properties of the Critical Care Family Needs Inventory. *Heart and Lung, 20,* 236–244.

Lewandowski, W., & Jones, S. L. (1988). The family with cancer: Nursing interventions throughout the course of living with cancer. *Cancer Nursing, 11,* 313–321.

Loveland-Cherry, C. J. (1986). Personal health practices in single parent and two parent families. *Family Relations, 35,* 133–139.

Loveland-Cherry, C. J., Youngblut, J. M., & Leidy, N. K. (1989). A psychometric analysis of the family environment scale. *Nursing Research, 38,* 262–266.

Lund, D. A., Feinhauer, L. L., & Miller, J. R. (1984). Living together: Grandparents and children tell their problems. *Journal of Gerontological Nursing, 11*(11), 29–33.

Lynn-McHale, D. J., & Bellinger, A. (1988). Need satisfaction levels of family members of critical care patients and accuracy of nurses' perceptions. *Heart and Lung, 17,* 447–453.

Macey, B. A. & Bouman, C. C. (1991). An evaluation of validity, reliability, and readability of the Critical Care Family Needs Inventory. *Heart and Lung, 20,* 398–403.

McCubbin, M. (1988). Family stress, resources and family types: Chronic illness in children. *Family Relations, 37,* 203–210.

McCubbin, M., & McCubbin, H. (1987). Family stress theory and assessment: The T-Double ABCX Model of Family Adjustment and Adaptation. In H. McCubbin & A. Thompson (Eds..), *Family assessment inventories for research and practice* (pp. 3–32). Madison, WI: University of Wisconsin.

McCubbin, H., & Patterson, J. (1983). The family stress process: The Double ABCX Model of Adjustment and Adaptation. In H. McCubbin, S. Sussman, & J. Patterson (Eds.), *Social stress and the family: Advances and developments in family stress theory and research* (pp. 7–37). New York: Haworth.

McCubbin, H., & Thompson, A. (1987). *Family assessment inventories for research and practice*. Madison: University of Wisconsin.

Meister, S. B. (1984). Family well-being. In J. Campbell & J. Humphreys (Eds.), *Nursing care of victims of family violence* (pp. 53–73). Reston, VA: Reston.

Mercer, R. T., & Ferketich, S. L. (1990). Predictors of family functioning eight months following birth. *Nursing Research, 39,* 76–82.

Mercer, R., Ferketich, S., DeJoseph, J., May, K., & Sollid, D. (1988). Effect of stress on family functioning during pregnancy. *Nursing Research, 37,* 268–275.

Mercer, R. T., May, K. A., Ferketich, S., & DeJoseph J. (1986). Theoretical models studying the effect of antepartum stress on the family. *Nursing Research, 35,* 339–346.

Mirr, M. P. (1991). Factors affecting decisions made by family members of patients with severe head injury. *Heart and Lung, 20,* 228–235.

Mishel, M., & Murdaugh, C. (1987). Family adjustment to heart transplantation: Redesigning the dream. *Nursing Research, 36,* 332–338.

Molter, N. C. (1979). Needs of relatives of critically ill patients: A descriptive study. *Heart and Lung, 8,* 322–329.

Moos, R. H. (1979). Evaluating family and work settings. In P. I. Ahmed & G. V. Coelho (Eds.), *Toward a new definition of health: Psychosocial dimensions*. New York: Plenum Publishing.

Moos, R. H., Insel, P. M., & Humphrey, B. (1974). *Preliminary Manual for Family Environment Scale, Work Environment Scale, Group Environment Scale*. Palo Alto, CA: Consulting Psychologists Press.

Moos, R. H., & Moos, B. S. (1986). *Family Environment Scale manual* (2nd ed). Palo Alto, CA: Consulting Psychologists Press.

Murphy, S. (1986). Family study and nursing research. *Image: Journal of Nursing Scholarship, 18,* 170–174.

Norris, L. O., & Grove, S. K. (1986). Investigation of selected psychological needs of family members of critically ill adult patients. *Heart Lung, 15,* 194–199.

Pett, M. A., & Vaughan-Cole, B. (1986). The impact of income issues and social status on post-divorce adjustment of custodial parents. *Family Relations, 35,* 103–111.

Pratt, L. (1976). *Family structure and effective health behavior: The energized family.* Boston: Houghton Mifflin.

Price, D. M., Forrester, D. A., Murphy, P. A., & Monaghan, J. F. (1991). Critical care family needs in an urban teaching medical center. *Heart and Lung, 20,* 183–188.

Pridham, K., & Zavoral, J. (1988). Help for mothers with infant care and household tasks: Perceptions of support and stress. *Public Health Nursing, 5,* 201–208.

Rose, L., Finestone, K., & Bass, J. (1985). Group support for the families of psychiatric patients. *Journal of Psychosocial Nursing and Mental Health Services, 23*(12), 24–29.

Siebert, K. D., Ganong, L. H., Hagemann, V., & Coleman, M. L. (1986). Nursing students' perceptions of a child: Influence of information on family structure. *Journal of Advanced Nursing, 11,* 333–337.

Sigsbee, M., & Geden, E. A. (1990). Effects of anxiety on family members of patients with cardiac disease learning cardiopulmonary resuscitation. *Heart and Lung, 19,* 662–665.

Smith, C. E., Mayer, L. S., Parkhurst, C., Pertkins, S. B., & Pingleton, S. K. (1991). Adaptation in families with a member requiring mechanical ventilation at home. *Heart and Lung,* 20, 349–356.

Stuart, G., Laraia, M., Ballenger, J., & Lydiard, R. (1990). Early family experiences of women with bulimia and depression. *Archives of Psychiatric Nursing, 4,* 43–52.

Sund, K., & Ostwald, S. K. (1985). Dual-earner families' stress levels and personal and life-style-related variables. *Nursing Research, 34,* 357–361.

Titler, M. G., Cohen, M. Z., & Craft, M. J. (1991). Impact of adult critical care hospitalization: Perceptions of patients, spouses, children, and nurses. *Heart and Lung, 20,* 174–182.

Uphold, C. R., & Strickland, O. L. (1989). Issues related to the unit of analysis in family nursing research. *Western Journal of Nursing Research, 11,* 405–417.

Webster-Stratton, C. (1989). The relationship of marital support, conflict, and divorce to parent perceptions, behaviors, and childhood conduct problems. *Journal of Marriage and the Family, 51,* 417–430.

Whall, A. L. (1981). Nursing theory and the assessment of families. *Journal of Psychiatric Nursing and Mental Health Issues, 19,* 30–36.

Whall, A. L., & Fawcett, J. (1991). *Family theory development in nursing: State of the science and art.* Philadelphia: Davis.

Wilk, J. (1988). Family environments and the young chronically mentally ill. *Journal of Psychosocial Nursing and Mental Health Services, 26*(10), 15–20.

Williams, P. D., Elder, J. H., & Griggs, C. (1987). The effects of family training and support on child behavior and parent satisfaction. *Archives of Psychiatric Nursing, 1,* 89–97.

Youngblut, J. M., Loveland-Cherry, C. J., & Horan, M. (1991). Maternal employment effects on family and preterm infants at three months. *Nursing Research, 40,* 272–275.

Chapter 11

Opiate Abuse in Pregnancy

CATHY STRACHAN LINDENBERG
COLLEGE OF NURSING
UNIVERSITY OF MASSACHUSETTS

ANNE B. KEITH
SCHOOL OF NURSING
UNIVERSITY OF SOUTHERN MAINE

CONTENTS

The social, economic, and human costs from drug abuse are incalculable. Many of its tragic effects are seen in the estimated 200,000 to 300,000 women who are addicted to narcotics and in the 5,000 to 10,000 children to whom they give birth each year (Edelin et al., 1988). Between 8% to 14% of pregnant women abuse some form of drug, whether alcohol, cigarettes, or other prescription or illicit drugs. Two to 3% are believed to use cocaine and opiates, and these numbers have been growing (The Organization for Obstetric, Gynecologic, & Neonatal Nurses, NAACOG, 1988). Approximately .05% of childbearaing women are believed to use opiates (heroin or methadone) during pregnancy.

This chapter includes a review of the primary research on heroin and methadone use in pregnancy published between 1982 and 1990. It provides a synthesis of current research regarding the effects of maternal opiate abuse during pregnancy on fetal and infant health and development. Its purpose is to contribute to the compilation of a comprehensive body of literature and provide direction for further research efforts.

RESEARCH CHARACTERISTICS

One hundred articles pertaining to opiate use in pregnancy were identified and obtained through an on-line computer search. The selection criteria for review were that each article be published between 1982 and 1990; present primary research findings (i.e., reports of original research as prepared by the investigator who conducted the study); and involve heroin or methadone use during pregnancy. Key words used in the computer search were "heroin, methadone, opiate, and pregnancy." Case studies (anecdotal descriptions of individual cases) or animal studies were not included in this literature review.

Sixty-eight of the articles identified met the selection criteria. Ninety-two percent of these articles were published in medical journals and 4.2% in nursing journals. A physician was the primary author in 68% of the articles. In no research article was a nurse the primary author, although a nurse was among the authors in 7% of the research articles. In more than half of the research articles, specialists from other disciplines were contributors, suggesting multidisciplinary research participation.

Most of the research reviewed is being carried out in eight regions of the United States and in four other countries by researchers in a dozen academic institutions affiliated with clinical settings. Thus the articles reviewed were not 68 independent studies but essentially multiple reports of studies describing a limited population. Many of the studies are based on inner-city, public assistance, and often minority-based populations.

Ninety-six percent of studies were clinical observational and correlational surveys on the obstetric, neonatal, or child development outcomes of opiate use in pregnancy. The studies provide information on social, behavioral, and environmental variables to a much lesser extent. Ten percent of the studies describe drug users only; 20% compare cases of opiate-exposed subjects to subjects exposed to other types of drugs (case comparison); and the remainder of the studies compare opiate-exposed subjects to nonexposed controls. A few of the studies were quasi-experimental in nature, that is, investigators evaluated the effect of a treatment or an intervention (Archie, Lee, Sokol, & Norman, 1989; Carin, Glass, Parekh, Solomon, & Wong, 1983; Finnegan, Michael, Leifer, & Desai, 1983a, 1983b; Giles et al., 1989; Kandall,

Doberczak, Mauer, Strashun, & Korts, 1983; Suffet & Brotman, 1984). Archie et al. (1989) evaluated the effect of methadone on the nonstress test; Finnegan et al. (1983a, 1983b), Carin et al. (1983), and Kandall et al. (1983) evaluated differing medication treatments for withdrawal in neonatal abstinence syndrome (NAS); Giles et al. (1989) evaluated inpatient and outpatient methadone intervention modalities; and Suffet and Brotman (1984) evaluated general pregnancy outcomes of a prenatal drug abuse program. One article was methodologic, comparing the validity and usefulness of meconium and urine assays for drug screening (Ostrea, Brady, Parks, Asencio, & Naluz, 1989).

In all the studies researchers used nonprobability sampling procedures with the exception of the Habel, Kaye, and Lee (1990) and Kaye, Elkind, Goldberg, and Tytun (1989) New York City population-based studies of infant birth and death certificates. The most frequent samples were comprised of mothers and infants who met specific selection criteria and were enrolled in health programs, whereas nonexposed controls were selected for studies as they became available. In nine studies, controls were matched to cases according to variables suspected to influence outcomes, such as age, racial, and socioeconomic characteristics (Chasnoff, Hunt, Kletter, & Kaplan, 1989; Fiks, Johnson, & Rosen, 1985; Gillogley, Evans, Hansen, Samuels, & Batra, 1990; Hans, 1989; Hans & Marcus, 1983; Neville, McKellican, & Foster, 1988; Oro & Dixon, 1987; Rosen & Johnson, 1982). The ethnic composition of the subjects within studies differed greatly from center to center, which means that even the results of the better designed studies may not be directly comparable.

The independent variable of chief concern was drug use, although confirmation of drug use and operational definitions for drug use, dosage, and frequency varied. In approximately one third of the studies, drug use was confirmed through urine analysis, and in the remaining through documented self-reports. Infant physiologic and developmental outcomes were dependent variables in two thirds of the studies, whereas maternal outcomes were dependent variables in about a fifth of the studies.

RESEARCH FINDINGS

Maternal Correlates

Demographic and Other Characteristics. The research literature does not delineate any demographically consistent patterns associated with opiate use in pregnancy, primarily because of the convenience of study samples. Most studies were based on inner-city populations enrolled in public-assistance programs. A disproportionate number of these populations are low income and of minority ethnic distribution and thus are not representative of the population at large. Nonetheless, Edelin et al. (1988) in their study of an inner-city Boston population (N = 779), found a disproportionate number of white women in a methadone maintenance program despite the fact that the majority of the population served in the prenatal clinics was black. Oro and Dixon's (1987) California-based study (N = 140) also found opiate use was more likely among whites and Hispanics, whereas cocaine was more predominant among urban blacks. Similarly, in a New York City metropolitan hospital population (N = 1170), Kaye et al. (1989) found that among opiate users there were a larger percentage of Hispanics and a smaller percentage of blacks than among cocaine abusers. Gillogley et al., in a 1990s California hospital-based study (N = 1643), found a disproportionately higher number of blacks and a lower number of Hispanics with positive prenatal drug toxicologies when compared with the general population. Fulroth, Phillips, and Durand (1989), in an Oakland, California, general hospital population study (N = 1107), found no difference in age, sex, and race among drug abusers and controls. Rosen and Johnson (1988) (N = 111) found no significant differences in race. The relationship of age to opiate use was likewise equivocal. Several studies reported no age differences among opiate users and nonopiate users (Chasnoff, Burns, Schnoll, & Burns, 1985; Fulroth et al., 1989; Oro & Dixon, 1987), whereas some studies suggested that methadone users are older (Edelin et al., 1988; Giles et al., 1989; Gillogley et al., 1990; Hagan, 1988; Kaye et al., 1989; Little, Snell, Klein, et al., 1990; Rosen & Johnson, 1988). In summary, the lack of large population-based surveys prohibits generalizations about the differential demographic characteristics of opiate use among pregnant women.

Most studies reported that opiate abusers are *more likely to abuse other drugs* than are nonabusers (Edelin et al., 1988; Giles et al., 1989; Gillogley et al., 1990; Johnson & Rosen, 1982; Little, Snell, Gilstrap, & Johnson, 1990; Rosen & Johnson, 1982, 1985; Wilson, 1989). Rosen and Johnson (1982) found the majority of women in their study used other drugs in addition to methadone during pregnancy, and Wilson (1989) reported more than 90% of the women in the study to be polydrug abusers. Chasnoff et al. (1985), however, found no significant differences in cigarette, alcohol, and marijuana use among methadone, polydrug abusers, cocaine, and opiate-free controls.

Psychosocial and Parenting Experiences. Few studies provided information about the differences in psychosocial and parenting experiences of drug and nondrug users (Colten, 1982; Edelin et al., 1988; Hagan, 1988;

Johnson, Glassman, Fiks, & Rosen, 1990; Lifschitz, Wilson, Smith, & Desmond, 1985; Marcus, Hans, & Jeremy, 1984a; Rosner, Keith, & Chasnoff, 1982; Wilson, 1989). Although a variety of psychosocial variables are explored, the operational measures vary in focus and definition among these studies, making results not easily comparable.

Colten (1982), in a cross-sectional comparative study (N = 145), found little difference among drug (n = 70) and nondrug users (n = 75) in their perceptions of how having children changes one's life, what are the nicest and worst things about having children, reasons for having children, perceptions about their own children, and activities engaged in with their children. She also found similar social supports among these two groups, although there was a nonsignificant trend for heroin users to rely more on their own mothers. Heroin users expressed more doubts about their adequacy as mothers and their ability to control or influence their children. Rosen and Johnson (1988) compared methadone-maintained women (n = 25), polydrug abusers (n = 42), and drug-free mothers (n = 44); the drug-dependent mothers scored higher on depression and lower on self-esteem.

Hagan's (1988) smaller comparative study (N = 44) of etiologic factors related to substance abuse found the following risk factors associated with substance abuse: greater chemical abuse in family of origin, early sexual abuse (<16 years), lack of expression and cohesion in families, greater familial conflict and control issues, and lack of ego center. Marcus, Hans, and Jeremy (1984a) found methadone users more likely to receive public assistance, have psychiatric dysfunction, and have decreased levels of education than nonexposed controls. These researchers reported that two thirds of drug abusers were in stable relationship with a male partner, but that methadone users had adequate but poorer resources for maternal functioning. Lifschitz et al. (1985) found an increased incidence of low-average and mildly retarded intellectural performance among drug-exposed infants (n = 51) versus nonexposed controls (n=41) associated with high prenatal risk scores and deficient home environmental scores, but not significantly associated with maternal narcotic use per se.

In a comparative study of methadone users (n = 62) and nonexposed controls (n = 31) matched for socioeconomic status (SES), race, and infant Apgar scores, Fiks et al. (1985) found that the methadone users required more assistance in parenting, were more socially isolated, and were less likely to pursue vocational and educational activities. Interpersonal and environmental impact of poor parenting may further interact with and compound the effects of drug exposure.

In contrast with the studies associating drug abuse with psychologic disorders, in Neville, McKellican, and Foster's (1988) general practice Australian population study (N = 72), no higher frequency in psychiatric disorders or disturbed family backgrounds was found among heroin users. Wilson (1989) compared untreated heroin users (n = 29), methadone-maintained women (n = 39), and a nonexposed control group (n = 57) matched for age, race, SES, and marital status. She found that the children of untreated heroin users experienced more substitute parents, but that no difference existed among the maternal groups in education, occupation, home environmental scores, income, and family stability. These findings highlight the need for greater understanding of the antecedent psychosocial factors that may influence a woman's decision to initiate or escalate opiate use. The development and use of valid and reliable measures for these constructs is likewise essential for comparative analysis and interpretation of these studies.

Use of Health Care System. These indicators of drug abusers have been described in a few of the studies (Chan, Wingert, Wachsman, Schuetz, & Rogers, 1986; Edelin et al., 1988; Ellwood, Sutherland, Kent, & O'Connor, 1987; Giles et al., 1989; Gregg, Davidson, & Weindling, 1988; Hogan, Collins, Di Giusto, & Harbutt, 1986; Mark, 1983; Neville et al., 1988; Oro & Dixon, 1987). In a British comparative study of heroin users and controls, matched for sex, age, and social class, higher yearly doctor-patient consultation rates were noted for the heroin users. More heroin users failed to attend appointments. When consultations related to heroin and its effects were excluded, the consultation rates were similar (Neville et al., 1988). In Australia, antenatal and postnatal hospital admissions and costs were greater among narcotic-abusing mothers than among controls (Ellwood et al., 1987; Giles et al., 1989). In a descriptive study of 62 Danish drug-abusing women, few had sought prenatal care (PNC), 38.6% had incomplete infant vaccinations, 41% had incomplete postpartum newborn examination, and only 47% had received hepatitis vaccine (Mark, 1983).

Opiate abusers have also been found to be less likely to receive PNC or to initiate it late (Giles et al., 1989; Gregg et al., 1988; Kaye et al., 1989). In Giles et al.'s (1989) Australia hospital-based prospective study of methadone-maintained (n = 12), heroin-exposed (n = 24), and drug-free controls (n = 52), they found that methadone-maintained women initiated PNC earlier than other drug users, but that all drug-using groups had significantly fewer PNC visits and longer hospital stays than nonexposed controls. Conversely, Oro and Dixon's (1987) matched study (N = 140) found no difference in PNC among cocaine, amphetamine, heroin, methadone, and nonexposed women. The short- and long-term costs and benefits of health care use patterns among drug users warrent further study.

Obstetric Characteristics. The studies reviewed provided almost no information on the contraceptive practices of opiate users and nonusers, although gravidity rates might suggest less contraceptive use among these women. Both Giles et al. (1989) and Gillogley et al. (1990) found higher fertility rates among drug users versus nondrug users. In one study of 54 cases of heroin use, in which about one half were HIV seropositive, data indicated that these women were continuing to become pregnant subsequent to the onset of heroin use and seroconversion (Robertson & Bucknall, 1986). Oro and Dixon (1987) found no statistically significant difference in gravidity among a group of cocaine and amphetamine abusers and controls, but did find that opiate abusers had greater maternal gravidity than either cocaine and amphetamine users or controls. Similarly, Kaye et al. (1989) found cocaine- and crack-abusing mothers had lower parity (1.4) than somewhat older opiate and polydrug abusers (1.9 and 2.0). Chasnoff et al. (1985) (n = 53) did not find significant differences in gravidity among cocaine users, methadone users, and nonexposed controls.

Researchers suggested that numerous obstetric complications were associated with opiate abuse including increased rates of anemia (Ellwood et al., 1987), abruptio placentae (Chasnoff et al., 1986; Chasnoff, Burns, & Burns, 1987; Oro & Dixon, 1987; Rosen & Johnson, 1982), spontaneous (SAB) and induced (TAB) abortions (Chasnoff et al., 1985; Gillogley et al., 1990; Mark, 1983), preterm labor (PTL) or delivery (PMD) (Chasnoff et al., 1986, 1987; Giles et al., 1989; Gillogley et al., 1990; Little et al., 1990; Oats, Beischer, Breheny, & Pepperell, 1984; Oro & Dixon, 1987; Rosen & Johnson, 1988), premature rupture of membranes (PROM), and infectious diseases. Chasnoff et al. (1987) (N = 125) found that cocaine abusers had a high incidence of labor and delivery complications, whereas the opiate group did not differ from the general population.

The relationship of opiate abuse and abruptio placentae has not been clearly demonstrated. Two reports associated cocaine alone, or in combination with opiates, with increased rates of abruptio placentae (Chasnoff et al., 1986, 1987). Yet in the Oro and Dixon (1987) (N = 104) and the Gillogley et al. (N = 598) matched control studies of economically and ethnically diverse obstetric populations, no significant difference in the incidence of placental hemorrhage was observed among opiate and nonexposed controls, but a significantly greater incidence was observed in cocaine-abusing women. Similarly, Finnegan et al. (1982) found cocaine-using women to experience significantly greater rates of abruptio placentae than either drug noncocaine-dependent women and nondrug-dependent women.

Prenatal anemia: Nutritional status as measured by prepregnancy weight or prenatal anemia is a potential variable that may interact with the outcomes of neonatal growth and development. The incidence of poor nutritional status as measured by prenatal anemia was a variable of concern in a few of the studies. Ellwood et al. (1987) (N = 370) found increased rates of anemia (12%) in narcotic-abusing women versus nonexposed controls. However, Oro and Dixon (N = 140), in a study matched for known maternal risk factors, did not find significant differences in anemia among opiate-abusing and nonexposed controls, but did find significantly more anemia in cocaine/amphetamine-abusing women. Edelin et al. (1988) found methadone users had less anemia than a group of polydrug users.

PTL and PMD: These were reported in a few of the studies. Alroomi, Davidson, Evans, Galea, and Howat (1988) found a 28% rate of PTD; Ellwood et al. (1987) a 25% rate; Oats et al. (1984) a 27% rate; and Selwyn et al. (1989) a 32% to 33% rate. In a comparative study ($N = 111$) of methadone-exposed, polydrug-exposed, and nonexposed infants, methadone-exposed infants had highest rates of prematurity. Similarly, in a comparative study of drug-exposed (cocaine and amphetamines and opiates) and a nonexposed matched group, both cocaine- and opiate-exposed infants had higher rates of prematurity than controls (Oro & Dixon, 1987). Chasnoff et al. (1986, 1987), however, found significantly greater rates of PTL and precipitous labor among cocaine-using women as compared with opiate-using women. Little et al. (1990a, 1990b) report a longer course of pregnancy in a methadone detoxification group of women versus a group of heroin users.

Abortion: Opiate abusers were reported to have excess histories of SAB and TAB abortions when compared with controls (Chasnoff et al., 1985; Ellwood et al., 1987; Giles et al., 1989; Gillogley et al., 1990; Mark, 1983). In a descriptive study of 62 Danish drug-abusing women, 11.7% had experienced a SAB, 28% a TAB (Mark, 1983). Ellwood et al.'s (1987) Australia-based population demonstrated greater abortion rates among known drug abusers than control clinic patients. Chasnoff et al. (1985) reported a 38% rate of SABs among cocaine users, 46% among methadone and cocaine users, 16% among methadone-only users, and none among controls. Although greater rates of abortion among drug users versus controls was a finding among the studies reviewed, the underlying reasons that contribute to this phenomenon have not been elucidated.

Other complications: An increased rate of respiratory diseases such as asthma, pneumonia, or bronchitis, major trauma such as motor vehicle accidents and assault, and greater rates of sexually transmitted diseases (STDs), and hepatitis was found in narcotic-abusing mothers versus drug-free antenatal controls in Australia (Ellwood et al., 1987). Little et al. (1990a, 1990b) in their Texas hospital-based study ($N = 124$) did not find a significant difference in STDs between heroin users and nonexposed controls, whereas Chasnoff et al. (1986) reported greater rates of infectious diseases, hepatitis, and venereal disease among cocaine abusers versus opiate users.

In summary, numerous obstetric complications have been found to be associated with opiate use; however, the pathophysiologic basis for many of these complications and the complex interaction of potentially confounding variables or effect modifiers has not been clearly elucidated.

Fetal, Neonatal, and Infant Correlates

Neonatal Complications. A wide variety of neonatal complications, such as fetal distress, congenital malformations, strabismus, anemia, otitis media, and sudden infant death (SIDS), has been reported to be associated with opiate use. These findings, however, have had limited replicability across studies.

Factors associated with opiate abuse indicative of fetal distress included fetal monitoring abnormalities, increased duration of premature rupture of membranes (PROM), meconium staining, and low Apgar scores. Ellwood et al. (1987) reported an increased frequency and duration of PROM in narcotic-abusing mothers versus controls. Edelin et al. (1988) found significantly greater rates of meconium staining (46%–50%) among methadone and polydrug-abusing women than a nonexposed group (12.3%), as did Little et al. (1990a, 1990b). Similarly, a greater duration of PROM was found among these groups when compared with nonexposed controls, although no significant differences in Apgar scores were observed. Chasnoff et al. (1985) (N = 122); Chasnoff, Hatcher, and Burns (1982) (N = 85); and Little et al. (1990a, 1990b) (N = 124) found no significant differences in Apgar scores in their comparative study of various types of drug abusers and controls. On the contrary, Gillogley et al. (1990) (N = 598) found significantly lower Apgar scores among drug-exposed versus nondrug-exposed infants. Chasnoff et al. (1987), however, did find significantly greater rates of fetal monitoring abnormalities among cocaine-exposed infants than among methadone-exposed infants (15.3% vs. 9.5%) and greater meconium staining (25% vs. 8.2%).

The relationship of a variety of physiologic complications and opiate use has been explored. In a general obstetric population in urban Australia, rates of congenital malformations were not found to differ between narcotic abusers and the general population (Oats et al., 1984). This was likewise true in Gillogley et al.'s (1990) California-based study (N = 598) and Little et al.'s Texas-based study (N = 124). The prevalence rate of strabismus in a drug-exposed group of infants was significantly greater than in the general population (Nelson, Ehrlich, Calhoun, Matteucci, & Finnegan, 1987). The incidence of otitis media was significantly greater among methadone-exposed infants when compared with polydrug users, and nonexposed infants, at 12 and 18 months (Rosen & Johnson, 1982, 1988). Anemia was also reported to be more likely in methadone-exposed infants at 12 months than among nonexposed controls (Rosen & Johnson, 1988). Hogan et al.'s (1986) study reported that at 18 and 24 months, no statistically significant diferences were noted in parental rating of child's health, history of past illnesses, periods of hospitalization, and reported visits to physicians among infants exposed and nonexposed to substance abuser in utero, yet a greater incidence of chronic illness was reported among narcotic-exposed infants.

Pulmonary function studies from birth to 24 hours among infants of drug-dependent women show a transient decrease in lung compliance and tidal volume when compared with normal controls. By 3 days of age, lung compliance and tidal volume return to normal despite persistent tachypnea among exposed infants (Finnegan, Lin, Reeser, Shaffer, & Delivoria-Papadopoulos, 1982). Ward et al. (1986) found that infants exposed to opiates have a decreased ventilatory response to carbon dioxide. In their comparative study of pneumograms of opiate-exposed infants and nonexposed controls they found that drug-exposed infants had a longer total sleep time, greater durations of apnea, a higher total duration of apnea, more periodic breathing, a higher mean respiratory rate, and a lower mean heart rate. The authors suggest that these abnormal sleeping ventilatory patterns may be related to an increased risk for SIDS. Three studies found higher than expected rates of SIDS among opiate-exposed infants (Alroomi et al., 1988; Chasnoff et al., 1986, 1987; Habel, Kaye, & Lee, 1990). Habel's New York City probability population-based study found death rates from SIDS and acquired immune deficiency syndrome (AIDS) were especially higher for drug-exposed infants versus infants in the general population, and rates were similar for opiate- and cocaine-exposed infants. These findings, however, are not consistent with the Boston-based study, which found no statistically significant differences in the incidence of SIDS in a prospective analysis of infants of cocaine-exposed and nonexposed infants (Bauchner et al., 1988). Once again, the discrepancies in study findings point to the difficulties in controlling for potentially confounding variables and effect modifiers. Repeated studies of population-based samples that assess multiple variables are crucial to evaluating the nature and extent of the relationship of drug users and SIDS.

Numerous authors report neonatal abstinence syndrome (NAS) in opiate and other drug-exposed infants. NAS withdrawal is manifested by a wide variety of central nervous system symptoms such as irritability, restlessness, incessant shrill crying, inability to sleep, increased muscle tone, hyperactive reflexes, tremors, and in severe cases, generalized convulsions. The incidence of mild or untreated NAS observed in opiate-exposed infants ranged from 87% to 21% (Fulroth et al., 1989; Wilson, 1989) while the incidence of treated or severe NAS reported ranged from 76% to 14% (Fulroth et al., 1989; Weinberger, Kandall, Doberczak, Thornton, & Bernstein, 1986).

Several studies compared the incidence of NAS among opiate-exposed and other drug-exposed infants (Finnegan, 1984; Finnegan et al., 1982; Fulroth et al., 1989; Kaye et al., 1989; Livesay, Ehrlich, Ryan, & Finnegan, 1989; Oro & Dixon, 1987; Rosen & Johnson, 1988). These studies suggested that the incidence of NAS among opiate-exposed infants is greater than among nonopiate-exposed infants (58% vs. 36% [Finnegan et al., 1982]; 14% in heroin-exposed vs. 6% in cocaine-exposed infants [Fulroth et al., 1989]; 33% in opiate-exposed vs. 3% in polydrug-exposed infants [Rosen & Johnson, 1988]). Gregg, Davidson, and Weindling (1988) found signs and symptoms of NAS in 33% of infants exposed to the mothers who inhaled heroin in contrast to 70% to 85% of those infants who were exposed to injected heroin. In general, symptomatology in infants exposed to inhaled heroin was less severe than in infants exposed to injected heroin. Maas, Kattner, Weingart-Jesse, Schafer, and Obladen (1990) compared 58 women in a methadone detoxification program to 17 opiate users. Although 63% of all infants developed NAS, the incidence was significantly lower in the methadone detoxification group (55% vs. 88%).

The highest incidences of NAS were found among the infants exposed to opiates and other drugs (70% [Finnegan et al., 1982] and 35% [Fulroth et al., 1989]). In Finnegan et al.'s 1982 study of 300 infants, an incidence of 58% NAS was found among infants exposed to opiates alone in utero; 70% in infants exposed to opiates combined with nonopiates in utero; and 36% in infants exposed to nonopiates alone. Fifty-nine percent of infants exposed to opiates alone or with nonopiates were treated for NAS. An average of 7.6 days of treatment were required to control signs and symptoms of NAS, and the average duration of treatment was 38.6 days. Paregoric was the most effective drug used in the treatment of NAS (Finnegan et al., 1982; Finnegan, 1984). Oro and Dixon (1987) assessed and compared differences among cocaine/amphetamine-exposed infants and opiate-exposed infants. The cocaine/amphetamine group was characterized by later onset of NAS, a higher percentage of infants demonstrating clinical signs until day 2, and lower NAS score. Peak severity occurred on days 2 and 3 in both groups. The cocaine/amphetamine group had significantly lower maximum NAS scores than the opiate-exposed group, although their scores were abnormal. In a study of infants exposed to cocaine or heroin during pregnancy, Fulroth et al. (1989) found that mild symptoms of withdrawal occurred in 26% of the cocaine exposed, 21% of the heroin exposed, 47% of cocaine and heroin combined, and in 30% of infants with a history of cocaine exposure. Withdrawal requiring treatment occurred in 6% of the cocaine group, 14% of the heroin group, and 35% in the combined cocaine and heroin-exposed group. Thus these studies indicate that the use of heroin with cocaine may heighten an infant's risk for NAS. In their retrospective reviews of New York birth certificates, Kaye et al. (1989) found that opiate-exposed infants were significantly more likely to show adverse neurologic signs and need intensive care than these exposed only to cocaine.

Somatic growth: Effects of opiate exposure on infant growth in utero are reported by numerous authors. The measures most frequently provided were intrauterine growth retardation (IUGR), small for gestational age (SGA), gestational age (GA), birth weight (BW), birth length (BL), and head circumference (HC). It is important to keep in mind, that although in many of the following studies researchers have found statistically significant differences in somatic growth measures among drug-exposed and nondrug-exposed infants, only a few used multivariate techniques (Hans, 1989; Kaye et al., 1989; Lifschitz et al., 1985) or matching (Chasnoff et al., 1986; Chasnoff et al., 1989; Fiks et al., 1985; Giles et al., 1989; Gillogley et al., 1990; Hans, 1989; Marcus et al., 1982a; Neville et al., 1988; Oro & Dixon, 1987; Rosen & Johnson, 1982) to evaluate the potentially confounding effects of other factors known to influence growth, such as genetic factors, maternal nutrition, and prenatal weight gain. Likewise it may be important to ask whether statistically significant findings are clinically significant.

Several authors found that opiate-exposed infants were significantly smaller than nonexposed controls (Chasnoff et al., 1985; Ellwood et al., 1987; Giles et al., 1989; Lifschitz, Wilson, Smith, & Desmond, 1983, 1985; Oats et al., 1984; Oro & Dixon, 1987; Rosen & Johnson, 1982). Oats et al.'s (1984) Australia-based study found increased rates of IUGR (27%) in known narcotic abusers versus nonexposed controls. Rosen and Johnson's (1982) comparative study of methadone-exposed and nonexposed infants found that drug-exposed neonates had higher rates of SGA not associated with alcohol or tobacco. Lifschitz et al. (1983, 1985) and Wilson (1989) compared untreated heroin-exposed infants, methadone-exposed, and nonexposed controls. Both the heroin and methadone infants were significantly smaller despite similar GA. The heroin group was smaller for gestational age at birth than the methadone group, and both were significantly SGA compared with the controls. However, when adjusting for infant sex, race, prenatal care, maternal weight gain, PNC risk score, maternal education, and smoking, the differences related to drug use were eliminated. Ellwood et al. (1987) and Giles et al. (1989) also reported increased SGA parameters in narcotic-abusing mothers versus controls.

In a few studies researchers compared opiate exposure to that of other drugs (Chasnoff, 1985; Fulroth et al., 1989; Giles et al., 1989; Gillogley et al., 1990; Oro & Dixon, 1987). Chasnoff et al.'s (1985) Chicago-based studies (N = 122) reported that IUGR and shorter GA were greater among infants exposed to opiates than those exposed to other drugs (sedatives/stimulants, pentazocine and tripelennamine [Ts and Blues], phencyclidine piperdine [PCP]) and nonexposed infants. Similarly, in a California-based comparative study (N = 140) of drug-exposed (cocaine and amphetamines and opiates) compared with a nonexposed matched group, drug-exposed infants had higher rates of IUGR and shorter GA (Oro & Dixon, 1987). Conversely, Fulroth et al. (1989) (N = 1107) did a comparative analysis of cocaine, heroin, cocaine/heroin, and cocaine history subjects and controls, and only found a significant higher incidence of IUGR in the cocaine group. Chasnoff et al. (1986) found also that cocaine users had shorter mean GA than polydrug noncocaine users. Green, Ehrlich, and Finnegan (1988) compared methadone-exposed infants and infants exposed to an antidepressant and methadone. The infants exposed to the antidepressant and methadone had significantly shorter GA and lower BW than those exposed only to methadone.

Neonatal growth measures: Many studies evaluate the relationship of opiate abuse and somatic growth measures. Low birth weight (LBW) was a common finding among opiate-exposed infants when compared with nonexposed controls (Chasnoff et al., 1982; 1984, 1985; 1986; Edelin et al., 1988; Fulroth et al., 1989; Giles et al., 1989; Gillogley et al., 1990; Hans, 1989; Lifschitz et al., 1983, 1985; Little et al., 1990a, 1990b; Livesay et al., 1989; Rosati, Noia, Conte, DeSantis, & Mancuso, 1989; Rosen & Johnson, 1982). Among these studies, the statistically significant LBW reported ranged from an average 677 g (Chasnoff et al., 1982) to 274 g. (Edelin et al., 1988). Lifschitz et al. (1983) compared infants of untreated heroin users, methadone users, and nonexposed mothers. They found the untreated heroin-exposed infants to have the smallest BWs and both drug-exposed groups to be significantly smaller than nonexposed controls. Habel et al.'s (1990) New York population-based study found that drug-exposed infants were more than 3 times as likely to be of LBW as infants in the general population.

In a number of studies researchers found statistically significant BL differences among heroin/methadone-exposed infants and nonexposed controls (Chasnoff et al., 1982, 1984, 1985, 1986; Giles et al., 1989; Gillogley et al., 1990; Lifschitz et al., 1983, 1985; Little et al., 1990a, 1990b; Livesay et al., 1989). Among these studies, the statistically significant shorter BL reported ranged from an average 3.2 cm (Chasnoff et al., 1982) to 2.1 cm (Lifschitz et al., 1983). In a study comparing methadone-maintained, untreated heroin addicts, and nonexposed controls, the BL of drug-exposed infants was significantly below controls, yet group means were similar after adjustment for sex, race, PNC, pregnancy weight gain, obstetric risk, maternal education, and smoking (Lifschitz et al., 1983).

HC differences were demonstrated between opiate-exposed neonates and nonexposed controls (Chasnoff et al., 1982, 1985, 1986; Giles et al., 1989; Gillogley et al., 1990; Green et al., 1988; Lifschitz et al., 1983; 1985; Livesay et al., 1989; Rosen & Johnson, 1988). Among these studies, the statistically significant difference in HC reported ranged from an average 2.5 cm (Chasnoff et al., 1985) to 1.5 cm (Lifschitz et al., 1985). Lifschitz et al. (1985) found that smaller HC correlated with poor maternal nutritional status and poor BW.

In a few studies researchers did not find statistically significant differences in BW, BL, and HC among exposed and nonexposed neonates. Chasnoff et al. (1985) compared cocaine-exposed, cocaine-and-methadone–exposed, methadone-exposed, and nonexposed controls. They found that the methadone-exposed neonates tended to be smaller on all parameters, but that the differences were not statistically significant. Similarly, Rosen and Johnson (1985) found no difference in BW among methadone-exposed and nonexposed controls. Little et al. (1990a, 1990b) found no difference in HC among heroin-exposed and nonexposed controls.

In several studies investigators compared the effects of opiate exposure and other drugs of abuse on BW, BL, and HC (Chasnoff et al., 1982, 1985, 1987; Edelin et al., 1988; Kaye et al., 1989; Livesay et al., 1989; Rosen & Johnson, 1988). Opiate-exposed neonates demonstrated smaller growth on all somatic growth parameters when compared with nonexposed controls and polydrug-exposed neonates (Chasnoff et al., 1982; 1986; Edelin et al., 1988; Rosen & Johnson, 1988). Polydrug users fell between methadone and controls on most outcomes but did not differ statistically from controls (Rosen & Johnson, 1988). Ts-and-Blues–exposed neonates had significantly lower somatic growth rates than nonexposed neonates and were similar to methadone-exposed infants. Neonates exposed to sedatives, stimulants, or PCP did not differ from nonexposed controls in somatic growth measures (Chasnoff et al., 1985). Kaye et al. (1989) (N = 1,170) compared opiate, cocaine, crack, and polydrug abusers, and found the combined cocaine-and-opiate–exposed group of neonates to have the smallest BWs and shortest GA. This suggests a heightened risk for these somatic growth effects when cocaine is combined with opiates. In a comparative study of cocaine and amphetamines, involving an opiate-exposed and a nonexposed matched group, both cocaine and opiate groups were negatively associated with BW, BL, and HC (Oro & Dixon, 1987). Gillogley et al.'s (1990) study found that BW, BL, HC, and GA were significantly lower in toxicology positive groups as compared with controls, but that the difference was most marked for cocaine and polydrug use groups. The group that was positive for opiates alone had outcomes similar to controls. Differences persisted even when controlling for prenatal care, smoking, and prior preterm births. Little et al. (1990a, 1990b) found normalized BW and HC among a detoxified group of women when compared with heroin users.

Conversely, in their 1985 and 1987 studies, Chasnoff et al. found no significant difference in GA, BW, BL, and HC in cocaine, opiate-exposed neonates and nonexposed neonates. Likewise, no statistically significant differences in fetal growth parameters were demonstrated between cocaine- and heroin-exposed groups of infants (Chasnoff, 1987). Chasnoff et al. (1986) also found that BW was similar for cocaine users and polydrug noncocaine users. The inconsistency of these findings may well be due to methodologic issues such as sample size or disparate group assignments and to failure to evaluate uncontrolled confounding variables that are known to influence growth and development.

Infant/child growth measures: Longitudinal studies of the long-term effects of opiate exposure on somatic measures are reported by several authors (Chasnoff et al., 1986; Hogan et al., 1986; Lifschitz et al., 1983; Rosen & Johnson, 1982, 1985). These studies found short-term differences in weight, height, and HC among drug-exposed and control groups, but with increasing age these differences tended to disappear with the possible exception of HC. Hogan et al. (1986) reported on a comparative study of the infants of narcotic-addicted ($N = 79$) and nonaddicted women ($N = 61$) at 18 and 24 months of age. There was no statistically significant difference between narcotic-exposed and nonexposed infants in weight or physical examination, yet HC was significantly smaller in the narcotic-exposed children. This difference was not accounted for by maternal height, GA, maternal smoking, or SES. Rosen and Johnson (1982) compared methadone-exposed infants ($N = 62$) and nonexposed controls ($N = 32$). At 18 months a significant incidence in HC below the 3rd percentile persisted among methadone-exposed infants, but by 84 months there were no statistically significant differences in height and weight (Rosen & Johnson, 1985). In a longitudinal study of untreated heroin-exposed ($N = 22$), methadone-exposed ($N = 21$) and nonexposed infants ($N = 28$) Lifschitz et al. (1983) found that at 3 years of age, height was comparable for all three groups. However, when adjusted for birth length, parental height, and smoking, methadone-exposed children were significantly shorter than heroin-exposed children, and nonexposed comparisons were intermediate in height. Likewise by 3 years of age, head size did not differ significantly among the groups (Lifschitz et al., 1985), however; factors associated with HC measures were BW, intrapartum risk score, and race. These studies by and large, do not support the notion that there are long-term teratologic effects of drug abuse on somatic growth, with the possible exception of HC. Once again, more evidence is needed to understand the long-term effects of opiates on somatic growth and development.

Neurobehavioral and Developmental Effects. The effects of opiate exposure at birth were assessed by Chasnoff et al. (1982, 1985, 1986, 1987), and Marcus et al. (1982b). Neonatal neurobehavioral assessments were done using Brazelton's Neonatal Behavioral Assessment Scale (BNBAS) (Brazelton & Spastics International Medical Publications, 1984). The BNBAS is a tool that provides guidelines for assessing the newborn's state changes, temperament, and individual behavior patterns. The scale includes 27 behavioral items that are scored on a 9-point scale and 20 elicited reflexes that are scored on a 3-point scale.

In a comparative study of opiate-exposed (heroin, methadone, and Ts and Blues), and other nonopiate drug exposure (sedatives and stimulants, and PCP), Chasnoff et al. (1985, 1986) ($N = 122$) found differences in the interactive ability, motor maturity, inanimate and animal visual and auditory orientation, consolability, and state control of all drug-exposed infants when compared with nonexposed controls. Although infants born to women addicted to sedatives/stimulants or PCP did not show statistically significant differences in orientation and motor maturity responses from the nonexposed controls, opiate-exposed infants were differentiated from other drug-exposed infants (sedatives/stimulants, T's and Blues, and PCP) and nonexposed controls by poorer motor control, and poorer visual and auditory orientation (Chasnoff et al., 1985). In a comparative study of drug-exposed (cocaine and amphetamines and opiate) and a nonexposed matched group, drug-exposed infants had altered neonatal behavioral patterns characterized by abnormal sleep patterns, poor feeding, tremors, and hypertonia (Oro & Dixon, 1987). Similarly, in a comparative study of newborns exposed to opiates and a nonexposed control group, a significant decrease in quiet sleep and an increase in active sleep were found (Pinto, Torrioli, Casella, Tempesta, & Fundaro, 1988). The same alterations, although less marked, were observed in a follow-up recording during the second month of life (Pinto et al., 1988).

Three U.S. metropolitan clinical sites (Chicago, New York, Texas) and an international site (Australia) provided most longitudinal follow-up data on the long-term neurobehavioral effects of opiates. In all of the studies researchers compared women with opiate use with nonexposed controls. In addition the Chicago-based Northwestern studies provided comparative information of the effects of opiates and other drugs (Chasnoff et al., 1982, 1985, 1986, 1987). Longer-term neurobehavioral effects of opiates and other drugs on infants and preschool children were assessed primarily using Bayley's Scales (1969). The Bayley is a widely used standardized infant assessment tool and consists of a motor scale (motor, state control, and social indicators) and a mental scale (cognitive indicators). The studies most frequently report on four types of behavior: motor, state control, cognitive, and social, and results were consistently equivocal.

Motor behaviors include variables such as coordination, muscle tonus, and activity. The Chicago-based studies that compare methadone-exposed infants and nonexposed controls ($N = 40$) found that methadone-exposed infants differed on motor functioning when compared with nonexposed controls at 4 months (Bernstein, Jeremy, Hans & Marcus, 1984; Marcus et al., 1982b). Infants were more tense, active, and poorly coordinated. A significant correlation between day-1 and 4-month motor function was found, and methadone-exposed infants showed poorer motor functioning at both ages (Marcus et al., 1982b). A study by Hans (1989) that followed children up to 2 years of age revealed that methadone-exposed infants lagged behind unexposed infants in motor development and poor fine motor coordination.

However, differences were not statistically significant at 24 months when the effects of SES, maternal intelligence quotient (IQ), and pregnancy birth complications were controlled.

The New York City population-based studies (Johnson & Rosen, 1982; Rosen & Johnson, 1982, 1988) (N = 64 and N = 111, respectively) reported that at both 6 and 18 months, a significantly higher incidence of developmental delays and poor fine motor coordination were observed in the methadone-exposed infants when compared with nonexposed controls. Likewise, at 36 months, methadone-exposed infants were less responsive to rattle decrement, less responsive to inanimate visual orientation, less alert, less cuddly, and less consolable. These infants had increased tone, less motor maturity, and increased pull to sit, and were more tremulous. Furthermore, drug-exposed infants had increased obstetric complications that correlated with maternal methadone dose and duration, severity of NAS, and birth weight. On the contrary, Chasnoff et al. (1985, 1986) reported that drug-exposed infants were comparable with nonexposed infants at 2 years of age, but that environmental factors and subsequent lack of stimulation may have a greater influential factor on development than maternal drug use during pregnancy.

State control behaviors include such variables as irritability, self-regulation, and energy level. The New York population-based studies found that both motor and state control were poorer in methadone-exposed infants than controls, yet Marcus et al. (1982a) found that individual profiles revealed an orthogonal relationship between motor functioning and state functioning, with motor functioning being a much clearer discriminator between methadone-exposed infants and controls. With age, both groups generally improved, but the nonexposed infants maintained some of their advantage in motor functioning. Chasnoff et al. (1985), found that infants born to women addicted to sedatives/stimulants or to PCP showed significantly poorer state organization and consolability than the nonexposed controls. PCP-exposed infants had more lability of state and poorer consolability than all other groups (sedative/stimulant, Ts and Blues) of drug-exposed neonates. Infants exposed to cocaine versus opiates had significant depressed state organization and increased irritability (Chasnoff et al., 1987). Methadone-exposed infants showed more depression of interactive behaviors and state controls than polydrug-exposed or control groups (Chasnoff et al., 1982).

Social behaviors include such variables as responsiveness to persons and quality of attachment to mother. In the New York City population-based studies, no statistically significant differences in social/psychomotor developmental indices were found at 4 months of age between methadone-exposed and nonexposed controls (Bernstein et al., 1984; Hans & Marcus, 1983; Marcus et al., 1982b, 1984b). Differences among infants were found to be associated with maternal interactive performance, psychopathology, and psychological and psychosocial resources, not with length or dosage of narcotic use.

Chasnoff et al. (1985, 1986) likewise reported on infant social development at 3, 6, 12, 18, and 24 months. Groups were similar in race, maternal education, gravidity, PNC, nutrition, cigarette, and alcohol exposure. They compared opiate-exposed, nonopiate (other drug)-exposed, and nonexposed infants. Using Bayley's (1972) psychomotor development indices, no significant differences were seen at 3 and 6 months among opiate-exposed infants, but significant differences were seen among nonopiate (other drug)-exposed infants at 3 months when compared with nonexposed controls. In general all three groups scored within the normal range, but a downward trend was evidenced among all groups by 24 months, suggesting that environmental factors may contribute significantly.

On the contrary, Rosen and Johnson's (1982, 1985, 1988) New York population-based studies (N = 64–93) found that at 6 months there were no statistically significant differences in psychomotor scores between methadone-exposed and nonexposed infants. However, at 12 and 18 months, there was a significant incidence of lower psychomotor scores. Hogan et al. (1986) and Di Giusto, Collins, Hurbutt and Hogan (1986) also found that among 18- and 24-month-old infants, narcotic-exposed infants were significantly less socially mature than nonexposed comparisons. Adjustments for maternal education, GA, number of times in foster care, and home inventory score did not change these findings. No intergroup differences in other measures such as SES, self-esteem ratings, or stress scores were reported. The variance found was associated with poorer environments and with caregivers having greater self-ratings of hopelessness.

When comparing opiate exposure with cocaine exposure, cocaine-exposed infants demonstrated significantly more depression of interactive behavior and poorer state organization than cocaine-and-heroin–exposed, methadone-exposed, and nonexposed infants (Chasnoff et al., 1985, 1986). All drug-exposed groups (Heroin/methadone maintenance [H/MM] sedatives/stimulants, Ts and Blues, and PCPs) exhibited abnormal neurobehavior, but psychomotor development was comparable with control infants at 2 years.

Johnson et al.'s (1990) New York City prospective study compared a group of 36-month-old methadone-exposed toddlers (n = 62) and a nonexposed control group (n = 31). They found no statistically linear association between maternal drug abuse history, perinatal characteristics, and maternal functioning with a child's developmental course. However, using qualitative cluster analysis (based on a composite of HC percentile, Merrill-Palmer Scale score, neurologic examination, and referrals for developmental problems), they distinguished three patterns of development and identified a group of resilient children coming from homes that provided nurturance and stability despite maternal drug abuse.

Cognitive behaviors include variables such as perception, attention, and memory. In the New York City–based population studies, no statistically significant differences were found at 4 months of age between methadone-exposed and nonexposed controls in cognitive behaviors (Bernstein et al., 1984; Hans, 1989). At 12 months, methadone-exposed infants showed poorer attention spans as a group than controls. Family risk factors did modulate the strength and direction of differences (low SES, maternal psychopathology, low IQ, absence of father). Poorer early use of medical resources (prenatal and perinatal complications) heightened group differences at an early age but by the end of 1 year no longer played a role (Hans, 1989; Marcus et al., 1984b). These findings persisted up to 2 years of age when controlling for SES, maternal IQ, and pregnancy birth complication index. Differences in cognitive development among infants was found to be associated with maternal interactive performance, psychopathology, psychological and psychosocial resources, and not with length or dosage of narcotic use.

In their Chicago-based population studies (Chasnoff et al., 1985, 1986) also reported on infant cognitive development at 3, 6, 12, 18, and 24 months. They compared opiate-exposed, nonopiate exposed, and nonexposed infants. On Bayley's mental development indices (MDI) significant differences were seen at 3 and 6 months among both drug-abusing groups when compared with nonexposed controls, but by 12 months differences became comparable among all three groups. MDI scores of narcotic and controls were within normal range, exhibiting downward trends in all groups by 24 months. All other drug-exposed groups (sedatives/stimulants, Ts and Blues, and PCPs) exhibited abnormal neurobehavior, but mental development was comparable with control infants at 2 years. Additionally, methadone-exposed infants were differentiated from other drug-exposed (sedatives/stimulants, Ts and Blues, and PCPs) infants and nonexposed controls by poorer visual and auditory orientation responses.

The Texas studies (Lifschitz et al., 1983, 1985; Wilson, 1989) (N = 71–125) compared methadone- and heroin-exposed infants and nonexposed matched (age, race, SES, and marital status) controls. The two drug-exposed groups were similar in educational background, age, and obstetric risk factors. Cognitive function was measured by the Bayley Scales of Infant Development (1972) and McCarthy Scales of Children's Abilities (1972). With the exception of lower performance by the heroin-exposed group at 18 months, there were no significant differences in cognitive function between drug-exposed and nonexposed children. However, there was a pattern of gradual decline over time consistent with the performance of a disadvantaged population. Despite the lack of statistically significant differences, at 3 years of age they reported an increased incidence of low to average and mildly retarded intellectual performance in the drug-exposed groups. The variables of PNC, prenatal (PN) risk score, and home environment were most predictive of intellectual performance, and the degree of maternal narcotic use was not found to be a significant factor. In a subsample of heroin-exposed infants, there was a 30% rate of grade repetition, 35% needed special educational services, and many had weak visual-motor perception and skills associated with disadvantaged families (Lifschitz et al., 1983, 1985; Wilson, 1989).

On the contrary, Rosen and Johnson's (1982, 1985, 1988) New York–based population studies (*N* = 64–93) found statistically significant cognitive differences among opiate-exposed and nonexposed infants at 6, 12, and 18 months. They also found significant neurologic abnormalities in opiate-exposed infants at 6, 12, and 18 months of age, and a significantly higher incidence of neurologic findings of tone discrepancy and abnormal eye findings.

The Australia-based studies (*N* = 140) comparing opiate-exposed and nonexposed infants at 18 to 24 months of age found opiate-exposed infants performing less well on tests of cognitive function than a comparison nonexposed group of infants. Adjustments for maternal education, GA, number of times in foster care, and home inventory scores did not alter these findings. There were no intergroup differences in other measures such as SES or self-esteem ratings or stress scores (Hogan et al., 1986; Di Giusto et al., 1986).

To date findings on the long-term consequences of maternal drug abuse on neurobehavioral development are not conclusive but suggest that no long-term developmental sequelae are directly associated with opiate exposure. The studies, however, underscore a number of methodologic issues inherent in this research. Substance abuse is a dynamic and multifactorial problem interacting with and confounded by not only physiologic but psychosocial and environmental factors. The varying types, doses, and duration of drug use further confound these relationships, as well as does smoking and alcohol consumption, found to be prevalent among drug users. More refined measures need to be developed to track the multifactorial variables interacting with and influencing substance abuse. Most of these studies have been based on a main-effects model of development that assumes a cause-and-effect relationship between specific risk factors and outcome. The underlying assumption is that impairment or dysfunction is the result of the biologic insult of narcotic exposure in utero. Development is highly dependent not only on the characteristics of the infant but the caretaking environment and their mutual influence on each other. Thus we need more information regarding not just medical factors but psychosocial and environmental factors.

These measures need to be evaluated not only over time, but with multivariate qualitative and quantitative statistical models.

Intervention Studies

When one considers the short- and long-term importance of drug use prevention, treatment, and rehabilitative interventions for pregnant and childbearing women and their children, it is surprising what little intervention research is reported in the literature. Although preventive interventions in the area of smoking and alcohol for pregnant and childbearing women are well known, such efforts in the area of illicit drug use prevention are almost nonexistent. In clinical practice preventive efforts are limited primarily to early detection through physical history, urine toxicology, and information on known effects of drug use. Treatment or management of pregnant drug users generally includes control and support of withdrawal and methadone maintenance therapy for narcotics. Other aspects of care that are often provided, but for which little evaluative research is evidenced, are offering support services (nursing, social worker, addiction counselor, dietitian, psychologists, psychiatrists, etc.), providing nutrition education and monitoring, monitoring for sexually transmitted diseases and interrenal illness, and monitoring fetal growth and well-being. Follow-up and rehabilitation continues to include inpatient-outpatient detoxification or methadone maintenance, health education, postnatal supportive counseling, contraceptive counseling, public health nurse visits and training in parenting skills, neonatal developmental testing, and follow-up. The authors found a paucity of studies in which researchers evaluated the individual and/or combined contribution of these treatment and rehabilitative intervention strategies directly targeted at pregnant women.

Only 11 articles included reports of the results of interventions in which comparative data from two or more groups were used to evaluate the effectiveness of outcomes or methods for managing the care of pregnant women with opiate addiction (Archie et al., 1989; Carin et al., 1983; Chan et al., 1986; Edelin et al., 1988; Finnegan et al., 1983a, 1983b, 1984; Giles et al., 1989; Kandell et al., 1983; Maas et al., 1990; Suffet & Brotman, 1984). Treatment variables studied were prenatal care, urine toxicologies, methadone maintenance, and pharmacologic treatments for NAS. Outcome variables assessed were initial and subsequent numbers of prenatal care visits; obstetric and neonatal complications; infant BW and other developmental measures; incidence, severity, and duration of neonatal abstinence syndrome; and numbers of pediatric visits during infancy. Other independent variables included sociodemographic characteristics of the mothers and their substance habits. No researchers focused on nursing interventions, although nurses were coauthors and were identified as caregivers. The subjects in all the studies consisted of women with opiate use in pregnancy who used methadone clinics and prenatal clinics or delivery services in urban hospitals. Comparisons were made between groups of mother-infant dyads with varying degrees of heroin, methadone, and polydrug exposure, and groups of nonexposed mother-infant dyads from the same prenatal population.

Prenatal Care Outcomes. Edelin et al. (1988) found that women in the methadone prenatal program ($n = 26$) were more likely to receive adequate prenatal care than street drug users not in the methadone program ($n = 37$), but less likely than all prenatal clinic users at the same Boston hospital ($N = 716$). The number of prenatal visits was the same for methadone users and nonexposed women, but was significantly less for heroin-using women not in the methadone program. Giles et al. (1989) found similar results in New South Wales, with women using only street drugs getting the latest start on care and having the fewest visits, women on methadone receiving more and earlier care, and controls receiving the most adequate care. Suffet and Brotman (1984) studied 219 births to New York City women in a comprehensive prenatal methadone program with no comparison groups and explored the effect of prenatal care adequacy on neonatal outcomes. Their regression analysis indicated that earliness of care, number of visits, and number of days in prenatal care all contributed to higher gestational age at birth and to BW. Methadone dose (at delivery) was not significantly associated with either.

Maternal Outcomes. These studies did not in general identify many maternal complications in the methadone treatment prenatal group. Edelin et al. (1988) found a lower rate of anemia in the methadone group compared with the women continuing on street drugs only. Giles et al. (1989) found more hyperemesis in the methadone group compared with street drug users and controls and more hypertension in the control groups compared with both methadone and street drug users. The West German program reported by Maas et al. (1990) included a group ($n = 17$) that was put on methadone and then detoxed down to none at delivery without a reported incidence of maternal complications. Archie et al. (1989) studied the impact of maternal methadone doses on the fetal results of nonstress tests, an important test for detecting signs of fetal distress in late pregnancy. They reported that maternal methadone administered immediately before the test was associated with decreased fetal movement and decreased fetal heart acceleration, and warned that this temporary effect could confound the interpretation of the test when it was used to make perinatal treatment decisions.

Edelin (1988) and Giles et al. (1989) reported that women in the methadone and street drug groups had much higher rates of smoking than control groups, and that most women used multiple drugs and alcohol regardless of methadone treatment. Urine toxicologies were used to screen pregnant women and to monitor compliance with methadone treatment. Edelin et al. found 17% cocaine use in the controls, and Giles et al. found heroin users in the general clinic population where they screened all patients for several months (after informing them). However, only 0.6% of the women were "unknown" heroin users, suggesting that this broad screening was not justified as an efficient method for finding opiate addicts.

Neonatal Outcomes. Edelin et al. (1988) and Maas et al. (1990) both reported higher rates of meconium aspiration and respiratory insufficiency in infants exposed to methadone compared with street drug or control groups. This is an undesirable effect of methadone. Differences in GA and BW were significant and reasonably consistent across all the studies. Edelin reported a total of 30% low birthweight (less than 2,500 g) among drug-exposed infants as compared to a 17% rate among the controls. Among the methadone-exposed group there were no very low-birthweight (less than 1,500 g) infants, although 30% had moderately low-birthweight (1,501 to 2,499 g) infants. The infants of mothers using street drugs during pregnancy and not enrolled in a methadone-treatment program experienced a 22% rate of moderately low birthweight (1,501 to 2,499 g) and an 11.4% rate of very low birthweight.

NAS was studied by Giles et al. (1989), Maas et al. (1990), and Suffet and Brotman (1989). Giles et al. (1989) showed that the women on methadone had lower rates of infants with NAS (74%) than street drug users (92%). Maas et al. (1990) found NAS rates of 88% among the heroin-exposed infants, 55% among the methadone-exposed infants, and less than 10% among the infants whose mothers had been detoxified. The methadone-maintained and -detoxified women were helped to achieve the lowest dose levels possible. Suffet and Brotman (1989) found this same effect, with increasing methadone dose associated with increasing severity of NAS.

The management of NAS in the neonate was the subject of several studies in the early 1980s, all focused on the pharmacologic control of withdrawal symptoms from fetal opiates with and without other drugs. Finnegan et al. (1983a) in Philadelphia reported on a series of 139 infants scored for severity of NAS and randomized to paregoric or phenobarbital if treatment was needed. Paregoric was found to be more effective in reducing major symptoms in infants of women with opiate use alone, and phenobarbital was more effective if opiates and other CNS depressants were combined. Diazepam was found to be much less effective. In a companion report, Finnegan et al. (1983b) analyzed the same data further and reported that phenobarbital used to treat infants exposed fetally to opiates combined with nonopiates produced faster results if given in a larger loading dose than if titrated based on the NAS severity score. In other reports from related studies, Finnegan et al. (1984) reported that a larger group of 300 infants had similar results and added information that the mean number of days to achieve control of symptoms of abstinence was 7.6 and mean days of treatment was 38.6. Also in 1983, Kandall et al. reported from New York City on a randomized trial of paregoric versus phenobarbital for 153 infants exposed in utero to opiates and other drugs. They found an increased rate of seizures in the phenobarbital group and did not find that this was related to maternal drug use or other factors. One other investigation later in 1983 by Carin et al. in Brooklyn, New York, studied multiple laboratory and physiologic measures in 31 infants exposed to methadone in utero and randomly assigned to paregoric or phenobarbital if treatment was needed based on the same NAS severity scale used by Finnegan et al. (1983a, 1983b). They found no obvious short-term outcome differences in choosing between phenobarbital and paregoric to treat NAS. Infants on phenobarbital received fewer days of treatment, probably because of the longer half-life of phenobarbital as treatment was ending. None of the infants had seizures in this small sample.

Infant Outcomes. Suffet and Brotman (1989) used the Bayley Scales (1972) to assess child development up to age 2 and interpreted the results to suggest that maternal methadone doses may be negatively associated with Bayley scores in boys only. Chan et al. (1986) studied a pediatric clinic population in California where the mothers had all been pregnant addicts. This researcher identified characteristics of active participants and dropouts in the first year of infancy. The dropout mothers were significantly different on the following characteristics: number with no prenatal care, no other children at home, smoking, several maternal complications, lower BW, and shorter gestation. They conclude that these variables may help identify a group that needs more careful follow-up and attention to special problems.

In summary, in the intervention studies, researchers suggested that women on methadone are spared some complications of those who use only street drugs but that results are not truly satisfactory and that methadone itself has undesirable consequences, especially for the infant. In general, the methadone prenatal programs were feasible and acceptable to clients. Few interventions were described beyond methadone and careful prenatal monitoring, and other associated problems such as smoking and continued polydrug use were not addressed.

DISCUSSION AND CONCLUSIONS

Health care providers everywhere are facing the mounting problems associated with drug abuse in pregnant women and its impact on their infants. The most obvious conclusions reached by this review is that research to date is almost exclusively descriptive and correlational. It provides very limited understanding as to the etiology of drug abuse in pregnancy and provides limited assistance on how to prevent and manage these problems. Current studies emphasize characteristics of the users and some of the short- and long-term physiologic effects on mothers and infants. Although deleterious effects on the morbidity and mortality of both mothers and infants appear to be multiple, the independent and interactive effects of opiate abuse and other variables are not well understood. Likewise the real and potential long-term effects are not clearly delineated. A theoretic basis for integrating and explaining the multiple variables and their interrelationships is almost nonexistent.

Methodologic Issues

Four key methodologic problems were encountered in this review of the literature. First, difficulties in accurately measuring the independent variable of type, dose, and frequency of drug abuse. This problem is exacerbated by the widespread incidence of polydrug use. One possibility for simplifying the measurement of drug use may be to use levels of severity of drug use (e.g., alcohol + smoking + heroin = highest level, etc.). Second, the difficulties in controlling so as not to potentially confound the variables and effect modifiers. Assessing the individual effect of any drug or health variable requires carefully designed studies with samples large enough to allow multivariate data analysis and statistical control for confounding variables. Unless confounding variables are controlled, study findings may either overestimate the magnitude of a specific substance or demonstrate a significant association where none exists. There are several variables such as ethnicity; socioeconomic, nutritional, and health status of the mothers; amount and adequacy of prenatal care; and life-style characteristics, to name only a few, that exacerbate or influence many of the outcomes being associated with drug use. It is difficult to isolate and measure the independent, combined, and cumulative effects of these variables. Multivariate statistical techniques must be encouraged to assist in evaluating the individual and combined influences of this complex drug use phenomenon. Third, the difficulties in obtaining, for comparison, representative and comparable samples. Random selection of subjects is not readily possible in this area of research, and studies are limited in their population scope. Women are generally accepted into studies as they become available, and controls are often assigned at best by matching on key variables known or suspected to influence outcomes. These issues limit both internal and external validity of the studies. Fourth, there were limitations of instrumentation and measurement. The validity and reliability of the instruments used to evaluate the multiple independent and dependent variables are of constant concern. This review suggests that an increasing number of studies are using established instruments and facilitating comparison of findings among studies; however, more attention needs to be given to the validity of the tools and the reliability of the data-gathering procedures. The development of new and more refined or sensitive tools may be required to truly differentiate some of the long-term effects of drug abuse.

RECOMMENDATIONS FOR FUTURE RESEARCH

Further research is essential if we are going to curb the initiation and escalation of drug abuse effectively. The studies reviewed overwhelmingly described the outcomes of opiate abuse and exposure on mothers and infants. More studies are needed in all aspects of drug abuse: prevention, early detection, treatment, and rehabilitation. Studies must progress from simple description and correlation to evaluation of the outcome costs and benefits of various prevention and treatment interventions.

Studies in which investigators explore the etiologic determinants of drug use are key to developing effective preventive programs. More attention needs to be given to etiologic factors that determine a woman's initial decision to use drugs and to continue their use. These studies must assess social, familial, genetic, biologic, and environmental factors such as stress, social influences, social supports, and psychologic competencies of pregnant and childbearing women. Sampling procedures in preventive research need to be more representative of the general population, and research designs must be prospective and longitudinal. To date, prevention research is largely and appropriately targeted at adolescents and carried out within the school systems. However, the etiology and development of drug abuse habits among adults and particularly among childbearing and pregnant women, is little understood. The health care system may provide a key arena for prevention interventions among this vulnerable population, and the transition to parenthood may provide a special window of opportunity not only for prevention and early drug use detection but a motivational window for teaching and learning healthy attitudes and life-styles.

More studies are needed that include evaluation and monitoring of the variety of treatment interventions currently being provided. Intervention studies are almost nonexistent. We must be able to answer questions as to what interventions are most efficient and cost-effective in early detection, treatment, and rehabilitation. Treatment or management of pregnant drug users generally includes control and support of withdrawal and methadone maintenance therapy for narcotics. Other aspects of care that are often provided, but for which little evaluative research is evidenced, are providing support services (nursing, social worker, addiction counselor, dietitian, psychologists, psychiatrists, etc.); offering nutrition education and monitoring; monitoring for sexually transmitted diseases and interrenal illness; and monitoring fetal growth and well-being. Follow-up and rehabilitation continues to include inpatient-outpatient detoxification or methadone maintenance; health education; postnatal supportive counseling; contraceptive counseling; public health nurse visits; and training in parenting skills, neonatal developmental testing, and follow-up. Evaluation research of the individual and combined contribution of these treatment and rehabilitative intervention strategies directly targeted at pregnant women is needed.

There is also a growing need for more longitudinal studies. The long-term growth and developmental effects of opiate exposure on infants is not clearly determined. Because the drug-addicted population is highly mobile, follow-up assessment of the mothers and infants over a long period is not easily accomplished, yet it is this information that is key to understanding the real, long-term human and economic costs of prenatal drug abuse to our society.

In summary, what is required is not only more research, but research that is more carefully designed and carried out. Specifically, more research is needed that includes exploration of the etiology of drug abuse in pregnancy, more research that is longitudinal, and more research that includes evaluation of the effectiveness and cost of interventions being used to prevent, detect early, and treat and rehabilitate pregnant substance abusers. These studies need to incorporate in their designs appropriate and well-defined experimental and control groups; a prospective methodology; and documentation of frequency, dose, and type of drug intake. These studies need to measure and control for a broader number of psychosocial, environmental, as well as physiologic variables that may be influencing the use of drugs, as well as the effect of drugs. Nurses are primary providers in the care of these women and children. Nurses are key health care providers serving in all aspects of health care to pregnant and childbearing women. The challenge and opportunity to address these research needs are great.

ACKNOWLEDGMENTS

Support for this literature review was provided by a Joseph Healey Grant from the University of Massachusetts, Boston. The authors express their appreciation to two colleagues who have provided consultation to this effort: Sylvia C.

Gendrop PhD, RN, and Helen Reiskin, PhD, RN, and acknowledge the research assistance of Elizabeth McDaniel-Alexander, BSN.

REFERENCES

Alroomi, L. G., Davidson, J., Evans, T. J., Galea, P., & Howat, R. (1988). Maternal narcotic abuse and the newborn. *Archives Diseases of Children 63,* 81–83.

Archie, C. L., Lee, M. I., Sokol, R. J., & Norman, G. (1989). The effects of methadone treatment on the reactivity of the nonstress test. *Obstetrics and Gynecology, 74,* 254–255.

Bauchner, H., Zuckerman, B., McClain, M., Frank, D., Fired, L. E., & Kayne, H. (1988). Risk of sudden infant death syndrome among infants with in utero exposure to cocaine. *Journal of Pediatrics, 11,* 831–834.

Bayley, N. (1972). *Bayley scales of infant development.* New York: Psychological Corp.

Bernstein, V., Jeremy, R. J., Hans, S. L., & Marcus, J. (1984). A longitudinal study of offspring born to methadone maintained women: II. Dyadic interaction and infant behavior. *American Journal of Drug and Alcohol Abuse, 10,* 161–193.

Brazelton, T. B., & Spastics International Medical Publications. (1984). *The Neonatal Behavioral Assessment Scale* (2nd ed.). Philadelphia: Lippincott.

Carin, I., Glass, L., Parckh, A., Solomon, N., Steigman, J., & Wong, S. (1983). Neonatal methadone withdrawal. *American Journal of Diseases of Children, 137,* 1166–1169.

Chan, L., Wingert, W. A., Wachsman L., Schuetz, S., & Rogers, C. (1986). Differences between dropouts and active participants in a pediatric clinic for substance abuse mothers. *American Journal of Drug and Alcohol Abuse, 12,* 89–99.

Chasnoff, I. J. (1985). Effects of maternal narcotic versus nonnarcotic addiction on neonatal neurobehavior and infant development. *National Institute on Drug Abuse Research Monograph, 59,* 84–95.

Chasnoff, I. J. (1987). Cocaine and methadone-exposed infants: A comparison. *National Institute Drug Abuse Research Monograph, 76,* 278.

Chasnoff, I. J., Burns, K. A., & Burns, W. J. (1987). Cocaine use in pregnancy: Perinatal morbidity and mortality. *Neurotoxicology and Teratology, 9,* 291–293.

Chasnoff, I. J., Burns, W. J., & Schnoll, S. H. (1984). Perinatal addiction: The effects of maternal narcotic and nonnarcotic substance abuse on fetus and neonate. *National Institute Drug Abuse Research Monograph, 49,* 220–226.

Chasnoff, I. J., Burns, W. J., & Schnoll, S. H. (1986). Prenatal drug exposure: Effects on neonatal and infant growth and development. *Neurobehavioral Toxicology and Teratology, 8,* 357–362.

Chasnoff, I. J., Burns, W. J., Schnoll, S. H., & Burns, K. A. (1985). Cocaine use in pregnancy. *New England Journal of Medicine, 313,* 666–669.

Chasnoff, I. J., Hatcher, R., & Burns, W. J. (1982). Polydrug and methadone addicted newborns: A continuum of impairment? *Pediatrics, 70,* 210–213.

Chasnoff, I. J., Hunt, C. E., Kletter, R., & Kaplan, D. (1989). Prenatal cocaine exposure is associated with respiratory pattern abnormalities. *American Journal of Diseases of Children, 142,* 583–587.

Colten, M. E. (1982). Attitudes, experiences, and self-perceptions of heroin addicted mothers. *Journal of Social Issues, 38,* 77–92.

Di Giusto, J., Collins, E., Harbutt, S., & Hogan, M. (1986). Children exposed antenatally to narcotic drugs: Developmental status at 18–24 months of age. *Australian Pediatric Journal, 22,* 238–239.

Edelin, K. C., Gurganious, L., Golar, K., Oellerich, D., Kyei-Aboagye, K., & Adel Hamid, M. (1988). Methadone maintenance in pregnancy: Consequences to care and outcome. *Obstetrics and Gynecology, 71,* 399–404.

Ellwood, D. A., Sutherland, P., Kent, C., & O'Connor, M. (1987). Maternal narcotic addiction: Pregnancy outcome in patients managed by a specialized drug dependency antenatal clinic. *Australian New Zealand Journal of Obstetrics & Gynecology, 27*(2), 92–98.

Fiks, K. B., Johnson, H. L., & Rosen, T. S. (1985). Methadone maintained mothers: 3-year follow up of parental functioning. *International Journal of Addictions, 20,* 651–660.

Finnegan, L. (1984). Maternal drug abuse during pregnancy and pharmacotherapy for neonatal abstinence syndrome. *National Institute on Drug Abuse (NIDA) Research Monograph, 55,* 158.

Finnegan, L. P., Lin, T. H., Reeser, D. S., Shaffer, T. H., & Delivoria-Papadopoulos, M. (1982). The effects of perinatal addiction on pulmonary function in the newborn. *National Institute on Drug Abuse (NIDA) Research Monograph, 41,* 319–326.

Finnegan, L. P., Michael, H., Leifer, B., & Desai, S. (1983a). An evaluation of neonatal abstinence treatment modalities. *Pediatric Research, 17,* 370–375.

Finnegan, L. P., Michael, H., Leifer, B., & Desai, S. (1983b). The pharmacotherapeutic efficacy of neonatal abstinence treatment modalities. *Pediatric Research, 17,* 371–373.

Fulroth, R., Phillips, B., & Durand, D. J. (1989). Perinatal outcome of infants exposed to cocaine and/or heroin in utero. *American Journal of Diseases of Children, 143,* 905–910.

Giles, W., Patterson, T., Sanders, F., Batey, R., Thomas, D., & Collins, J. (1989). Outpatient methadone programme for pregnant heroin using women. *Australian New Zealand Journal of Obstetrics and Gynecology, 29,* 225–229.

Gillogley, K. M., Evans, A. T., Hansen, R. L., Samuels, S. J., & Batra, K. K. (1990). The perinatal impact of cocaine, amphetamine and opiate use detected by universal intrapartum screening. *American Journal of Obstetrics and Gynecology, 163,* 1535–1542.

Green, L., Ehrlich, S., & Finnegan L. (1988). The use of tricyclic antidepressants in methadone-maintained pregnant women and infant outcome. *National Institute on Drug Abuse Research Monograph, 81,* 266–272.

Gregg, J. E. M., Davidson, D. C., & Weindling, A. M. (1988). Inhaling heroin during pregnancy: Effects on the baby. *British Medical Journal, 12,* 296, 754.

Habel, L., Kaye, K., & Lee, J. (1990). Trends in reporting of maternal drug abuse and infant mortality among drug-exposed infants in New York City. *Women Health, 16*(2), 41–48.

Hagan, T. (1988). A retrospective search for the etiology of drug abuse: A background comparison of a drug-addicted population of women and a control group of nonaddicted. *National Institute on Drug Abuse Research Monograph, 81,* 254–261.

Hans, S. L. (1989). Developmental consequences of prenatal exposure to methadone. *Annals of the New York Academy of Sciences, 562,* 195–207.

Hans, S. L., & Marcus, J. (1983). Motoric and attentional behavior in infants of methadone-maintained women. *National Institute on Drug Abuse Research Monograph, 43,* 287–293.

Hogan, M., Collins, E., Di Giusto, J., & Harbutt, S. (1986). Children exposed antenatally to narcotic drugs: Health and growth at 18–24 months of age. *Australian Pediatric Journal, 22,* 238.

Johnson, H. L., Glassman, M. B., Fiks, K. B., & Rosen, T. S. (1990). Resilient children: Individual differences in developmental outcome of children born to drug abusers. *Journal of Genetics and Psychology, 151,* 523–539.

Johnson, H. L., & Rosen, T. S. (1982). Prenatal methadone exposure: Effects on behavior in early infancy. *Pediatric Pharmacology, 2,* 113–120.

Kandall, S. R., Doberczak, T. M., Mauer, K. R., Strashun, R. H., & Korts, D. C. (1983). Opiate & CNS depressant therapy in neonatal drug abstinence syndrome. *American Journal of Diseases of Children, 137,* 378–382.

Kaye, K., Elkind, L., Goldberg, D., & Tytun, A. (1989). Birth outcomes for infants of drug abusing mothers. *New York State Journal of Medicine, 89,* 256–261.

Lifschitz, M. H., Wilson, G. S., Smith, E. O., & Desmond, M. M. (1983). Fetal and postnatal growth of children born to narcotic dependent women. *Journal of Pediatrics, 102,* 686–691.

Lifschitz, M. H., Wilson, G. S., Smith, E. O., & Desmond, M. M. (1985). Factors affecting head growth and intellectual function in children of drug addicts. *Pediatrics, 75,* 269–274.

Little, B. B., Snell, L. M., Gilstrap, L. D., III, & Johnston, W. L. (1990a). Patterns of multiple substance abuse during pregnancy: Implications for mother and infant. *Southern Medical Journal, 83,* 507–509.

Little, B. B., Snell, L. M., Klein, V. R., Gilstrap, L. C., III, Knoll, K. A., & Breckenridge, J. D. (1990b). Maternal and fetal effects of heroin addiction during pregnancy. *Journal of Reproductive Medicine, 35,* 159–162.

Livesay, S., Ehrlich, S., Ryan, L., & Finnegan, L. P. (1989). Cocaine and pregnancy: Maternal and infant outcomes. *Annals of the New York Academy of Sciences, 562,* 358–359.

Maas, U., Kattner, E., Weingart-Jesse, B., Schafer, A., & Obladen, M. (1990). Infrequent neonatal opiate withdrawal following maternal methadone detoxification during pregnancy. *Journal of Perinatal Medicine, 18,* 111–118.

Marcus, J., Hans, S. L., & Jeremy, R. J. (1982a). Differential motor and state functioning in newborns of women on methadone. *Neurobehavioral Toxicology and Teratology, 4,* 459–462.

Marcus, J., Hans, S. L., & Jeremy, R. J. (1982b). Patterns of 1 day and 4 month motor functioning in infants of women on methadone. *Neurobehavioral Toxicology and Teratology, 4,* 473–462.

Marcus, J., Hans, S. L., & Jeremy, R. J. (1984a). A longitudinal study of offspring born to methadone maintained women: I. Design, methodology and description of women's resources for functioning. *American Journal of Drug and Alcohol Abuse, 10,* 135–160.

Marcus, J., Hans, S. L., & Jeremy, R. J. (1984b). A longitudinal study of offspring born to methadone maintained women: III. Effects of multiple risk factors on development at 4, 8 and 12 months. *American Journal of Drug and Alcohol Abuse, 10,* 195–207.

Mark, I, (1983). The newborn addict: Ante-and postnatal care. *Scandinavian Journal of Social Medicine, 11,* 11–16.

McCarthy, . (1972). *McCarthy Scales of Children's Abilities*. New York: Psychological Corp.

Nelson, L. B., Ehrlich, S., Calhoun, J. H., Matteucci, T., & Finnegan, L. P. (1987). Occurrence of strabismus in infants born to drug dependent women. *American Journal of Diseases of Children, 141,* 175–178.

Neville, R. G., McKellican, J. F., & Foster, J. (1988). Heroin users in general practice: Ascertainment and features. *British Medical Journal, 296,* 755–758.

Oats, J. N., Beischer, N. A., Breheny, J. E., & Pepperell, R. J. (1984). The outcome of pregnancies complicated by narcotic drug addiction. *Australian New Zealand Journal of Obstetrics and Gynaecology, 24,* 14–16.

The Organization for Obstetric, Gynecologic and Neonatal Nurses. (1988, October). Looking for answers. *NAACOG Newsletter, 16,* 4.

Oro, A. S., & Dixon, S. D. (1987). Perinatal cocaine and methamphetamine exposure: Maternal and neonatal correlates. *Journal of Pediatrics, 111,* 571–578.

Ostrea, E. M., Jr., Brady, M. J., Parks, P. M., Asencio, D. C., & Naluz, A. (1989). Drug screening of meconium in infants of drug-dependent mothers: An alternative to urine testing. *Journal of Pediatrics, 115,* 474–477.

Pinto, F., Torrioli, M. G., Casella, G., Tempesta, E., & Fundaro, C. (1988). Sleep in babies born to chronically heroin addicted mothers: A follow-up study. *Drug Alcohol Dependency 21,* 43–47.

Robertson, R. J., & Bucknall, A. B. (1986). Pregnancy and HTLVIII-LAV transmission in heroin users. *Health Bulletin, 44,* 364–366.

Rosati, P., Noia, G., Conte, M., DeSantis, M., & Mancuso, S. (1989). Drug abuse in pregnancy: Fetal growth and malformations. *Panminerva Medicine, 31,* 71–75.

Rosen, T. S., & Johnson, H. L. (1982). Children of methadone-maintained mothers: Follow-up to 18 months of age. *Journal of Pediatrics, 101,* 192–196.

Rosen, T. S., & Johnson, H. L. (1985). Long term effects of prenatal methadone maintenance. *National Institute on Drug Abuse Research Monograph, 59,* 73–83.

Rosen, T. S., & Johnson, H. L. (1988). Drug addicted mothers, their infants, and SIDS. *Annals of the New York Academy of Science, 533,* 89–96.

Rosner, M. A., Keith, L., & Chasnoff, I. J. (1982). The Northwestern University Drug Dependence Program: The impact of intensive prenatal care on labor and delivery outcomes. *American Journal of Obstetrics and Gynecology, 144,* 23–27.

Selwyn, P. A., Schoenbaum, E. E., Davenny, K., Robertson, V. J., Feingold, A. R., Shulman, J. F., Mayers, M. M., Klein, R. S., Friendland, G. H., & Rogers, M. F. (1989). Prospective study of human immunodeficiency virus infection and pregnancy outcomes in intravenous drug users. *Journal of American Medical Association, 261,* 1289–1294.

Suffet, F., & Brotman, R. (1984). A comprehensive care program for pregnant addicts: Obstetrical, neonatal, and child development outcomes. *International Journal of the Addictions, 19,* 199–219.

Ward, S. L., Schuetz, S., Krishna, V., Bean, X., Wingert, W., Wachsman, L., & Keene, T. G. (1986). Abnormal sleeping ventilatory pattern in infants of substance abusing mothers. *American Journal of Diseases of Children, 140,* 1015–1020.

Weinberger, S. M., Kandall, S. R., Doberczak, T. M., Thornton, J. C., & Bernstein, J. (1986). Early weight-change patterns in neonatal abstinence. *American Journal of Diseases of Children, 140,* 829–832.

Wilson, G. S. (1989). Clinical studies of infants and children exposed prenatally to heroin. *Annals of New York Academy of Sciences, 562,* 183–194.

Chapter 12

Alcohol and Drug Abuse

Eleanor J. Sullivan
School of Nursing
University of Kansas
Medical Center

Sandra M. Handley
School of Nursing
University of Kansas
Medical Center

CONTENTS

Alcohol and drug abuse are important topics for nurses. The National Institute of Alcohol Abuse and Alcoholism (NIAAA) estimates that 25% of all hospitalized patients have problems related to alcohol abuse (NIAAA, 1990). The National Institute on Drug Abuse reports that 6% of the general population is currently using some type of illicit drug, and another 2% are abusing prescription drugs (NIDA, 1991). However, nurses have only recently begun to address the addictions. Most of the research by nurses on this important problem has been developed in the last 10 years.

This chapter includes a review of research by nurses on alcohol and other drug abuse from 1980 to 1991. According to DSM-III-R, the appropriate diagnostic terms are *psychoactive substance dependence* and *psychoactive substance abuse* (American Psychiatric Association, 1987). *Dependence* is defined diagnostically as impaired control of substance use and continued use despite adverse consequences. *Abuse* is defined as maladaptive patterns of substance use. In this chapter, we have used the terms *alcohol* and *drug abuse* and *substance abuse* to refer to both abuse and dependence to facilitate readability.

Studies were identified by a computer search of the CINAHL supplemented by a manual search for those years not computer indexed. The topics searched were substance use, substance dependence, alcohol, and alcoholism. Also, two leading journals in the field, the *Journal of Studies on Alcohol* and the *International Journal of Addictions,* were searched manually for nurse authors. Current texts and studies were reviewed for relevant citations.

Published research was included if a nurse was first or second author, and if sufficient methodologic detail was reported to evaluate the study. Studies by nurses from other English-speaking countries, primarily Great Britain and Canada, were included when the topic was applicable. Studies by nonnurse authors were selectively included when the subjects were nurses and the content was related to topics of concern in nursing.

Four categories of research emerged from the research topic and the study population. They were (a) prevalence; (b) alcohol and drug abuse clients; (c) alcohol and drug abuse in the clinical specialties; and (d) nurse attitudes, behaviors, and education. Research on alcohol and drug abuse in nurses was reviewed previously (Sullivan & Handley, 1992).

Forty-four studies were reviewed from 32 journals. Twenty-four studies (55%) were published in nursing journals, 15 (34%) were in alcohol and drug abuse journals, and 5 (11%) were in other professional journals.

Eleven studies included specification of a theoretic framework that underpinned the study. Because the alcohol and drug abuse field lacks a generally accepted theory, these studies included application of existing theories to alcohol and drug abuse. The most frequently used frameworks were self-esteem (3 studies: Bennett, 1988; Byers, Raven, Hill, & Robyak, 1990; Gibson, 1980) and stress (2 studies: Rosenfield & Stevenson, 1988; Shelley & Anderson, 1986). Theories used in single studies were Jellinek's theory of alcoholism (Fortin & Evans, 1983), locus of control (Huckstadt, 1987), cognitive dissonance (Forchuk, 1984), Erikson's ego development (Talashek, 1987) and Fishbein's behavioral intention model (London, 1982). In the remainder of the studies (34), no theoretical framework was specified or clearly implied.

In terms of research design, twenty-five (57%) were descriptive, ten

(23%) were correlational, six (14%) were quasi-experimental and three (7%) were experimental studies. Research by nurses on alcohol and drug abuse is in the early stages of development, primarily at the exploratory stage. This early level of development also may be due to the limited number of nurses with research preparation or experience in the alcohol and drug field.

PREVALENCE

In several studies investigators used survey techniques to determine the prevalence of alcohol and drug use among specific populations. Trinkoff, Ritter, and Anthony (1990) studied cocaine abuse in more than 14,000 subjects through a secondary analysis of National Institute of Mental Health data. Prevalence rates were high in white males in two age-work categories: young and unemployed, and educated and professionally employed. This study is an excellent example of secondary analysis of an existing data set.

Engs developed a program of research examining alcohol use in college students. A survey of 6,115 college students from 112 colleges revealed that 20% were heavy drinkers, and more than two thirds had experienced side effects of drinking (Engs & Hanson, 1985). Furthermore, heavy drinking was inversely related to grade-point average.

A subsample from this 1985 study was compared with an earlier sample of college students (Engs, 1977). The percentage of heavy drinkers had increased, more students were experiencing drinking-related problems, and heavy drinking among female students had tripled in the intervening years. Engs and Hanson (1986) also found drinking problems were more frequent in students ($N = 4266$) from states with lower drinking ages. Contradictory to other well-known studies in the alcohol abuse field that demonstrated the genetic propensity for alcoholism (Cloninger, Bohman, & Siguardsson, 1981; Engs 1990; Goodwin, Schulsinger, Hermansen, Guze, & Winokur, 1973) found no correlation between family background of alcohol abuse and drinking among male or female students. Potential explanations are that drinking practices of college students may differ from those of the general adult population or that the survey questions used to determine family background (whether a parent or grandparent drinks too much) was unreliable.

ALCOHOL AND DRUG ABUSE CLIENTS

Most studies of alcohol and drug abuse clients used subjects in inpatient treatment settings. The settings included both psychiatric units and general hospital alcohol/drug treatment units. This research was subdivided into research on client characteristics and interventions (10 studies) and research on recovering clients (7 studies).

Characteristics and Interventions

These studies were focused on identifying characteristics of clients in alcohol and drug treatment settings that could become the basis for interventions. Two nurse researchers studied women. Fortin and Evans (1983) interviewed 50 female alcoholics regarding the length of time between first intoxication and loss of control over drinking, which represents the rate of progression of the disease (Jellinek, 1946). Employment, number of children at home, and higher education were associated with a longer progression of the disease, whereas parental alcoholism was related to a shorter progression. The subject to variable ratio was only 5 to 1 rather than the minimum 10 to 1 recommended for the multivariate analyses used. It is also not clear that Jellinek's 1946 criteria for progression are the state of the science today.

Anderson (1980) used a chart review to identify the health needs of drug abusers in treatment and found women had more unmet health needs than men. Anderson then developed and tested a nursing intervention for women drug abusers (Anderson, 1982; 1986). Drug-dependent women (N = 155) who sought emergency department care for drug-related health problems and who refused referral for drug treatment were randomly assigned to experimental or control groups. Experimental subjects received individual therapy for 8 weeks by a nurse who focused on client-identified issues. The experimental treatment did not affect perceived stress or emotional distress. The experimental group initially reported a lower daily drug cost (Anderson, 1982), but this difference was short-lived (Anderson, 1986). These subjects may have been particularly resistant to improvement because of their prior refusal of treatment, the treatment may not have been appropriately conceptualized for their needs, or the length/frequency of treatments may have been inadequate.

Two studies investigated self-esteem with all-male or primarily male subjects. Gibson (1980) examined the effect of reminiscence groups on self-esteem in 61 male alcoholics on a detoxification unit. Experimental subjects participated in a nurse-led group designed to elicit significant memories. When these subjects were compared with controls with no intervention, there were no differences in self-esteem; however, pretest scores indicated that the groups differed at baseline. Because the patients were in detoxification, changes in self-esteem may not be feasible in such a short time.

An intervention to enhance self-esteem was tested with 50 alcoholics (48 men, 2 women) in treatment (Byers et al., 1990). Experimental subjects were paired with nursing home clients as companions during the last 2 weeks of treatment. Little change in self-esteem occurred.

Both of these studies attempted to define and measure a therapeutic intervention based on the perceived importance of increasing self-esteem in alcoholics, presumably to increase the potential for sustained recovery. The lack of significant results suggests a need for reconsideration of the theory, the type and dosage of the intervention, or the design of the experiment.

Using locus-of-control theory, Huckstadt (1987) found that active alcoholics scored higher on the belief in external control than nonalcoholics. The authors suggest that the belief that external factors control drinking behavior may contribute to difficulty in achieving sobriety and, conversely, to the success of Alcoholics Anonymous (AA), which uses a directive approach.

Using cognitive dissonance as the conceptual framework, Forchuk (1984) examined denial, self-concept, and the alcoholic stereotype in 116 Canadian subjects of both sexes. All subjects rated alcoholics in general more negative than themselves. Subjects who denied alcoholism (6%) reported the greatest differences between alcoholics and themselves. The findings are consistent with the conceptual framework and suggest that subjects' negative perceptions of alcoholics in general may reinforce their own denial. Further research on the role of denial in resistance to recovery could be fruitful because denial is an important concept in alcohol dependence.

One study tested the effectiveness of L-Tryptophan, a nonprescription nutrient, as a means to reduce sleep disturbance and depression in 76 male patients in alcohol treatment (Asheychik et al., 1989). Three control groups and two treatment groups with varying medication schedules, including placebos, were established. Depression decreased for all subjects (experimental and control); however, L-Tryptophan appeared to accelerate the rate of improvement. Sleep disturbances decreased for all subjects, but L-Tryptophan had no effect on sleep. Few subjects, however, reported sleep disturbances initially. It is therefore not possible to draw any conclusions about L-Tryptophan. Several more rigorously controlled studies would be needed.

Conlon and Radinsky (1981) used a chart review to study the effect of type of referral on completion of referral in alcoholic clients. Referrals with a specific appointment and contact person were most often completed by the client. Other factors that could impact referral (e.g., aspects of the referral process, client characteristics, and organizational variables) were not examined.

In these studies of client characteristics and interventions, investigators explored some potential intervention strategies, but none found very large, if any, effects. None of the studies built on one another resulting in isolated, unrelated findings. Only Anderson's work used a nursing paradigm. This lack of a unique nursing perspective may be due to the interdisciplinary nature of alcohol and drug treatment. Differences in the experience of alcohol and drug abuse between men and women also is an understudied area with potential for exploration.

Characteristics of Recovery

Studies by nurses of clients in recovery from alcohol or drug abuse were focused on identifying characteristics associated with recovery and the nature of recovery itself. Two researchers examined recovering subjects using qualitative methodologies. Banonis (1989) used a phenomenologic perspective to explore awareness of recovery in three subjects. The author conceptualized recovery as "moving from darkness to light."

Kus (1988a) interviewed 20 recovering gay men to determine factors contributing to alcoholism in this group. No subject identified gay bars as a factor in his alcoholism, which the author suggests supports his hypothesis that nonacceptance of gayness is the etiology of alcoholism in this population. Such conclusions are unsubstantiated by these findings and inconsistent with the grounded theory technique reported to have been used. Kus (1988b) then interviewed 30 gay men in AA who reported that through the AA steps they were able to accept their own homosexuality. Questionable rigor in implementing the qualitative method and possible researcher bias limit usefulness of the findings.

Another approach to studying recovery was taken by Hoffman and Estes, who developed the Body and Behavioral Experience Inventory (BBE) to measure the physiologic and psychologic symptoms experienced during early recovery (Hoffman & Estes, 1986). More behavioral than body symptoms were reported by all subjects, and female subjects reported a higher incidence and frequency of problems on almost all scales. Alcohol severity correlated positively with BBE symptoms (Hoffman & Estes, 1987). Information about body and behavioral symptoms could provide the basis for interventions to assist clients with the difficult experiences of recovery.

Rosenfield and Stevenson (1988) studied the relationship between drinking, eating behaviors, and stress in 37 normal-weight, 37 overweight, and 23 recovering alcoholic women. Desire for alcohol was higher in recovering alcoholic women under high stress conditions; however, alcoholic women craved alcohol more under all stress conditions. The study identifies interesting relationships between food, alcohol, and stress that could be further explicated. Further study of craving and its relationship to recovery would be of great interest.

Bennett (1988) studied the effects of stress and social support on self-esteem in 45 young male alcoholics in recovery. Self-esteem correlated positively with both length of abstinence and with the presence of social support. Social support contributed to self-concept directly rather than indirectly through buffering (Cohen & Wills, 1985). This study found a more meaningful self-esteem relationship than other studies (Byers et al., 1990; Gibson, 1980) and suggests that self-esteem increases with the length of abstinence. It is difficult to know whether this finding has any relevance for treatment. It may just be that abstinence over time leads to better mental health.

Research in the nursing clinical specialties includes both alcohol and drug abuse in clients with other primary diagnoses and alcohol and drug-related knowledge and abilities of nurses in the clinical specialties. Reflecting a broad spectrum of alcohol and drug abuse interest, studies were found in all clinical areas except mental health nursing.

Medical-Surgical Nursing

Only two studies were found of alcohol and drug abuse in medical-surgical clients. This is surprising because medical-surgical nursing is the largest nursing specialty area and a high percentage of patients in medical and surgical units have alcohol or drug-related problems (NIAAA, 1990).

In one study, 101 medical-surgical nurses were randomly selected and asked to identify the most frequent nursing diagnoses for alcoholic patients and then to rank the diagnoses according to their difficulty of care (Bartek, Lindeman, Newton, Fitzgerald, & Hawks, 1988). The most difficult physiologic diagnoses were potential for injury, alteration in elimination, and fluid volume deficit. The most difficult psychosocial nursing diagnoses were ineffective individual or family coping and noncompliance. Strengths of this descriptive study are the identification of the problems nurses encounter in caring for alcohol- or drug-abusing clients, and the use of nursing diagnoses. The next steps would be to determine the prevalence of these diagnoses and to investigate effective nursing interventions.

An Australian study used a nurse-administered assessment scale to detect withdrawal symptoms in general hospital patients suspected of being at risk for such symptoms (Foy, March, & Drinkwater, 1988). Half (54%) of the high-risk patients had scores indicating a need for medical treatment. Using the scale to guide treatment, withdrawal symptoms were prevented in most patients. This study validated the use of the scale, the importance of nursing assessment in withdrawal, and the value of assessing alcohol and drug use in *all* hospitalized patients.

Nursing Care of Women

Two studies examined alcohol or drug abuse in gynecologic clients. Over 30% of women in a private gynecology practice with the diagnosis of infertility or pelvic pain had a potential problem with alcohol or drugs, a rate much higher than the 5% population estimate for women (Busch, McBride, & Benaventura, 1986). Although the low response rate (36%) limits generalizability, the findings suggest questions about a clinical population that merits further investigation.

Shelley and Anderson (1986) found that alcoholic women ($N = 100$) had more menstrual distress than nonalcoholic subjects ($N = 100$). Although conclusions are limited by convenience sampling and the use of self-reports, further study of the relationship between menstrual distress and alcoholism is indicated. It would be important to determine whether menstrual discomfort was a precursor to excessive drinking or an effect of it.

Pediatric Nursing

Two research themes appeared in pediatric nursing: children of alcoholics, and the incidence of alcohol or drug abuse in children or adolescents. Surprisingly, no studies were found by nurses of either substance abuse or treatment in adolescents.

Scavnicky-Mylant (1986) studied the drawings of children of alcoholics aged 5 to 11. Identified themes were poor self-image, sense of powerlessness, denial, and feelings of responsibility for parental drinking. The subjects were emotionally and socially immature. Although small, the study involved an innovative method of studying younger, less verbal clients, and its findings included themes on which intervention strategies could be based.

Talashek (1987) examined ego identity in adolescent Alateen members matched with controls. Subjects with alcoholic parents were significantly lower on ego identity and more likely to have had extended school absences. Both findings could be the basis for further investigation and development of research-based interventions.

Two studies were focused on nursing knowledge about children of alcoholics. Arneson, Triplett, Schweer, and Snider (1983) surveyed school nurses on their ability to identify and manage children of alcoholics. Almost all subjects (93%) had identified children of alcoholics in their practice. Their interventions primarily were directed toward enhancing the student's self-esteem and referring students to other resources. Subjects indicated they needed more information on early identification and help with intervention strategies.

In a subsequent study, Arneson, Schultz, and Triplett (1987) surveyed nurses on their knowledge of the impact of parental alcoholism on children. Many (40%) of the 265 respondents had contact with children of alcoholics in their work. These subjects were knowledgeable about the immediate effects of parental alcoholism but less knowledgeable about the long-term impact. Experience, rather than formal education, provided their information. Both studies identify knowledge deficits about alcohol and drug abuse that could be the basis for interventions with school and other community-based nurses. The work also demonstrates the frequency with which nurses come in contact with subjects at high risk for alcohol-related difficulties.

Using Fishbein's behavioral intention model, London (1982) studied intended drinking behavior in 650 5th- and 7th-grade students from an urban, largely minority, school system. Seven percent indicated they intended to become intoxicated in the next 2 weeks. Students with positive beliefs about intoxication were more likely to intend to become intoxicated. Although the large sample size is a strength, low variation in the outcome measure (intention) and characteristics of the sample (i.e., minority, urban) limit generalization to other student populations. Also, intention, in an age group characterized by impulse, may not predict actual behavior.

Community Health Nursing

One study of nurses in a community health setting was found. Reynolds and Ried (1985) examined the effects of education and experience on perceived skill with alcohol or drug assessment, and referral in 55 community health nurses. Although most (60%) rated themselves as skilled in assessment and referral, actual referrals in the previous year varied from none (41%) to one or two (38%). Continuing education and work experiences, rather than nursing education, were associated with higher referral rates. Although self-report may not accurately measure skill, this study is consistent with other reports that nursing education contributes little to skill in caring for alcohol and drug abuse clients. Given community health nurses' potential for case finding and intervention, they are an important group to educate about abuse problems.

NURSE ATTITUDES, BEHAVIORS, AND EDUCATION

Research in this area includes attitudes of nurses and nursing students, nurse behaviors, and nursing education. Three studies by nonnurse researchers examined the attitudes of students. In a study of 1,106 subjects, Wechsler and Rohman (1982) found that nursing and medical students were more interested in caring for clients with alcohol-related problems (21% and 24%, respectively) than social work students (12%) or counseling students (10%). This study documented negative attitudes and beliefs about alcohol problems among professional students, although nursing students were among the least negative.

Attitudes toward drug abusers rather than alcoholics were examined by Meiderhoff, Ray, and Talarchek (1986). When nursing students ($N = 166$) were compared with subjects in an earlier study (Meiderhoff & Ray, 1980), nursing students' attitudes toward drug abusers were less punitive than students in the physical sciences, but more punitive than students in the social sciences and humanities.

Reisman and Schrader (1984) found that nurses ($N = 27$) with higher referral rates to an employee alcohol program were more knowledgeable about the disease and had more personal experience with alcoholism. Although this study is limited by its single site and small sample size, it identifies a relationship between attitudes and practice behavior that should be investigated further.

Three studies by nurses examined attitudes of nursing students or nurses. In a study of 1,449 Australian students, Engs (1982) found that nursing students scored higher than students in human services on beliefs in psychologic and physical-genetic etiologies. Low instrument reliabilities and cultural differences, however, must be considered before generalizing the results of this study.

Sullivan and Hale (1987) found that a sample of 1,026 nurses who were members of the American Nurses Association (ANA) scored high on beliefs in psychologic and physical-genetic etiologies and on belief in medical treatment. Because only about 10% of nurses belong to the ANA and the response rate was low (30%), these results cannot be generalized to the nursing population.

Similar to Engs (1982), but contrary to Wechsler and Rohman (1982), Cannon and Brown (1988) found that nurses ($N = 396$) scored somewhat lower than other health professionals on substance abuse attitudes, particularly permissiveness and nonmoralism. These reports of conflicting views of nurses' attitudes may be related to the choice of instruments or measurement differences. Using the same instrument, both Engs (1982) and Sullivan and Hale (1987) found that nursing students' and nurses' attitudes were similar regarding etiologies of alcoholism. Using another instrument, Cannon and Brown (1988) found nurses' attitudes to be more moralistic and less permissive than other health professionals. Both the dimensions being measured and the reliability and validity of the instruments should be considered in future studies of attitudes. If nurses' attitudes influence their behavior with alcohol- or drug-abusing clients (as Reisman and Shrader [1984] found), then accurately determining attitudes and identifying characteristics associated with negative attitudes are the first steps toward improving them.

Educational interventions designed to change attitudes in nursing students have been tested by several researchers. Tamlyn (1989) studied the effect of a 3-hr seminar on attitudes toward alcohol on 96 randomly selected Canadian nursing students. One week later, the experimental group expressed more positive attitudes toward alcoholics, and those attitudes remained 2 months later. The intervention appeared to affect attitudes; however, the lack of a pretest attitude measurement and a low subject-to-variable ratio limits conclusions.

Harlow and Goby (1980) replicated a study of nursing student attitudes (Ferneau, 1967). They found that 25 students with a clinical experience in an alcohol treatment program were significantly more knowledgeable and had more positive attitudes toward alcoholics than 20 students from another school without the experience. Additionally, the experimental groups' positive attitudes were sustained over 1 year. Although the students in both programs were similar in age, race, and religion, other possible differences in students, faculty, or programs were not examined. Farnsworth and Bairan (1990) also replicated the Ferneau study using a different attitude scale. After their clinical experience, students increased their satisfaction in working with alcoholics and their positive perceptions of alcoholics. The subjects in this study, however, were not compared with controls.

The impact of a course about addictions on nursing students' attitudes was evaluated by Jack (1989). Students taking the course ($n = 46$) were compared with a control group ($n = 36$) that did not take the course. The experimental group developed stronger antidrug attitudes toward tobacco and opiates, but attitudes toward alcohol and other drugs did not change. Students scored high on the scale initially so there is a potential ceiling effect, that is, the students had little room to improve. Also, the experimental group self-selected the course, which may indicate greater enthusiasm for the topic. Random assignment or crossover designs would improve the validity of study findings in future educational intervention studies.

These few studies suggest that clinical and classroom content increases students' knowledge about the problem and may improve their attitudes toward such clients. Identification of the specific factors associated with attitude changes would be of great interest. An evaluation of the different attitude scales also would advance attitude measurement.

Improving nursing practice through education has not been addressed in the research literature in the United States. Only one study, in Great Britain, explored the impact of a continuing education program on nursing practice

(Rowland & Maynard, 1989). Three months after participating in a program designed to teach medical-surgical nurses to screen their clients for alcoholism and to educate high-risk clients on drinking sensibly, only half of the nurses used the screening tool regularly, and only half thought educating clients was useful. No client outcomes were reported, and no reasons for the nurses' reluctance to screen were given. Although this study lacks scientific rigor, it raises important questions about nurses' roles in screening for alcoholism and in patient education that should be investigated.

Three surveys uncovered similar results in identifying the amount of alcohol and drug abuse content in professional nursing education. In surveying 55 graduate psychiatric–mental health nursing programs, Bush and Svanum (1983) found that the majority (74%) included such content, albeit minimally. Carter (1983) found that most (82% to 98%) baccalaureate, master's, and nurse practitioner programs (*N* = 275) offered alcohol and drug abuse content, averaging a total of 3 to 5 class hours during the program. More recently, Hoffman and Heinemann (1987) surveyed 335 diploma, associate-degree, and baccalaureate nursing programs on the curriculum time devoted to alcohol and drug abuse. Again, all schools included content, but the majority (63%) devoted less than 5 class hours to the combined subjects. Similar results were found in baccalaureate programs in New York State and associate-degree programs had even less content (Long, Gelfand, & McGill, 1991). These reports consistently demonstrate the minimal amount of content on alcohol and drug abuse in nursing education.

RECOMMENDATIONS FOR FUTURE RESEARCH

Initial investigative work in alcohol and drug abuse by nurse researchers has begun. Unfortunately, little of the research relates to or builds on other studies. The exceptions are those on prevalence (most notably by Engs and colleagues) with a body of knowledge on alcohol abuse in college students and on education.

Studies have not been replicated, and systematic knowledge building, based on a sound theoretic foundation, is lacking. Most of the studies are descriptive or retrospective (Arneson et al., 1983, 1987; Bartek, Lindeman, Newman, Fitzgerald, & Hawks, 1988; Bennett, 1988; Busch et al., 1986; Fortin & Evans, 1983; London, 1982; Shelley & Anderson, 1986; Talashek, 1987) that have identified characteristics of clients with alcohol and drug problems. It is difficult, however, to determine if these charcteristics can be the basis for actual interventions or even if the research justifies this approach. Some studies (Fortin & Evans, 1983; Tamlyn, 1989) used multivariate techniques with small subject-to-variable ratios, thereby decreasing the stability of the findings.

Research on actual nursing interventions is sparse and inconclusive. Interventions were found to be only minimally effective in some studies (Anderson, 1986; Asheychik et al., 1989), although Foy's intervention improved patient outcomes (Foy et al., 1988). Also, Conlon and Radinsky (1981) demonstrated that specific appointments and contacts improved completion of referrals for alcohol follow-up. The major concern in this field, the relationship between variables and the positive outcomes of abstinence and improved functioning, have not been pursued by nurse researchers. Only one study (Hoffman & Estes, 1987) was longitudinal. Gender as a variable in treatment and recovery has not been consistently explored.

Several studies examined attitudes and, in some cases, attempted to change attitudes using educational and clinical experiences with generally positive results. Nursing education, both undergraduate and graduate, was found to be inadequate in preparing nurses to care for clients with one of this country's major health care problems.

No research on nursing care or roles in treatment settings was found, which may be due to the frequently constricted role of nursing practice in such settings. Investigations of nursing roles in treatment and a demonstration of their effectiveness would be welcome additions to the nursing literature.

It is particularly interesting that no studies by nurse researchers were found in the mental health nursing literature, other than the subspecialty of alcohol and drug abuse itself. Substance abuse and dependency are recognized as psychiatric diagnoses according to DSM III-R (American Psychiatric Association, 1987), and many substance abuse clients are treated in psychiatric units. Of particular interest in the field today are studies of comorbidity and dual diagnosis of substance abuse and psychiatric illness. Because of this absence of work, now is an especially opportune time for mental health nurse researchers to consider this area.

Because so little research has been done and there is such a need to examine ways in which nursing care of alcohol and drug abuse clients can be improved, the field offers almost unlimited opportunities for nurse investigators. In addition, alcohol and drug abuse are the focus of attention today by the public and government. The "war on drugs," federal requirements mandating drug and alcohol workplace policies, and increasing attention to the social consequences of abuse (e.g., crime, homicides, drunk driving, drug-exposed newborns) indicate the country's concern about the problem. In fiscal year 1992, the NIAAA and the National Institute on Drug Abuse (NIDA) allocated $481.9 million to research, increases of 5% and 9% over the previous year.

Nursing education, along with medical education, has lagged behind in including substantial content on this vital health care problem. Thus, it is not surprising that nurses have not identified the potential research opportunities in the field. Recognizing this deficiency, NIAAA and NIDA have sponsored model curricula development and faculty development initiatives. Both offer the opportunity to increase faculty knowledge regarding substance abuse and to improve both knowledge and skills in future nurses. Thus, interest in the topic should be generated among both faculty and future graduate students.

Alcohol and drug abuse results in costs to society in billions of dollars; loss of jobs, lives, and health; and untold human suffering. Nurses have the opportunity and the responsibility to identify and offer assistance to alcohol and drug abuse clients in their care as well as the many others affected by the substance abuser (e.g., family members, employers, innocent victims). To offer such assistance, extensive and substantial research is needed to determine the most effective nursing interventions with substance abuse clients, their families, and communities to provide the knowledge, skills, and positive attitudes that nurses need to offer this care. Nurses in all clinical specialties in nursing need to be able to identify alcohol and drug abuse in their clients, to intervene and refer them for assistance, and to care for recovering clients appropriately. Previous significant studies need to be replicated to validate their findings. Most important, nurse researchers need to develop programs of research in this field so that each study builds on prior work in order that the resulting body of knowledge can provide a foundation for nursing practice.

REFERENCES

American Psychiatric Association. (1987). *Diagnostic and statistical manual of mental disorders* (3rd ed., rev.) Washington, DC: Author.

Anderson, M. (1980). Health needs of drug dependent clients: Focus on women. *Women and Health, 5*(1), 23–33.

Anderson, M. (1982). Personalized nursing: A unique approach to drug dependent women. *Journal of Emergency Nursing, 8,* 225–231.

Anderson, M. D. (1986). Personalized nursing: An effective intervention model for use with drug-dependent women in an emergency room. *International Journal of Addictions, 21,* 105–122.

Arneson, S. W., Schultz, M., Triplett, J. L. (1987). Nurses' knowledge of the impact of parental alcoholism on children. *Archives of Psychiatric Nursing, 1,* 251:257.

Arneson, S. W., Triplett, J. L., Schweer, K. D., & Snider, B. C. (1983). Children of alcoholic parents: Identification and intervention. *Children's Health Care, 11,* 107–112.

Asheychik, R., Jackson, T., Baker, H., Ferraro, R., Ashton, T., & Kilgore, J. (1989). The efficacy of L-Tryptophan in the reduction of sleep disturbance and depressive state in alcoholic patients. *Journal of Studies on Alcohol, 50,* 525–532.

Banonis, B. C. (1989). The lived experience of recovering from addiction: A phenomenological study. *Nursing Science Quarterly, 2,* 37–43.

Bartek, J. K., Lindeman, M., Newton, M., Fitzgerald, A. P., & Hawks, J. H. (1988). Nurse-identified problems in the management of alcoholic patients. *Journal of Studies on Alcohol, 49,* 62:70.

Bennett, G. (1988). Stress, social support, and self-esteem of young alcoholics in recovery. *Issues in Mental Health Nursing, 9,* 151–167.

Busch, D., McBride, A. B., & Benaventura, L. M. (1986). Chemical dependency in women: The link to OB-GYN problems. *Journal of Psychosocial Nursing and Mental Health Services, 24*(4), 26–30.

Busch, D., & Svanum, S. (1983). Alcoholism and drug abuse education in graduate psychiatric/mental health nursing: A survey. *Journal of Alcohol and Drug Education, 28*(2), 4–7.

Byers, P. H., Raven, L. M., Hill, J. D., & Robyak, J. E. (1990). Enhancing the self-esteem of inpatient alcoholics. *Issues in Mental Health Nursing, 11,* 337–346.

Cannon, B. L., & Brown, J. S. (1988). Nurses' attitudes toward impaired colleagues. *Image, 20,* 96–101.

Carter, A. J. (1983). Alcohol and drug abuse training in nursing schools. *Alcohol Health and Research World, 8,* 24–25, 29.

Cloninger, C. R., Bohman M., & Sigvardsson, S. (1981). Inheritance of alcohol abuse. *Archives of General Psychiatry, 38,* 861.

Cohen, S., & Wills, T. A. (1985). Stress, social support, and the buffering hypothesis. *Psychological Bulletin, 98*(2), 310–357.

Conlon, J. M., & Radinsky, R. L. (1981). Outcomes of referrals of alcoholics in crisis. *Issues in Mental Health Nursing, 3,* 271–281.

Engs, R. C. (1977). Drinking patterns and drinking problems of college students. *Journal of Studies on Alcohol, 38,* 2144–2156.

Engs, R. C. (1982). Drinking patterns and attitudes toward alcoholism of Australian human-services students. *Journal of Studies on Alcohol, 43,* 517–531.

Engs, R. C. (1990). Family background of alcohol abuse and its relationship to alcohol consumption among college students. *Journal of Studies on Alcohol, 51,* 542–547.

Engs, R. C., & Hanson, D. J. (1985). The drinking patterns and problems of college students: 1983. *Journal of Alcohol and Drug Education, 31,* 65–83.

Engs, R. C., & Hanson, D. J. (1986). Age-specific alcohol prohibition and college students' drinking problems. *Psychological Reports, 59,* 979–984.

Farnsworth, B., & Bairan, A. (1990). The difference in pre- and postaffiliation attitudes of student nurses toward alcohol and people with alcohol-related problems. *Addictions Nursing Network,* 2)3), 23–27.

Ferneau, E. W. (1967). What student nurses think about alcoholic patients and alcoholism. *Nursing Outlook, 15*(10), 40.

Forchuk, C. (1984). Cognitive dissonance: Denial, self concepts and the alcoholic stereotype. *Nursing Papers, 16*(3), 57–69.

Fortin, M. T., & Evans, S. B. (1983). Correlates of loss of control over drinking in women alcoholics. *Journal of Studies on Alcohol, 44,* 787–796.

Foy, A., March, S., & Drinkwater, V. (1988. Use of an objective clinical scale in the assessment and management of alcohol withdrawal in a large general hospital. *Alcoholism: Clinical and Experimental Research, 12,* 360–364.

Gibson, D. E. (1980). Reminiscence, self-esteem and self-other satisfaction in adult male alcoholics. *Journal of Psychiatric Nursing and Mental Health Services, 18*(3), 7–11.

Goodwin, D. W., Schulsinger, R., Hermansen, L., Guze, S. B., & Winokur, G. (1973). Alcohol problems in adoptees raised apart from alcoholic biological parents. *Archives of General Psychiatry, 28,* 238–243.

Harlow, P. E., & Goby, M. S. (1980). Changing nursing students' attitudes toward alcoholic patients: Examining effects of a clinical practicuum. *Nursing Research, 29,* 59–60.

Hoffman, A. L., & Estes, N. J. (1986). A tool for measuring body and behavioral experiences. *Alcohol Health and Research World, 11,* 26–29, 72.

Hoffman, A. L., & Estes, N. J. (1987). Body and behavioral experiences in recovery from alcoholism. *Rehabilitation Nursing, 12,* 188–192.

Hoffman, A. L., & Heinemann, M. E. (1987). Substance abuse education in schools of nursing: A national survey. *Journal of Nursing Education, 26,* 282–287.

Huckstadt, A. (1987). Locus of control among alcoholics, recovering alcoholics, and non-alcoholics. *Research in Nursing and Health, 10,* 23–28.

Jack, L. W. (1989). The educational impact of a course about addiction. *Journal of Nursing Education, 28,* 22–28.

Jellinek, E. M., (1946). Phases in the drinking history of alcoholics. *Quarterly Journal of Studies of Alcohol, 7,* 88.

Kus, R. J. (1988a). Alcoholism and non-acceptance of gay self: The critical link. *Journal of Homosexuality, 16,* 25–41.

Kus, R. J. (1988b). "Working the program": The Alcoholics Anonymous experience and gay American men. *Holistic Nursing Practice, 2*(4), 62–74.

London, F. B. (1982). Attitudinal and social normative factors as predictors of intended alcohol abuse among fifth- and seventh-grade students. *Journal of School Health, 52,* 244–249.

Long, P. Gelfand, G., & McGill, D. (1991). Inclusion of alcoholism and drug abuse content in curricula of varied health care professions. *Journal of the New York State Nurses Association, 22*(1), 9–12.

Meiderhoff, P. A., & Ray, S. (1980, July). *Attitudinal and behavioral changes resulting from participation in drug abuse educational courses.* Paper presented at the annual meeting of the American Association of Colleges of Pharmacy, Boston, MA.

Meiderhoff, P. A., Ray, S., & Talarchek, G. (1986). The constraints of professional-socialization: Nursing student attitudes toward drug abusers. *Research Communications in Substances of Abuse, 7,* 70–80.

National Institute on Alcohol Abuse and Alcoholism. (1990). *Alcohol and Health* (DHHS Publication No. ADM 88-0002). Washington, DC: U.S. Government Printing Office.

National Institute on Drug Abuse (1991). *National Household Survey on Drug Abuse* (DHHS Publication No. ADM 91-1732). Washington, DC: U.S. Government Printing Office.

Reisman, B. L., & Shrader, R. W. (1984). Effect of nurses' attitudes toward alcoholism on their referral rate for treatment. *Occupational Health Nursing, 32,* 273–275.

Reynolds, B., & Ried, L. D. (1985). Factors associated with public health nurses' perceptions of skill in chemical dependency assessment and referral. *Journal of Drug Education, 15,* 23–32.

Rosenfield, S. N., & Stevenson, J. S. (1988). Perception of daily stress and oral coping behaviors in normal, overweight, and recovering alcoholic women. *Research in Nursing and Health, 11,* 166–174.

Rowland, N., & Maynard, A. K. (1989). Alcohol education for patients: Some nurses need persuading. *Nurse Education Today, 9,* 100–104.

Scavnicky-Mylant, M. (1986). The use of drawings in the assessment and treatment of children of alcoholics. *Journal of Pediatric Nursing, 1,* 178–194.

Shelley, S., & Anderson, C. (1986). The influence of selected variables on the experience of menstrual distress in alcoholic and nonalcoholic women. *JOGNN: Journal of Obstetric, Gynecologic, and Neonatal Nursing, 15,* 484–491.

Sullivan, E. J., & Hale, R. E. (1987). Nurses' beliefs about the etiology and treatment of alcohol abuse: A national study. *Journal of Studies on Alcohol, 48,* 456–460.

Sullivan, E. J., & Handley, S. M. (1992). Alcohol and drug abuse in nurses. In J. Fitzpatrick, R. L. Taunton, & J. Q. Benoliel (Eds.), *Annual review of nursing research* (Vol. 10, pp. 113–125). New York: Springer Publishing Co.

Talashek, M. L. (1987). Parental alcoholism and adolescent ego identity. *Journal of Community Health Nursing, 4,* 211–222.

Tamlyn, D. L. (1989). The effect of education on student nurses' attitudes toward alcoholics. *Canadian Journal of Nursing Research, 21,* 31–47.

Trinkoff, A. M., Ritter, C., & Anthony, J. C. (1990). The prevalence and self-reported consequences of cocaine use: An exploratory and descriptive analysis. *Drug and Alcohol Dependence, 26,* 217–225.

Wechsler, H., & Rohman, M. (1982). Future caregivers' views of alcoholism treatment. *Journal of Studies on Alcohol, 43,* 939–955.

Chapter 13

Nursing Research on Patient Falls in Health Care Institutions

JANICE M. MORSE
SCHOOL OF NURSING
PENNSYLVANIA STATE UNIVERSITY

CONTENTS

Since the 1960s, research on patient falls has escalated. Once considered a normal and expected consequence of aging, of hospitalization and illness, or an unavoidable *accident,* patient falls now are considered both predictable and preventable. In the past 30 years, research agendas have changed from estimating the numbers of patient falls and the outcomes of those falls to predicting the patient's likelihood of falling and identifying and testing strategies for reducing and preventing falls. The purpose of this review is to examine research related to patient falls in health care institutions including the identification and evaluation of strategies to prevent patient falls, and to make recommendations for future research. It is important to note that the focus of the review is health care institutions; because falls that occur in the community are caused by different factors (Rubenstein & Robbins, 1989), they are beyond the scope of this review. Studies on falls from 1966 to 1991 were located through (a) MEDLINE, *PsychLit,* and *CINAHL* databases; (b) *Cumulative Index of Nursing and Allied Health Literature, Index Medicus,* and *Social Sciences Citation Index*; (c) hand searches of bibliography entries of published articles; and (d) personal communication with researchers active in the field.

SEVERITY OF THE PROBLEM

Falls have been identified as the second leading cause of accidental death in the United States, and 75% of those falls occurred in the elderly population (Rubenstein & Robbins, 1989). Furthermore, in elderly hospital patients, approximately 6% of falls result in serious injuries (Morse, Tylko, & Dixon, 1987). These injuries are estimated to cost billions of dollars (Baker & Harvey, 1985), and they often result in death from secondary causes. Furthermore, it has now been suggested that two-thirds of all falls that occur in the elderly population are preventable.

Patient falls that occur in acute care, long-term care, or in nursing homes have long been a nursing concern. Initially, comparison of institutional fall rates was difficult. Even though falls were considered an inevitable part of aging, nursing staff felt responsible and was ashamed when a patient fell. Consequently, incident reports were more likely to be filed or only required to be filed when an injury resulted from the fall. Fear of the large numbers of falls that might be revealed from accurate reporting or the fear of legal action resulted in administrative decisions to suppress institutional fall rates. As a result of these decisions, it was not until the early 1970s that the seriousness of the problem was identified. Even when institutional fall rates were published, different methods for reporting these statistics were used, making assessment of the severity of the problem difficult. Unfortunately, this continues to be a problem (Morse & Morse, 1988).

Today, it is understood that patient falls in an institution are not random events. Patient falls are a patterned and predictable event and, therefore, a preventable occurrence. However, disciplinary biases are evident in the search for factors contributing to falls and the recommended strategies for prevention. The purpose of this review is to examine various approaches to the identification of the fall-prone patients in health care institutions, to provide an in-depth review of the contribution of nursing research to this problem, and to describe the "state of the art" of fall prevention research in nursing.

Definition of a Fall

One of the greatest problems in research literature on patients falls appeared to be the problem of defining a fall. Morris and Isaacs (1980) defined a fall as "an untoward event in which the patient comes to rest unintentionally on the floor," but exceptions can be found that do not fit this definition. For example, was it considered a fall if a staff member broke the fall by "catching" the patient or the patient collapsed into a chair? Was it considered a fall if the patient managed to grasp onto a handrail and slid or eased himself or herself onto the floor? These issues have never been resolved, and they remain a methodologic problem.

A more important issue in the examination of patient falls is variation in the type of falls. In the medical literature, falls are first described as physiologic. Morse et al. (1987) identified physiologic falls as anticipated and unanticipated. Each type of fall is indicative of different etiology and requires different prevention strategies. Anticipated physiologic falls are predictable falls that occur in patients with impaired gaits, who may use a walking aid and are frequently disoriented. These falls constitute approximately 78% of all falls. Conversely, unanticipated physiologic falls, 8% of falls, occur in patients who are oriented, but who may faint, experience a seizure, or syncope, or who have knees that "give way." These unanticipated falls may not be preventable until the first fall has occurred and the physiologic cause is diagnosed. Thereafter, preventive measures should focus on preventing patient injury should another fall occur. The second group are accidental falls, which occur when the patient trips or slips. These falls (14% of all falls) occur in patients who are alert and have a normal gait, and they are prevented by ensuring a safe environment (Morse et al., 1987).

RESEARCH APPROACHES

A patient fall may be caused by myriad factors, such as pathophysiologic, psychologic, social, or environmental, or it may be caused from the cumulative effect of two or more factors within these categories. Patient falls have serious ramifications and the consequences of falls cross disciplinary boundaries. Thus, the problem of falling has become a research priority for nurses, gerontologists, physicians, physical therapists, bioengineers, psychologists, and social workers. From the 1960s to the late 1970s, falls researchers used epidemiologic methods and focused on the identification and seriousness of the problem; however, more recently, disciplinary and professional concerns have been reflected in the researchers' approach to the problem. For example, physicians now tend to focus on the etiology underlying the fall and the control of symptoms predisposing the fall; physical therapists primarily consider the biomechanics of the fall, the gait of fall-prone patients, and the prevention of weakness; bioengineeers concentrate on the reduction of environmental hazards such as the design of stairs, the height of handrails, and the creation of a safe environment; psychologists are interested in factors such as depression or confusion that predispose a patient to fall and in the psychologic consequences of falling; and social workers examine the ability of the fall-prone patient to maintain independence. Nurse researchers have concentrated on assessing the fall-prone patient to identify the cause of the fall, and these researchers have tended to use a comprehensive approach, incorporating physical, psychologic, social, and environmental factors, an approach that reflects the holistic philosophy of the nursing discipline. There has been less attention given to research evaluating recommended interventions. Nursing has tended to move directly to application, implementation, and evaluation of fall-prevention programs, usually consisting of multiple fall-prevention strategies (see, e.g., the review article by Whedon & Shedd, 1989), which reflects the pragmatic disciplinary values of care and praxis.

The clinical focus, the professional role, and the disciplinary bias of the major approaches provide a broad context in which patient falls are generally examined. The overall purpose of the research, from the researcher's disciplinary perspective, is to enhance his or her profession's ability to prevent or to manage the problem of patient falls. This disciplinary perspective and the associated domain of professional practice provide "blinders" that delineate the variables, research approaches, and methods that restrict or limit the broad application and the overall utility when implementing research findings.

Epidemiologic Approaches

The retrospective chart review is the most common method of identifying fall rates within an institution and the risk factors that contribute to the fall. Retrospective chart reviews provide an extensive amount of data about the fall-prone patient. In addition to how many patients fall, investigators using retrospective methods have identified patterns in patient falls by linking the fall with patient characteristics such as gender and age, the patient diagnosis and number of diagnoses, patient treatments, environmental characteristics, patient activity when the fall occurred, and the outcome or any injury that may have occurred as a result of the fall. Frequently, these studies are reported without comparison groups, and thus results are not compared with the patient population from which the samples were drawn. Consequently, erroneous conclusions are made and discrepant results are evident among published studies. Such a problem is found in Perry's (1982) study where it was concluded that gender of the patient is a variable that contributes to the patient's likelihood of falling. If the researcher obtains statistically significant differences between the number of males and females who fall and assumes that the population in the cohort consists of an equal number of males and females, then the conclusion is erroneous. In the elderly, longevity of females results in disproportionate female-to-male ratios, and the sample must be compared with appropriate age groups of the patient population for that particular institution (Morse et al., 1987). This error is important as results of such studies have been used to construct tools for identifying the patient at risk of falling that include variables such as gender of the patient as a risk factor. Finally, comparison of the fall group with the nonfall group frequently has been conducted using univariate statistics such as chi-square and *t*-tests, although more sophisticated statistical methods are available to detect and elicit differences between groups.

Despite the problems, the descriptive, retrospective research has made an important contribution to knowledge of patient falls by drawing attention to the seriousness and extensiveness of the problem, and it often provides baseline data for evaluation of a fall-prevention program. The studies have shown that falls increase exponentially with increasing age and that falls have correctly been labeled as a "disease of aging" (Lund & Sheafor, 1985; Manjam & MacKinnon, 1973). Repeatedly, researchers have reported that most falls occur between the patient's bed and the bathroom, that falls are frequently associated with incontinence, and that falls tend to occur at times when the staff is busy or unavailable (Lund & Sheafor, 1985; Manjam & MacKinnon, 1973). Finally, the majority of patients who fall have impaired mental status (Vlahov, Myers, & Al-Ibrahim, 1990; Warshaw et al., 1982).

Medical Approaches

In the medical perspective, a fall generally is considered a symptom of underlying pathology. Consequently, the identification and control or correction of the disease removes the symptom and therefore reduces the risk of the fall (Patel, 1976). This perspective has four important implications. First, the fall symptom must be evident before the patient is examined for underlying disease. This means that the patient must fall (or report having fallen) before the patient is recognized as fall prone, assessed, and labeled as fall prone, and prevention strategies are implemented. This approach may be problematic as the goal of medicine must inevitably be to prevent the reoccurrence of a fall rather than a fall per se. Thus, as the original fall experienced by the patient may result in injury, this approach is not predictive or entirely preventive. The second problem is that the cause of the fall may be iatrogenic, that is, the consequence of medical treatment. For example, a fall in an elderly patient may be traced to the poor absorption of or intolerance to drugs, to the prescribing of drugs that interact poorly, to the interactive effects of prescription drugs and alcohol, or to the administration of drugs to which the patient is sensitive (Stegman, 1983). Consequently, a fall may require modification of a treatment regime, or it may result in the decision to maintain the necessary treatments despite the continued risk of repeated falling. The third implication is that medicine is interested primarily in intrinsic, physiologic falls; accidental or extrinsic falls are not of interest as they are not considered preventable in the medical domain. If they are to be prevented, they are considered the domain of bioengineers who seek solutions to the fall problem by reducing environmental hazards. The last and serious limitation of the medical approach is that patients may not report the fall to the physician because they may fear reprisal, such as admission to a nursing home, or may forget the incident. In one study, 32% of the subjects with confirmed falls did not recall the event 3 months afterward (Cummings, Nevitt, & Kidd, 1988). Thus, when the onus is on the patient to report the fall, many patients who have fallen and are at risk of a repeated fall may not receive preventive treatment.

Symptoms and diseases that have been associated with an increased risk of falling are arthritis, heart disease, neurologic disorders, cardiac dysfunction (e.g., arrhythmias, valvar disease, and blocks) and depression (Robbins et al., 1989). Medical examination focuses on the identification of problems such as syncope, orthostatic hypotension, epilepsy, drop attacks, and neurologic conditions (e.g., brain tumors, hydrocephalus, and cerebral atrophy) (Botez & Hausser, 1982). Even when assessing gait, physicians conduct a detailed examination, assessing step length, stride width, speed, and the number of steps per minute, balance, sway, and muscle strength (Maki, Holliday, & Fernie, 1990; Ring, Nayak, & Isaacs, 1988). Following the development of a lengthy and detailed instrument, the Gait Assessment Rating Score, Wolfson, Whipple, Amerman, and Tobin (1990) concluded that a simple method of visual rating of gait features may be a "useful alternative to established methods of gait analysis" (p. M12). Similarly, Robbins et al. (1989) note that "three or four variables contained most of the predictive value" in their regression equation. Hip weakness, low balance score, and numbers of prescription medications taken accounted for predicting 76.6% of the falls with 89% sensitivity and 60% specificity. They made a plea for reducing the number of variables in instruments to predict patient falls, concluding that "basic risk assessment may be further abbreviated" (p. 1633).

Biomechanical Approaches

A cadre of researchers from physical therapy and neurology have investigated the patient fall from an ergonomic/kinetic perspective. These researchers attribute falling to gait disorders of orthopedic origin, diseases such as Parkinson's disease that result in gait disorders, cervical spondylosis (Whipple, Wolfson, & Amerman, 1987), or changes that occur with advancing age, such as weakness and changes in reflexes affecting balance and gait. When the cause of falls may be attributed to these physiologic causes, in addition to providing treatment when appropriate, the patient may be given physical therapy, instruction on how to avoid falling, and walking aids to reduce fall risk.

Environmental Approaches

Researchers who focus primarily on falls as an accidental event focus on reducing environmental hazards as a strategy to reduce falls. For instance, they examine floor surfaces to reduce slippage and glare (Tisserand, 1985), the height and location of handrails (Maki, Bartlett, & Fernie, 1984), and the position and type of lighting. Frequently, the environmental perspective is combined with the biomechanical approach (e.g., Maki et al., 1984) to ensure optimal safety for the disabled. For instance, Vlahov et al. (1990) observed that 82% of the falls occurred within 60 days of admission in the rehabilitation hospital and these falls occurred when patients were transferring to or from a wheelchair. These authors recommended that to prevent accidents, wheelchairs should be redesigned and the center of gravity changed to avoid tipping.

NURSING RESEARCH ON PATIENT FALLS

Nursing Approaches

In contrast to the preceding approaches, the nursing approach is more comprehensive and perhaps because of the nature of nursing practice (i.e., the provision of 24-hr care), it may incorporate a more multidisciplinary approach that includes biomechanical, environmental, and medical strategies. Nurse researchers have recognized the multivariate nature of the fall and have included physiologic, psychologic, and environmental causes and accepted responsibility for the nurse's role in the prevention of falls by providing quality care. Consequently, nurse researchers are concerned with identifying factors that predict the patient's risk of falling and are engaged in an aggressive search for nursing strategies to prevent the occurrence of falls.

Chart Reviews: Characteristics of Fallers. When examining patient falls, nurse researchers usually begin by conducting a literature review of the fall research to compile a checklist of significant variables. Next, a retrospective chart review of patients who have fallen in their institution over some preselected period is conducted (see Gross, Shimamoto, Rose, & Frank, 1990; Hendrich, 1988; Rainville, 1984; Tack, Ulrich, & Kehr, 1987). With few exceptions, these studies do not involve a comparison group. Once a profile of a fall-prone patient is "confirmed," usually by auditing charts of patients who have fallen and examining the number of patients with each of the characteristics, then interventions to prevent the fall are planned. The checklist frequently becomes an assessment tool that forms the basis of a care plan for ensuring the safety of patients at risk of falling or, more recently, to confirm the nursing diagnosis of "potential for injury."

A more sophisticated approach was used in a study by Janken, Reynolds, and Swieck (1986) who conducted a chart review with patients who fell and with a randomly selected comparison group. Six hundred thirty-one charts of patients 61 years and older were randomly selected from 17,392 patient charts; of these, 300 patients had not fallen, and 331 patients had fallen. Two periods were included in the analysis: the day of admission and the day prior to the fall. Comparison, using stepwise multiple regression, of those patients who had fallen with those who had not fallen revealed the standard risk factors contributing to patient falls. Significant differences were noted between the fall and comparison groups, but regression analysis explained only 22% of the variance with five dichotomous variables. These variables (or risk factors) were confusion, decreased mobility of lower extremities, general weakness, vertigo, and substance abuse. The authors indicated that a prospective study was necessary to confirm these findings as only data previously collected (i.e., information that is already recorded on the patient chart) were included in the analysis.

Identification of the Fall-Prone Patient

There are two types of scales to identify the fall-prone patient. The purpose of the first type of scale is to identify the patient's probability or risk of falling;

the second type of scale is used to assess factors that contribute to the patient's risk of falling. Although the first type of scale supplies information on the patient's likelihoood of falling, which is usually presented as a fall score, it supplies little information about interventions to reduce the patient's risk of falling, or prevent falls. Consequently, a more thorough assessment of the patient must be conducted for the purpose of reducing the patient's probability of falling. Conversely, instruments that identify factors contributing to the patient's risk of falling may give direction on how to reduce the patient's risk but supply little information on the patient's probability of falling. The first type of scale is quick and easy to use, sensitive to changes in the patient's condition, and should be used routinely and frequently; the second type of scale involves cumbersome assessment forms and is probably used only once or twice during the hospital stay, perhaps after admission or after a fall occurs.

Scales to Predict the Probability of Falling. Four of the scales to predict the patient's probability of falling were located in the nursing literature. The first was developed by Arsenault (1982). This scale consists of six variables (age, history of falling, medications, mobility, mentation, and sensory defects) and a weighted scoring system (of values from 1 to 10) for the presence of risk factors. The scale also is interesting because patient typologies for various risk levels are presented, with appropriate interventions. This work is promising, but no indices of reliability or validity were available.

The second scale, developed by Easterling (1990), was not developed from a research base, and the weightings for each item apparently were arbitrarily assigned. Although it was prospectively tested for 1 year, there was no reliability or validity data presented for this scale.

A third study listing predictive risk factors for stroke patients (Byers, Arrington, & Finstuen, 1990) is still in the process of development. Thus far, significant risk factors (e.g., history of falls, impaired decision-making, restlessness, generalized weakness, and fatigability) have been identified, but the final step of reducing these variables to a scale and developing weights has yet to be completed.

The fourth scale, the Morse Fall Scale (Morse, Morse, & Tylko, 1989), consists of six items: history of falling, secondary diagnosis, use of an ambulatory aid, intravenous, gait (as normal gait, patient on bedrest, weak, or impaired), and mental status (oriented to own abilities or overestimates ability and forgets limitations). As each item is scored in multiples of five, it is quick to use and easy to score. As a patient's fall proneness varies throughout the day and as nurses become familiar with the scale, they learn to identify changes in the patient's condition that affect the patient's fall score and to adjust the patient's risk of falling accordingly.

Data used in the development of the Morse Fall Scale were collected prospectively and included in a randomly selected group for comparison; thus, the Morse Fall Scale overcomes the problems of nonrandom selective and retrospective designs limiting other checklists. Normative scores have been developed for the scale for acute care, nursing home, and rehabilitation populations (Morse, Black, Oberle, & Donahue, 1989), and instructions are provided for determining risk score according to the patient setting (Morse, 1986). Reliability and validity testing have been conducted using discriminant analysis, with 80.5% of the patients correctly identified as fallers. Sensitivity of the scale is 78%, and specificity is 83%. The interrater reliability correlation was $r = .96$ (Morse, Morse, & Tylko, 1989). Finally, prospective testing of the scale in three patient care settings (long-term care, rehabilitation, and acute care) has been reported (Morse, Black et al., 1989). Thus, as a screening device for identifying the patient's probability of falling, the scale makes an important contribution. However, it is recommended that all patients at apparent high risk of falling be assessed for risk of falling. Thus, their risk of falling and subsequent fall risk may be reduced.

Instruments to Assess Factors Contributing to Fall Risk. Nine forms developed to assess factors that contribute to the patient's fall proneness have been published (Barbieri, 1983; Fife, Solomon, & Stanton, 1985; Hendrich, 1988; Llewellyn, Martin, Shekleton, & Firlit, 1988; Rainville, 1984; Spellbring, Gannon, Kleckner, & Conway, 1988; Tack et al., 1987; Young, Abedzadeh, & White, 1989). These forms have generally been constructed from the nursing literature or from a group meeting of expert nurses rather than from research that includes a control group of patients who have not fallen. Thus, most of the assessment forms contain items that were not significant in controlled research. For example, these assessment forms include gender (Rainville, 1984), orthostatic hypotension (Llewellyn et al., 1988; Spellbring et al., 1988), and age (Fife et al., 1985; Llewellyn et al., 1988; Rainville, 1984), all variables that have not been verified in controlled studies. These forms have included the following variables: age; gender; history of falls; secondary diagnosis; patient condition (weakness or dizziness); impaired gait; urinary incontinence or urgency; sensory deficiency (such as visual or auditory loss or the inability to communicate); impaired mental status, depression, or a "poor attitude"; the use of ambulatory aids; inappropriate footwear; and medications (especially the use of diuretics, analgesics, hypnotics, tranquilizers, laxatives, or cathartics). Environmental factors include poor lighting, shiny floors, or spilled water. There is inconsistency among forms regarding variables included, and those selected for inclusion appear to be based on investigator preference rather than on a research base.

The most comprehensive of these forms was developed by Spellbring and associates (1988), and this form includes 15 variables. Although most of these forms are checklists to guide future nursing care, the form developed by Innes and Turman (1983) includes a rating scale, indicating that attempts were made to combine the assessment form with a predictive fall-risk score. Further, forms may link the assessments with nursing diagnoses (e.g., Janken et al., 1986) or with intervention strategies for the nursing care plan. Until recently, there was little attempt to establish any form of reliability and validity, even interrater reliability, before implementation of these assessment forms (Spellbring, 1992). Although speed is necessary and these approaches promising, there is much work to do on the development of these scales.

Development and Testing of Fall-Prevention Strategies

Developing and testing fall-prevention strategies is the least developed research area. Falls are recognized as a problem that may be caused from a wide variety of physiologic, psychologic, environmental, and care factors, and efforts to prevent patient falls generally depend on the individual assessment of each patient at risk of falling. Recognizing the role and responsibility of nurses in the prevention of falls and the fact that the number of falls increases when units are short staffed (Llewellyn et al., 1988), increasing awareness of nursing staff by introducing safety awareness, usually as a fall-prevention program, is a common method of reducing patient falls. By giving regular inservices to staff about the factors that contribute to patient falls, providing staff with regular fall statistics, and reminding them of safety practices, safety precautions are used more consistently with individual patients. As a consequence, the fall rate is reduced. Several investigators have recommended that fall-prone patients be identified with colored dots placed on their beds, charts, and outside their door so that patient surveillance may be increased, and patients can be supervised or assisted with toileting and other activities (Whedon & Shedd, 1989). However, as Maciorowski and associates (1988) note, the effectiveness of these educational strategies for fall prevention has yet to be evaluated.

Intervention Checklists. To standardize intervention strategies and to ensure that interventions are not omitted from consideration, several checklists of strategies have been published. As with the fall-assessment checklists, there are discrepancies among these lists, and none is comprehensive. The interventions suggested range from those that are under the control of nurses, such as offering assistance with voiding to strategies that may be initiated by nurses, such as requesting a medical consultation to reevaluate the patient's medications.

Several comprehensive literature reviews (Maciorowski et al., 1988;

Whedon & Shedd, 1989) have been published recently. These review articles could be used to develop a more complete list of prevention strategies.

Changing attitudes of nurses. The most successful strategy to date appears to be changing attitudes of nurses. Increased awareness of patient falls increases supervision and perhaps reduces the response time for giving assistance or for answering call bells. Ironically, acceptance of patient falls as a reality if patient mobility is to be maintained is inherent in this model. Accepting the possibility that patients may fall if they are to be independent, the risk of injury must be weighed against the benefits of independent mobility. Further, muscle wasting and weakness are reduced with continued mobility, so that the actual probability of falling decreased in active patients. Interestingly, the use of patient restraints, often applied to prevent the patient from falling (Masters & Marks, 1990; Tinetti, Lui, & Ginter, 1992), paradoxically increased the risk of falling. Patient restraints inhibited the patient's movement in the bed or chair and, therefore, increase muscle wasting and weakness, which further contributed to a weak gait and increased the risk of falling. McHutchion and Morse (1990) note that if nurses are given a clear message from nursing administrators that they are prepared to accept the risk of injury from a fall rather than restrain a patient, the nurses' attitudes will change regarding the use of restraints, and the institution's fall rate will actually decrease (Tinetti et al., 1992).

Nursing-Biomechanical Engineering Solutions. In the past 5 years, several bed alarms have been developed as a means for facilitating nursing surveillance of the fall-prone patient. Two of these alarms have been described in the literature: the Bedcheck Alarm (Bedcheck Corporation, Tulsa, OK) and the Ambularm (Rigi Systems, Inc., Mill Valley, CA). The results of using these alarms have been reported in the literature (Widder, 1985), and they appear to be helpful in reducing the number of falls from beds or chairs. As an alternative to restraints, these alarms alert staff when confused patients attempt to leave the bed, and in one study (Llewellyn et al., 1988), patient falls were reduced by 60%.

However, given the implication of the number of falls from the patient's bed and the recognized importance of keeping the bed in the low position, it is interesting that a geriatric bed the same height as a domestic bed has not been developed. Because of the mechanism required for adjusting the height, tilting the bed, and so forth, the lowest deck height of a hospital bed currently on the North American market is 4 inches higher than a domestic bed, and it may be 6 or more inches higher in some models. This results in an unexpected drop for the patient when climbing out of bed. Full-lenth side rails contribute to patient injury when the patient climbs over the side rail or climbs out of bed by dropping over the foot of the bed. Three-quarter-length side rails that allow the patient a safe route to exit from the bed should be used. These problems are presently being addressed by this author in collaboration with a bioengineer, and a safe geriatric bed is being developed.* Such collaborative projects between nurses and engineers are beneficial, for nursing input into the design of hospital equipment improves design and increases patient safety.

EVALUATION OF FALL-PREVENTION PROGRAMS

Evaluation of fall prevention is both problematic and paradoxic as the very act of increasing awareness may result in an increase in the reporting of falls, possibly leading to the erroneous conclusion that the intervention has had no effect or even made the problem worse. In addition, the probability of occurrence is often too low to detect differences. One solution is to use the Poisson distributions or to use delayed cross-over designs to detect differences. It is therefore recommended that along with the number of falls, the number of injuries resulting from falls should be calculated. Although injuries may be a relatively rare event, this may be a more reliable measure to evaluate the effectiveness of a fall-prevention program (Morse & Morse, 1988).

ETHICAL IMPLICATIONS OF FALL RESEARCH

Researching patient falls introduces some interesting ethical problems. It introduces a dilemma into the identification of a patient's likelihood of falling and the responsibility of the researcher simultaneously to prevent the expected fall and to protect the patient from injury (i.e., to implement the preventive strategy) before the occurrence of the fall, that is, before the predicted event. In other words, if the goal of such a research program is the prevention of falls, clinicians, aware of consequences of falling for their patients and the legal ramifications of patients who have fallen (both for the institution and themselves as practitioners), are eager to introduce fall-prevention programs. Yet fall-prevention research programs must logically begin with identification of the characteristics of the fall-prone patient, developing predictive criteria for the identification of the fall-prone patient, and testing these criteria prospectively. The next phase is the development of strategies for fall prevention and testing these prevention strategies in the clinical area.

In this time-consuming research sequence, which extends over several

*Patent: Heinz, University of Alberta Hospitals, and Morse, University of Alberta, 1991.

years, the stage is inevitably reached between these two steps of identification and prevention where reliable, valid, and clinically practical means for the identification of the fall-prone patients are successfully developed, and yet strategies for prevention are not yet available. Publication of the means for identifying the fall-prone patient (e.g., the Morse Fall Scale) results in the immediate adoption of the scale into practice. In essence, this results in the identification of fall-prone patients before measures to prevent the recognized and inevitable falls have been developed. This conflict places the staff in an untenable position. Although such a position may provide documentation for assisting the staff in obtaining additional staff on the unit or for providing constant care for the patient at risk, there is the possibility of the increased use of restraints to ensure safety for such patients. It is important that variables such as fall proneness be entered into the calculation of staffing ratios. In short, it is of little use for staff and perhaps harmful to be able to recognize who will fall if there is little that can be done to prevent the fall.

An interesting "solution" to this problem is presently being tested by Maas and colleagues (1990), who are protecting patients from injury rather than falling. They are reducing injuries from falls by testing the use of pads to prevent a fractured hip. Even though fractured hips constitute less than 0.4% of all injuries (Morse, Prowse, Morrow, & Federspeil, 1985), the prognosis for a fractured hip is poor; this intervention will prevent the use of the strategies with severe iatrogenic effects, such as the use of restraints.

Another interesting problem occurs when both the means to predict patients falls and appropriate interventions to prevent falls have been developed. One cannot develop and test the means to predict the fall-prone patient without also simultaneously introducing fall-prevention strategies. Yet the implementation of fall-prevention strategies directly interferes with the evaluation of the criterion measure (i.e., the occurrence of a fall) used to test the predictive instrument. Because of the association of falls to morbidity and mortality, the concurrent evaluation of both a predictive instrument and fall-prevention strategies is morally essential. This strategy can only be partially successful, for in reality falls should not occur if the diverse prevention strategies are "successful." The only alternative to this dilemma is the cooperation of the staff to document "missed" or prevented falls qualitatively. As this documentation includes the prevention of falls by the successful triggering of alarms and falls prevented by nurses "catching" patients in precarious situations, the number of prevented falls is much higher than the number of falls without intervention strategies. This figure is further confounded by the implementation of fall-prevention strategies, such as offering a patient a bed pan at regular intervals. These strategies may indirectly reduce fall risk, but they cannot be directly linked to specific incidents.

DIRECTIONS FOR FUTURE RESEARCH

The present trend toward the nonresearch-based development of assessment forms from the intuitive "experience" of expert nurses and the immediate implementation of these forms in the practice setting without establishing validity and reliability is a problem. These forms are then used to develop care plans, intervention strategies, or nursing diagnoses without concern for the research process. Even when the research process is used, such as by Janken et al. (1986), research data tend to be obtained from retrospective chart reviews rather than prospectively in the clinical area. This results in the researcher being able only to include data that have been collected, and these variables may not necessarily be the ones that are most important or pertinent to the problem. There is a dearth of research using data collected at the time of the fall, and despite ethical dilemmas, research using prospective designs is critically needed.

Many of the fall-prevention strategies suggested in the literature are obvious, commonsense, simple interventions, and yet they have not been tested or implemented. For instance, researchers have recommended that rails be installed between the patient's bed and the bathroom, and that this distance be reduced so that safe independence is maintained. The cost of such modifications is relatively small when compared with the cost of injury. Numerous researchers have examined floors in hospitals and nursing homes and recommend that they not be highly polished to prevent glare and to prevent patients from slipping. Yet the use of such polish continues to be standard practice in many institutions. Many interventions that would increase safety in institutions are practical matters that do not need research skill, time, and money to "prove" their effectiveness, yet they are not implemented.

The future direction for nursing research on patient falls needs to be extended into the areas of assessment and intervention, but this research must be rigorously developed and tested with various patient populations. Further, there is a need for multidisciplinary research, with strong nursing input. For instance, at this time, there is not a safe geriatric bed available on the market with a mattress height that is low enough for elderly patients to climb into or out of unaided. The consultation of nurses in the design, construction, and testing of such devices is essential. Recognizing the multidisciplinary nature of patient falls, nurses should play a key role in the coordination of such research instead of trying to solve the problem alone or ignoring the simultaneous development of research in other disciplines. Programs in fall research should include coinvestigators from planning, engineering, and medicine so that innovative and practical prevention strategies may be realized.

REFERENCES

Arsenault, T. M. (1982) Slips and falls: Problem identification and resolution by a primary nurse. In *Nursing Research: Advancing clinical practice for the 80's* (pp. 386–398). Stanford: Department of Nursing Science, Stanford University Hospital, Stanford CA.

Baker, S. P., & Harvey, A H. (1985). Fall injuries in the elderly. *Clinics in Geriatric Medicine, 1*(3), 501–512.

Barbieri, E. B. (1983). Patient falls are not patient accidents. *Journal of Gerontological Nursing, 9*(1), 165–173.

Botez, M. I., & Hausser, C. O. (1982). Falls. *British Journal of Medicine, 28*, 494–503.

Byers, V., Arrington, M. E., & Finstuen, K. (1990). Predictive risk factors associated with stroke patients falls in acute care settings. *Journal of Neuroscience Nursing, 22,* 147–154.

Cummings, S. R., Nevitt, M. C., & Kidd, S. (1988). Forgetting falls: The limited accuracy of recall in falls in the elderly. *Journal of the American Geriatrics Society, 36,* 613–616.

Easterling, M. L. (1990). Which of your patients is headed for a fall? *RN, 53*(1), 56–59.

Fife, D. D., Solomon, P., & Stanton, M. (1985). A risk/fall program: Code orange for success. *Nursing Management, 15*(11), 50–53.

Gross, Y. T., Shimamoto, Y., Rose, C. L., & Frank, B. (1990). Why do they fall? Monitoring risk factors in nursing homes. *Journal of Gerontological Nursing, 16*(6), 20–25.

Hendrich, A. L. (1988). An effective unit-based fall prevention plan. *Journal of Nursing Quality Assurance, 3*(1), 28–36.

Innes, E. M., & Turman, W. G. (1983) Evaluating patient falls. *Quality Review Bulletin, 9*(2), 30–35.

Janken, J. K., Reynolds, B. A., & Swieck, K. (1986). Patient falls in the acute care setting: Identifying risk factors. *Nursing Research, 35,* 215–219.

Llewellyn, J., Martin, B., Shekleton, M., & Firlit, S. (1988). Analysis of falls in the acute surgical and cardiovascular surgical patient. *Applied Nursing Research, 1,* 116–121.

Lund, C., & Sheafor, M. L. (1985). Is your patient about to fall? *Journal of Gerontological Nursing, 11*(4), 37–41.

Maas, M. (1990). Reducing patient falls in a long-term care setting. *Canadian Nurse, 86,* 16–17.

Maciorowski, L. F. Munro, B. H., Deitrick-Gallagher, M., McNew, C. D., Sheppard-Hinkel, E., Wanich, C., & Ragan, P. A. (1988). A review of the patient fall literature. *Journal of Nursing Quality Assurance, 3*(1), 18–27.

Maki, B. E., Bartlett, S. A., & Fernie, G. R. (1984). Influence of stairway and handrail height on the ability to generate stabilizing forces and moments. *Human Factors, 26,* 705–714.

Maki, B. E., Holliday, P. J., & Fernie, G. R. (1990). Aging and postural control: A comparison of spontaneous- and induced-sway balance tests. *Journal of the American Geriatrics Society, 38*(9), 1–9.

Manjam, N. V. B., & MacKinnon, H. H. (1973). Patient, bed and bathroom: A study of falls occurring in a general hospital. *Nova Scotia Medical Bulletin, 52,* 23–25.

Masters, R., & Marks, S. F. (1990). The use of restraints. *Rehabilitation Nursing, 15,* 22–25.

McHutchion, G., & Morse, J. M. (1990). Releasing restraints: A nursing dilemma. *Journal of Gerontological Nursing, 15*(2), 16–21.

Morris, E. V., & Isaacs, B. (1980). The prevention of falls in a geriatric hospital. *Age and Ageing, 9,* 181–185.

Morse, J. M. (1986). Computerized evaluation of a scale to identify the fall-prone patient. *Canadian Journal of Public Health, 767*(Suppl.), 21–25.

Morse, J. M., Black, C., Oberle, K., & Donahue, P. (1989). A prospective study to identify the fall-prone patient. *Social Sciences and Medicine, 28,* 81–86.

Morse, J. M., & Morse, R. M. (1988). Calculating fall rates. *Quality Review Bulletin, 14,* 369–371.

Morse, J. M., Morse, R. M., & Tylko, S. J. (1989). Development of a scale to identify the fall-prone patient. *Canadian Journal on Aging/La Revue Canadienne du Vieillissement, 8,* 366–377.

Morse, J. M., Prowse, M., Morrow, N., & Federspeil, G. (1985). A retrospective analysis of patient falls. *Canadian Journal of Public Health, 76,* 116–118.

Morse, J. M., Tylko, S. J., & Dixon, H. A. (1987). Characteristics of the fall-prone patient. *Gerontologist, 27,* 516–522.

Patel, K. P. (1976). Falls and faints in the elderly: Look to their clinical history for clues. *Modern Geriatrics, 6,* 28–34.

Perry, B. C. (1982). Falls among the elderly: A review of the methods and conclusions of epidemiologic studies. *Journal of the American Geriatrics Society, 30,* 367–371.

Rainville, N. G. (1984). Effect of an implemented fall prevention program on the frequency of patient falls. *Quality Review Bulletin, 10,* 287–291.

Ring, C., Nayak, L., & Isaacs, B. (1988). Balance function in elderly people who have and who have not fallen. *Archives of Physical Medicine and Rehabilitation, 69,* 261–264.

Robbins, A. S., Rubenstein, L. Z., Josephson, K. R., Schulman, B. L., Osterweil, D., & Fine, G. (1989) Predictors of falls among elderly people: Results of two population-based studies. *Archives of International Medicine, 149,* 1628–1633.

Rubenstein, L. Z., & Robbins, A. S. (1989). Falling syndromes in elderly persons. *Comprehensive Therapy, 15*(6), 13–18.

Spellbring, A. M. (1992). Assessing elderly patients at high risk for falls: A reliability study. *Journal of Nursing Quality Assurance, 6*(3), 30–35.

Spellbring, A. M., Gannon, M. E., Kleckner, T., Conway, K. (1988). Improving safety for hospitalized elderly. *Journal of Gerontological Nursing, 14*(2), 31–37.

Stegman, M. R. (1983). Falls among elderly hypertensives—Are they iatrogenic? *Gerontology, 29,* 339–406.

Tack, K. A., Ulrich, B., & Kehr, C. (1987). Patient falls: Profile for prevention. *Journal of Neuroscience Nursing, 19,* 83–89.

Tinetti, M. E., Liu, W.-L., & Ginter, S. F. (1992). Mechanical restraint use and fall-related injuries among residents of skilled nursing facilities. *Annals of Internal Medicine, 116,* 369–374.

Tisserand, M. (1985). Progress in the prevention of falls caused by slipping. *Ergonomics, 28,* 1027–1042.

Vlahov, D., Myers, A. H., & Al-Ibrahim, M. S. (1990). Epidemiology of falls among patients in a rehabilitation hospital. *Archives of Physical Medicine and Rehabilitation, 71,* 8–12.

Warshaw, G. A., Moore, J. T., Friedman, S. W., Currie, C. T., Kennie, D. C., Kane, W. J., & Mears, P. A. (1982). Functional disability in the hospitalized elderly. *Journal of the American Medical Association, 248,* 847–850.

Whedon, M. B., & Shedd, P. (1989). Prediction and prevention of patient falls. *Image: Journal of Nursing Scholarship, 21,* 108–114.

Whipple, R. H., Wolfson, L. I., & Amerman, P. M. (1987). The relationship of knee and ankle weakness to falls in nursing home residents: An isokinetic study. *Journal of the American Geriatrics Society, 35*(1), 13–20.

Widder, B. (1985). A new device to decrease falls. *Geriatric Nursing, 6,* 287–288.

Wolfson, L., Whipple, R., Amerman, P., & Tobin, J. N. (1990). Gait assessment in the elderly: A Gait Abnormality Rating Scale and its relation to falls. *Journal of Gerontology: Medical Sciences, 45,* M12–M19.

Young, S. W., Abedzadeh, C. B., & White, M. W. (1989). A fall-prevention program for nursing homes. *Nursing Management, 20*(11), 80y–80ff.

Index

Contents of Previous Volumes

VOLUME II

VOLUME III

VOLUME IV

VOLUME V

VOLUME VI

VOLUME X

ORDER FORM

Save 10% on Volume 12 with this coupon.

___ Check here to order the ANNUAL REVIEW OF NURSING RESEARCH, Volume 12, 1994 at a 10% discount. You will receive an invoice requesting prepayment.

Save 10% on all future volumes with a continuation order.

___ Check here to place your continuation order for the ANNUAL REVIEW OF NURSING RESEARCH. You will receive a pre-payment invoice with a 10% discount upon publication of each new volume, beginning with Volume 12, 1994. You may pay for prompt shipment or cancel with no obligation.

Name ______________________________

Institution ______________________________

Address ______________________________

City/State/Zip ______________________________

Examination copies for possible adoption are available to instructors "on approval" only. Write on institutional letterhead, noting course, level, present text, and expected enrollment (include $3.00 for postage and handling). Prices slightly higher overseas. Prices subject to change.

Mail this coupon to:
SPRINGER PUBLISHING COMPANY
536 Broadway, New York, N.Y. 10012